Frontiers in Heart Failure

(Volume 1)

Clinical Issues

Edited by

Panagiotis Georgoulias

Nuclear Medicine Department

School of Medicine, University of Thessaly

Larissa

Greece

Bentham Science Publishers Ltd.
Executive Suite Y - 2
PO Box 7917, Saif Zone
Sharjah, U.A.E.
Email: subscriptions@benthamscience.org

BENTHAM
SCIENCE

CONTENTS

FOREWORD 1

When Dr. Georgoulias asked me to write this foreword, I was honored and thrilled to have the opportunity to introduce this outstanding work on the "Frontiers in Heart Failure – Molecular Imaging".

This book represents the collaborative effort of numerous talented physicians and scientists throughout Greece with expertise in heart failure to present this complex topic. This challenging task has been accomplished *via* a multidisciplinary approach in this well organized e-book that discusses all aspects of the disease. Heart failure is a very prevalent disease with high mortality and significant social and economic impact on societies. As such it is imperative to understand this silent epidemic, which affects all organs and systems of the body. We live in the era of personalized medicine where the potential exists to identify and in theory prevent factors that lead to heart failure as well as to slow the progression of disease.

The layout of this e-book follows a logical progression and thus gives the reader a comprehensive approach to the study of heart failure. The first several chapters discuss epidemiology, cardiac physiology and pathophysiology, genetics, clinical manifestations, laboratory variables and biochemical markers. The book goes on to address management of heart failure patients including the role of echocardiography, medical therapy, interventional and device therapy, as well as novel treatments for heart failure such as gene and cell therapy approaches. The second portion of the book is dedicated to imaging modalities for heart failure other than echocardiography. Computed tomography is first discussed as a fundamental method to delineate structural anatomy as well as to provide support for invasive techniques used in heart failure. Magnetic resonance imaging is then discussed as an imaging modality which can accurately establish the diagnosis of heart failure and which can also be used for quantification of ventricular function as well as tissue characterization. The bulk of the second portion of the book is a journey through the various imaging capabilities of Nuclear Medicine, which provide both functional and anatomic information. Myocardial Perfusion (SPECT) Imaging and Gated-SPECT are first highlighted, as they are particularly useful in the heart failure patient population, two thirds of which has ischemic heart disease as the underlying cause. The importance of identifying myocardium at risk, (ischemic yet viable), is emphasized in these chapters, as is the ability of these agents to assess myocardial viability and follow-up of left ventricular function after revascularization. Subsequent chapters discuss PET perfusion imaging, hybrid imaging, and assessment of viability with both SPECT and PET applications. More advanced topics such as cardiac neurotransmission SPECT and PET imaging, radiolabelled fatty acid metabolism imaging, and molecular imaging of: apoptosis, atheromatous plaques, and gene and stem cell therapies complete this section of the book. The final portion of this book discusses important related topics including: artifacts and pitfalls in cardiac molecular imaging, radiation safety, and technical advances such as the rapidly evolving role of PET/MRI and as yet only experimental SPECT/MRI in heart failure management.

I would like to thank my colleague Efrosyni Sfakianaki MD, Assistant Professor in Radiology/NM at UM for her cooperation in reviewing this great e-book.

In conclusion, I am very excited about this e-book, not only because of its superbly organized, well- illustrated and presented content, but also because as an e-book it can be carried and propagated throughout the community much more easily than a hard copy book. The editor and chapter authors have succeeded admirably in the endeavor to produce what promises to be an outstanding resource for the examination and therapy of the patients with Heart Failure both now and in the future.

Dr. George N. Sfakianakis
Department of Radiology
University of Miami, Miller School of Medicine
Miami
FL
USA

FOREWORD 2

Heart failure represents a global healthcare challenge. The severity of the problem is well established in the industrialized countries, where heart failure incidence, prevalence, morbidity and mortality have affected a large population with significant medical and economic demands of the society. Ischemic cardiomyopathy constitutes the most common cause of heart failure in western societies, whereas other causes, such as valvular cardiomyopathy and Chagas disease, may play a more important role in the rest parts of the world. However, as the developing nations also became more urbanized, an increase of heart failure rate has been observed, particularly cases with ischemic aetiology.

We have witnessed major advances in our diagnostic and therapeutic options for heart failure during the last decades. In particular, molecular imaging methods have broadened our understanding of the failing heart at the molecular and cellular level. The continual upsurge in research is promising but this increase in the available literature makes it difficult to stay informed with selected topics in the field. Therefore, it is my pleasure to write a foreword for this e-Book, entitled "Frontiers in Heart Failure – Molecular Imaging", (Editor Professor P. Georgoulias, Bentham Science Publishers). Experts providing crucial and updated information concerning all aspects of heart failure management wrote the chapters in this excellent book.

The e-Book is divided into two sections. The first section includes an update on the pathophysiological and clinical characteristics of the heart failure syndrome, and the therapeutic strategies that can be implemented for these patients. It would be useful not only for cardiologists, but also for any health professionals interested in state-of-the-art heart failure management. Additionally, novel therapies are presented, such as gene and cell therapies. The role of molecular imaging for the evaluation and follow-up of heart failure patients is approached in the second section. It allows the reader to understand better the wide range of molecular imaging methods, including myocardial perfusion imaging, viability assessment, cardiac remodelling evaluation, cardiac neurotransmission imaging, atheromatous plaques imaging and free fatty acids studies. The most advanced imaging modalities in heart failure are also presented, such as single photon emission tomography, positron emission tomography, computed tomography, magnetic resonance imaging and hybrid imaging systems. Finally, important relevant technical factors and advances are comprehensively addressed in the last part of the e-Book.

Based on its strong clinical orientation, I believe that most clinicians will find “Frontiers in Heart Failure – Molecular Imaging” of immediate practical interest. I consider this e-Book an excellent contribution for anyone involved in health failure patients’ care or research.

Dr. Javed Butler
Heart Institute
Stony Brook University
New York
USA

PREFACE

During the last decades, heart failure has become a main reason for health care utilization by patients living in western countries. It represents one of the leading causes of morbidity and mortality due to cardiovascular disorders, particularly in the elderly. Undoubtedly, heart failure can be regarded as a contemporary epidemic since the prevalence of the syndrome has steadily risen. Despite its clinical importance, various aspects of the pathophysiology of the failing heart seem to be inadequately understood. A better understanding of this complex syndrome, at the molecular and cellular level, is expected to have significant consequences for the patients at the clinical setting. Therefore, more accurate investigation of the disorder and effective management of heart failure patients remain primary objectives in the field of cardiovascular research.

This e-Book aims to present cutting edge heart failure diagnostic methods and therapies related to the major fields of interest of the authors, along with findings obtained through their research work. After providing clinically oriented information in the first part, the second part of the e-Book focuses on molecular imaging techniques. The first chapter by G Giamouzis *et al.* includes current definitions, epidemiology, cost and health care policies in the field of heart failure management. In the second chapter, I Aidonidis *et al.* present fundamental cardiac cellular and subcellular physiology concepts that could permit a better assessment of myocardial pathophysiology. The third chapter by F Triposkiadis *et al.* is devoted to molecular and cellular alteration in heart failure, while recent advances regarding the genetic basis of the syndrome are reported by D Koumbi *et al.* in the next chapter. J Skoularigis *et al.* focus on clinical manifestations, patients' investigation, co-existing diseases and prognosis estimation. Laboratory variables and biomarkers represent useful tools for clinicians when treating patients with heart failure clinical findings. This chapter by CA Zivlas and DV Cokkinos reviews well established and novel laboratory tests that may support clinical decision making. By assessing cardiac structure and function, echocardiography offers diagnostic and prognostic information. E Tsougos summarizes the role of echocardiography based on current applications and future developments. Three chapters are devoted to heart failure therapies. S Katsanos and JT Parissis present up-to-date medical therapy of the syndrome, while P Antonitsis *et al.* review available interventional and device therapies. The novel gene and cellular therapeutic strategies are discussed by E Papanikolaou and NP Anagnou in the last chapter of the first section of the e-Book.

The second section of the e-Book starts with computed tomography (CT) and magnetic resonance imaging (MRI) in heart failure that are reviewed by IA Chryssogonidis *et al.* and MA Mademli and NL Kelekis in the first two chapters, respectively. Radiopharmaceuticals and techniques used for myocardial perfusion single photon emission computed tomography (SPECT) imaging are presented in the next chapter by PA Georgoulias *et al.* Electrocardiographically gated SPECT (G-SPECT) combines assessment of myocardial perfusion and left ventricular function within a single study. Applications of G-SPECT for functional evaluation and remodelling investigation in the failing heart are discussed by S Tsiouris *et al.*, Positron emission tomography (PET) perfusion imaging is reviewed by S Chatziioannou *et al.*, based on its advantages, such as high diagnostic accuracy, short study time and lower radiation doses compared to SPECT. Hybrid imaging systems (SPECT/CT, PET/CT, PET/MRI) are reported in the chapter by DJ Apostolopoulos as the integration of structural and functional or metabolic information, achieved by multimodality imaging, offer valuable insights in heart failure syndrome. The presence of myocardial viability has been considered a significant determinant of patients' outcome. Two chapters are devoted to myocardial viability assessment; E Moralidis presents SPECT and PET techniques for these purposes, whereas VI Valotassiou and JV Malamitsi provide a comparison of radioisotopic and non-radioisotopic methods for viability identification. Furthermore, cardiac neurotransmission imaging in heart failure is reviewed by D Agostini *et al.*, based on SPECT techniques, and SI Koukouraki according to PET imaging. Cardiac metabolism is essential for myocardial contractility and maintenance of cardiomyocyte integrity. HJ Verberne presents various SPECT and PET tracers for the assessment of myocardial free fatty acids imaging. Moreover, A Doumas and I Iakovou focus on current and future applications of molecular imaging in heart failure regarding cell apoptosis and atheromatous plaques formation. Molecular imaging of the novel gene and cell therapies is presented by A Katsikis and M Koutelou. In the last three chapters of the e-Book, potential artifacts and pitfalls are reported by I Tsougos and PA Georgoulias, radiation protection considerations are reviewed by C Kappas and K Theodorou, and various technical advances in the field of cardiac molecular imaging are provided by GK Loudos.

In conclusion, the purpose of this e-Book is to capture and explore improvements towards the diagnosis and therapy of heart failure by established and novel strategies and procedures, focusing on molecular imaging methods.

This e-Book represents significant work of chapters' authors who deserve all appreciation. I would like to highlight the major contribution of G Angelidis and I Tsougos. Further, I wish to acknowledge the contribution of E Kapitsaki (SPEG Consulting Co., Athens, Greece) for the designing of the cover page of this e-Book. Finally, I would like to thank the excellent team of Bentham Science Publishers and especially Faryal Sami for the cooperation.

Dr. Panagiotis A. Georgoulias
Nuclear Medicine Department
School of Medicine, University of Thessaly
Larissa, Greece

List of Contributors

Andreas Xanthopoulos	Department of Cardiology, University Hospital of Larissa, University of Thessaly, Larissa, Greece
Antonios Ziakas	1st Department of Cardiology, AHEPA University Hospital, Thessaloniki, Greece
Chrissi Hatzoglou	Department of Physiology, School of Medicine, Faculty of Health Sciences, University of Thessaly, Larissa, Greece
Christos A. Zivlas	Biomedical Research Foundation of the Academy of Athens, Athens, Greece
Chrysovalantou Nikolaidou	1st Department of Cardiology, AHEPA University Hospital, Thessaloniki, Greece
Constantina Sambani	Laboratory of Health Physics, Radiobiology & Cytogenetics, NCSR "Democritus", Athens, Greece.
Daphne Koumbi	Laboratory of Health Physics, Radiobiology & Cytogenetics, NCSR "Democritus", Athens, Greece. Department of Genetics & Biotechnology, Faculty of Biology, National & Kapodistrian University of Athens, Athens, Greece
Dennis V. Cokkinos	Biomedical Research Foundation of the Academy of Athens, Athens, Greece
Eleni Papanikolaou	Laboratory of Cell and Gene Therapy, Biomedical Research Foundation of the Academy of Athens, Athens, Greece. Laboratory of Biology, National & Kapodistrian University of Athens, Medical School, Athens, Greece
Elias Tsougkos	2nd Cardiology Clinic (Heart Failure and Preventive Cardiology Section), Henry Dunant Hospital Center, Athens, Greece
Filippos Triposkiadis	Department of Cardiology, University Hospital of Larissa, University of Thessaly, Larissa, Greece
George P. Patrinos	Department of Pharmacy, University of Patras, Patras, Greece
Gregory Giamouzis	Department of Cardiology, University Hospital of Larissa, University of Thessaly, Larissa, Greece
Isaac Aidonidis	Department of Physiology, School of Medicine, Faculty of Health Sciences, University of Thessaly, Larissa, Greece
John Skoularigis	Department of Cardiology, University Hospital of Larissa, University of Thessaly, Larissa, Greece
John T. Parissis	Heart Failure Unit, Attikon University Hospital, Athens, Greece

Konstantinos Gourgoulianis	Department of Physiology, School of Medicine, Faculty of Health Sciences, University of Thessaly, Larissa, Greece
Nicholas P. Anagnou	Laboratory of Cell and Gene Therapy, Biomedical Research Foundation of the Academy of Athens, Athens, Greece. Laboratory of Biology, National & Kapodistrian University of Athens, Medical School, Athens, Greece
Panagoula Kollia	Department of Genetics & Biotechnology, Faculty of Biology, National & Kapodistrian University of Athens, Athens, Greece
Paschalis-Adam Molyvdas	Department of Physiology, School of Medicine, Faculty of Health Sciences, University of Thessaly, Larissa, Greece
Polychronis Antonitsis	Cardiothoracic Department, AHEPA University Hospital, Thessaloniki, Greece
Rodopi Stamatiou	Department of Physiology, School of Medicine, Faculty of Health Sciences, University of Thessaly, Larissa, Greece
Sotirios Zarogiannis	Department of Physiology, School of Medicine, Faculty of Health Sciences, University of Thessaly, Larissa, Greece
Spyridon Katsanos	Heart Failure Unit, Attikon University Hospital, Athens, Greece

"Everything that is really great and inspiring is created by the individual who can labor in freedom"

Albert Einstein

"Out of My Later Years", 1950

Frontiers in Heart Failure

(Volume 1)

Clinical Issues

CHAPTER 1

Definition, Epidemiology, Economic Cost and Health Policies

Gregory Giamouzis[*], **John Skoularigis** and **Filippos Triposkiadis**

Department of Cardiology, University Hospital of Larissa, University of Thessaly, Larissa, Greece

Abstract: Heart failure (HF) is a complex clinical syndrome that is a consequence of any functional or structural impairment of left ventricular filling or pumping of blood. It is considered as a crucial healthcare issue and has been called "the epidemic of the 21st century", namely because of its rising prevalence and the considerably high mortality, morbidity, and care expenditures it poses to the health care systems; HF prevalence is increasing with advancing age. 2-3% of the general population worldwide has HF, whereas among elderly individuals (≥80 years of age) about 12% of both genders have HF. Mortality is exceptionally high, since almost half of the patients will die 5 years after the establishment of diagnosis. The cost of HF care is high, mostly driven by the frequent hospitalizations for HF, and will remain an important concern for the healthcare systems. The estimated HF prevalence and cost of care will significantly increase in the near future, in part because of the longer survival of HF patients due to the continuous optimization of life-prolonging medical and interventional therapies, as well as the aging of the population in the developed countries, which eventually leads to a greater number of individuals at risk for incident HF. Therefore, strategies aiming to HF prevention and improvement of care efficiency are urgently needed. The purpose of this chapter is to provide an in-depth look at the current definitions, epidemiology, cost and health care policies regarding HF in the developed world.

Keywords: Decompensation, Economic cost, Epidemiology, Health care, Heart failure, Health policies, Hospitalization, Left ventricular dysfunction, Prevention, Structural heart disease, Telemonitoring.

[*] **Corresponding author Gregory Giamouzis:** Department of Cardiology, University Hospital of Larissa and University of Thessaly, Larissa, Greece; Tel: +30 2414 00 2721; Fax: +30 2410 67 0248; E-mail: grgiamouzis@med.uth.gr.

Panagiotis Georgoulias (Ed.)

INTRODUCTION

Heart failure (HF) is a complex clinical syndrome that is a consequence of any functional or structural impairment of left ventricular filling or pumping of blood [1]. It results in the inability of the heart to deliver oxygen at a rate commensurate with the metabolic needs of the tissues, despite normal filling pressures or to do so the left ventricle needs to work at the cost of elevated filling pressures [2]. The principal manifestations of the syndrome are i) dyspnea at exertion or even at rest and fatigue, which impair exercise capacity, and ii) water and sodium retention that may lead to pulmonary and peripheral congestion/edema. A proportion of patients show primarily exercise intolerance with no clinical evidence of congestion; others exhibit mainly signs and symptoms of fluid retention. Since not all patients manifest clinically significant volume overload, the term "chronic heart failure" is prefered over the previously used "congestive heart failure". The diagnosis of HF can be challenging and is mainly a clinical diagnosis based on a careful history and physical examination; therefore, there is no single diagnostic procedure for a definite diagnosis. However, many of HF symptoms are of limited diagnostic value since they are non-discriminating, therefore demonstration of an underlying cardiac cause is fundamental to the diagnosis [3]. In many cases, the underlying cause is myocardial disease leading to impaired systolic ventricular function. In the rest, impairment of ventricular diastolic function or pathologies of the valves and the pericardium, or even heart rhythm and conduction abnormalities are the main cause of HF. Identification of the underlying heart disorder is crucial, as the specific pathophysiologic mechanism usually dectates the optimal therapeutic intervention to be made. Notably, HF should not be confused with either cardiomyopathy or left ventricular (LV) dysfunction; these latter terms describe underlying structural etiology for incident HF.

DEFINITIONS

HF may be related to a wide spectrum of LV disorders, ranging from normal LV size and preserved ejection fraction (EF) to severe dilatation and markedly reduced EF [4]. In the majority of the patients, the consequences of systolic and diastolic dysfunction coexist, irrespectively of EF. EF has traditionally been given an important role in phenotyping HF patients; most clinical trials enrolled patients based on the EF, since such classification underscores differences in patient demographics, comorbidities, long-term prognosis, and responsiveness to therapeutic modalities. Nevertheless, one should take into account that EF measurements are significantly affected by the imaging technique used and the experience of the operator. Preferably, the terms "preserved" or "reduced EF" should be used over the terms "preserved" or "reduced systolic function", since systolic function disorders can be demonstrated among HF patients with preserved EF and vice versa. Below we present the terminology used by the European Society of Cardiology (ESC) in the 2012 HF Guidelines, based on the LVEF, the time-course and the symptomatic severity of the syndrome [2].

Terminology Related to Left Ventricular Ejection Fraction (LVEF)

Historically, the terminology that has been used to describe HF is based on LVEF values. EF mathematically represents the quotient of the stroke volume (end-diastolic volume minus the end-systolic volume) and the end-diastolic volume. In patients with systolic dysfunction, *i.e.* impaired contraction and therefore decreased active emptying of the LV, the stroke volume can be maintained by an increase in the end-diastolic volume (*i.e.* the LV dilates); consequently the heart ejects a smaller fraction of a larger volume. As the systolic dysfunction becomes more severe, the volumes of the left ventricle (end-diastolic and end-systolic) gradually increase and the EF decreases, a process known as "remodeling" of the left ventricle. Most of the major HF trials have enrolled patients with a reduced EF (HF-rEF), *i.e.* LVEF ≤35%, previously called "systolic HF", and it is only in these patients that effective therapies have been confirmed to date. Other, more recent, studies enrolled patients with HF and an EF >40-45% and no other causal cardiac abnormality (such as valvular or pericardial disease). Some of these patients did not have a normal EF (generally considered to be >50%) but also did not show a major reduction in systolic function either. Because of this, the term HF with 'preserved' EF (HF-pEF) was introduced to describe these patients. Patients with an EF in the range 40-50% therefore represent a 'grey area' and most probably suffer primarily from mild systolic dysfunction. The diagnosis of HF-pEF is more challenging than the diagnosis of HF-rEF because it is largely one of exclusion, *i.e.* other non-cardiac underlying causes of the patient's symptoms (such as anemia or chronic lung disease) must first be discounted [5].

Usually these patients have increased LV wall thickness and left atrial (LA) size but not LV dilatation. There is also evidence of diastolic dysfunction, which is generally accepted as the likely cause of HF in these patients (hence the term 'diastolic HF') [6]. Notably, more sensitive measures of systolic function may indicate abnormalities in patients with a preserved or even normal EF, hence the preference for stating preserved or reduced EF over preserved or reduced 'systolic function'.

Terminology Related to the Time-course of Heart Failure (HF)

Patients who have never exhibited the clinical features of HF are described as having asymptomatic LV dysfunction (systolic, diastolic or both depending on the underlying abnormality). To underscore the importance of preventability, the American College of Cardiology/American Heart Association (ACC/AHA) has taken a new approach to the classification of HF, emphasizing the evolution and progression of the disease (Fig. **1**) [7]. Individuals at high risk for incident HF and no structural cardiac abnormality are described as having stage A HF. Asymptomatic patients with structural abnormalities are now classified as stage B HF. Stage C includes patients with past or current symptoms of HF related to underlying structural heart disease, whereas stage D describes patients with end-stage disease who require specialized treatment approaches, such as mechanical circulatory support, continuous IV inotrope administration, cardiac transplantation, or hospice care. Only stages C and D meet the requirements for the traditional clinical diagnosis of HF. This classification is intended to complement, but not replace, the New York Heart Association (NYHA) Functional Classification (see below).

Patients who have showed evidence of HF for a period of time are often said to suffer from 'chronic HF'. Patients with unchanged signs and symptoms under treatment for at least a month are said to be 'stable'. Stable HF may deteriorate 'acutely' *i.e.* suddenly and require hospital admission, an event of considerable prognostic significance; then the patient may be described as 'decompensated'. The very first presentation of new HF is called '*de novo HF*' and may present either acutely, (*e.g.* acute myocardial infarction) or gradually (*e.g.* subclinical cardiac dysfunction). Although symptoms and signs may resolve ('compensation'), the underlying cardiac dysfunction usually does not; therefore, HF patients remain at risk of recurrent 'decompensation'. Occasionally, however, a patient may suffer from 'reversible' HF, *i.e.* due to a problem that may resolve completely, as in acute viral myopericarditis. There are particular HF subgroups (*e.g.* 'idiopathic' dilated cardiomyopathy) that may also show substantial or even complete recovery of LV systolic function with modern disease-modifying therapeutic strategies (including an angiotensin converting enzyme inhibitor, a beta-blocker, and a mineralocorticoid receptor antagonist). The term 'congestive HF' is still in use, especially in the USA, to describe HF, either acute or chronic, with findings of congestion due to water and sodium retention. Interestingly, depending upon a patient's stage of illness, many or all of these terms may accurately apply to the same patient at different times.

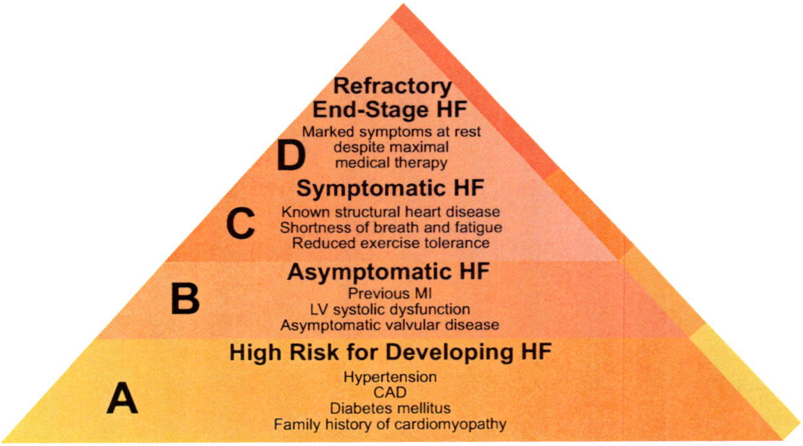

Fig. (1). American College of Cardiology/American Heart Association pyramid approach to heart failure stages [7].

Terminology Related to the Symptomatic Severity of Heart Failure (HF)

The terms used to describe different functional status at different time intervals are based on the NYHA functional classification (Table **1**). Patients in NYHA class I do not show heart disease - related symptoms; patients in NYHA classes II, III or IV experience mild, moderate or severe symptomatology, respectively. Although there is a clear relationship between symptom severity and mortality, there is poor correlation between symptomatology and ventricular function. It is not unusual for HF patients to experience a rapid change in symptoms; a stable chronic HF patient with mild symptoms can suddenly become dyspnoic at rest with the onset of an arrhythmia, whereas an acutely decompensated patient experiencing a hypertensive pulmonary edema with NYHA class IV symptoms may rapidly improve with the administration of vasodilators and diuretics. Symptom deterioration is associated with increased risk of death or hospitalization and requires prompt medical management. Apparently, the two major goals of HF treatment are: i) clinical improvement, preferably to the point of the patient becoming asymptomatic, and ii) reduction of morbidity and mortality.

Table 1. New York Heart Association functional classification based on severity of symptoms and physical activity.

Class I	No limitation of physical activity. Ordinary physical activity does not cause undue breathlessness, fatigue, or palpitations.
Class II	Slight limitation of physical activity. Comfortable at rest, but ordinary physical activity results in undue breathlessness, fatigue, or palpitations.
Class III	Marked limitation of physical activity. Comfortable at rest, but less than ordinary physical activity results in undue breathlessness, fatigue, or palpitations.
Class IV	Unable to carry on any physical activity without discomfort. Symptoms at rest can be present. If any physical activity is undertaken, discomfort is increased.

EPIDEMIOLOGY

Lifetime Risk

The lifetime risk of developing HF is 20% for Americans ≥40 years of age [8]. Data from the National Heart, Lung and Blood Institute (NHLBI) - sponsored Framingham Heart Study indicate that [9]:

a. HF incidence is about 10 per 1000 population after 65 years of age.
b. 75% of HF cases have prior hypertension.
c. The lifetime risk of developing HF for both men and women at the age of 40 years is 1 in 5.

d. At the age of 80 years, the remaining lifetime risk for development of new HF is still 20% for both genders, despite of the much shorter life expectancy.
e. At the age of 40 years, the lifetime risk of incident HF in the absence of a history of myocardial infarction is 1 in 9 for men and 1 in 6 for women.
f. The lifetime risk for people with arterial blood pressure higher than 160/90 mmHg is 2-fold higher of those with less than 140/90 mmHg.

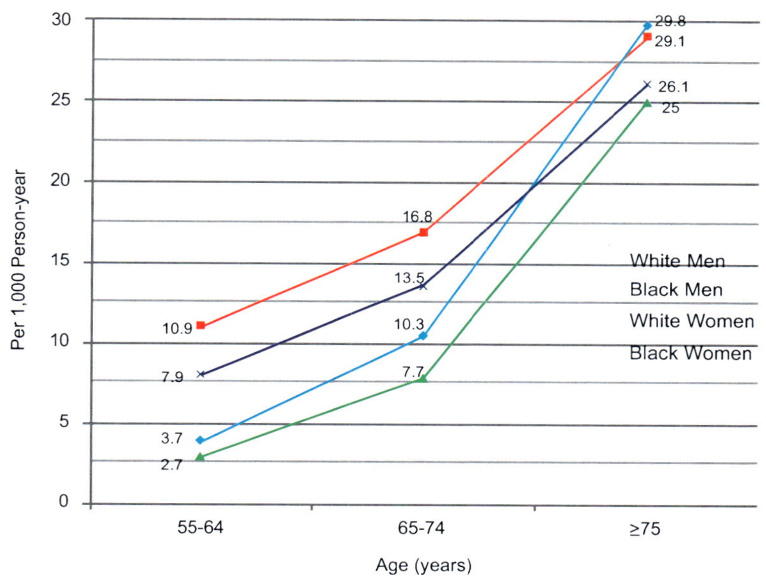

Fig. (2). Annual event rates (per 1000 person-years) for the first episode of acute decompensated HF (data from the Atherosclerosis Risk in Communities community surveillance 2005–2011) [10].

Incidence and Prevalence

HF incidence has increased over the past several decades, with almost 870,000 new HF cases diagnosed in the year 2014 in the United States [10]. HF is a disease of the elderly, since its incidence increases linearly with advance age, rising from approximately 20 per 1,000 individuals aged 65 to 69 years to >80 per 1,000 individuals among those aged ≥85 years [11]. Disparities, however, in the epidemiology of HF have been identified. In the Multi-Ethnic Study of Atherosclerosis (MESA) the relationship between congestive HF incidence and race/ethnicity were explored in a multiracial, population-based study. The highest incidence rate of HF was observed in African Americans (4.6 per 1000 person-years), followed by Hispanics (3.5 per 1000 person-years), whites (2.4 per 1000 person-years), and Chinese Americans (1.0 per 1000 person-years) [12]. In the Atherosclerosis Risk in Communities (ARIC) study, incidence rate per 1000 person-years was lowest among white women and highest among African American men, with African Americans having a greater 5-year mortality rate than whites (Fig. **2**) [13]. The mean age at diagnosis varies with race and ethnicity and ranges from 48.1 years for non-Hispanic African American males to 61.4 years for non-Hispanic white females (Fig. **3**) [14].

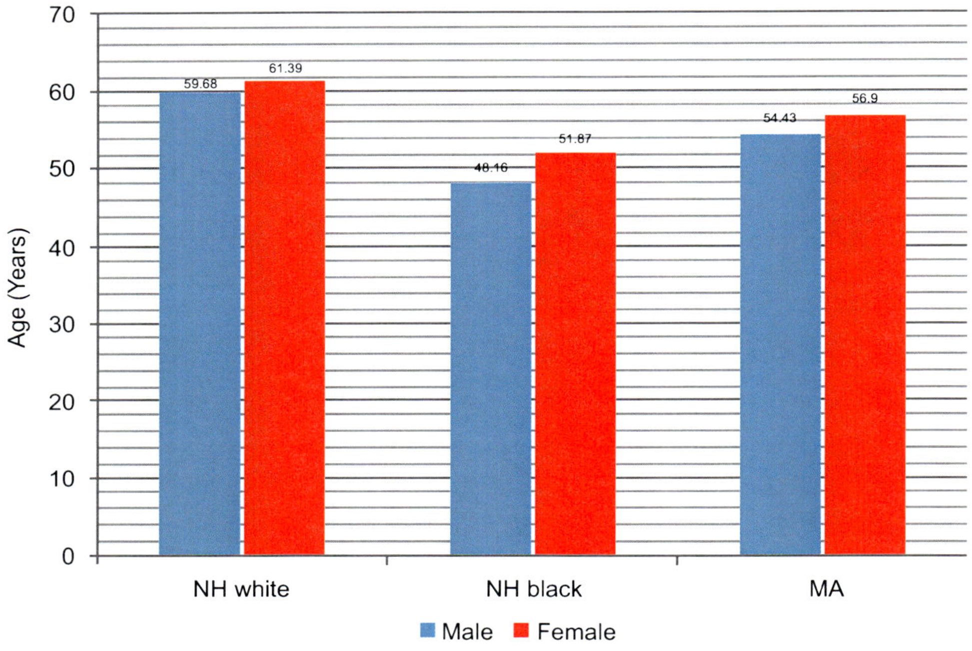

Fig. (3). Mean age at diagnosis of heart failure by race/ethnicity [14].
MA: Mexixan Americans; NH: non-hispanic.

The prevalence of subclinical LV systolic or diastolic dysfunction ranges from 6% to 21% and increases with age [15]. As was shown in the Left Ventricular Dysfunction Prevention study, patients with untreated asymptomatic LV dysfunction show an annual 10% risk for developing HF symptoms and 8% risk of death or HF hospitalization [16]. Data from the community show a prevalence of 21% for asymptomatic mild and 7% for moderate or severe LV diastolic dysfunction, linked to an increased risk of symptomatic HF and subsequent mortality [15]. Approximately 5.7 million persons in the United States have clinically manifest HF, and the prevalence continues to rise with the aging of the population in both genders (Fig. **4**) [10]. According to the latest ACC/AHA 2015 Heart Disease and Stroke Statistics, HF in non-Hispanic African American males and females has a prevalence of 2.8% and 3.2%, respectively, *versus* 2.2% in non-Hispanic white males and females (Table **2**) [10]. In the Medicare-eligible population, HF prevalence rose from 90 to 121 per 1000 beneficiaries from 1994 to 2003 [2]. HF-rEF and HF-pEF each make up about half of the total HF burden [17]. HF prevalence is highest in the elderly and, since life expectancy has risen constantly in the last 5 decades (it is estimated that one in 5 Americans will be >65 years of age by 2050), the number of Americans with HF is expected to significantly worsen in the future (Table **3**, Fig. **5**) [18].

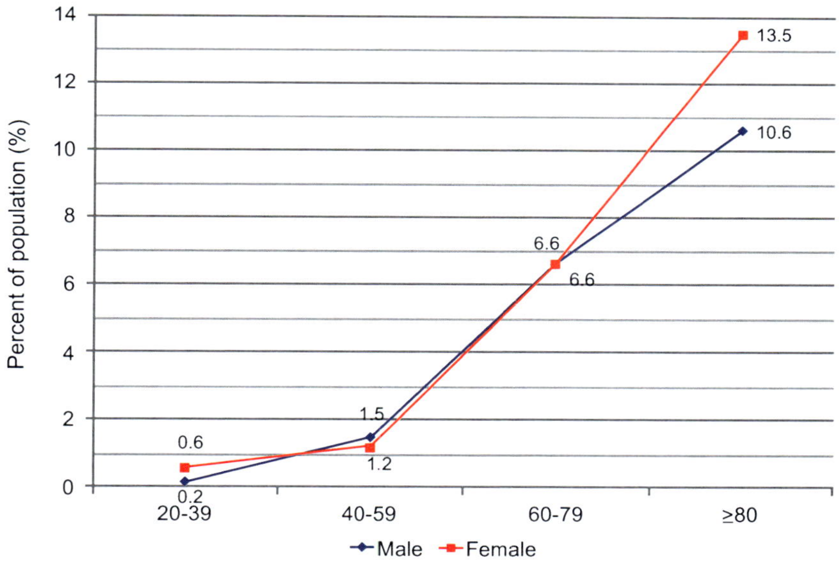

Fig. (4). Prevalence of heart failure by sex and age (National Health and Nutrition Examination Survey: (2009-2012) [10].

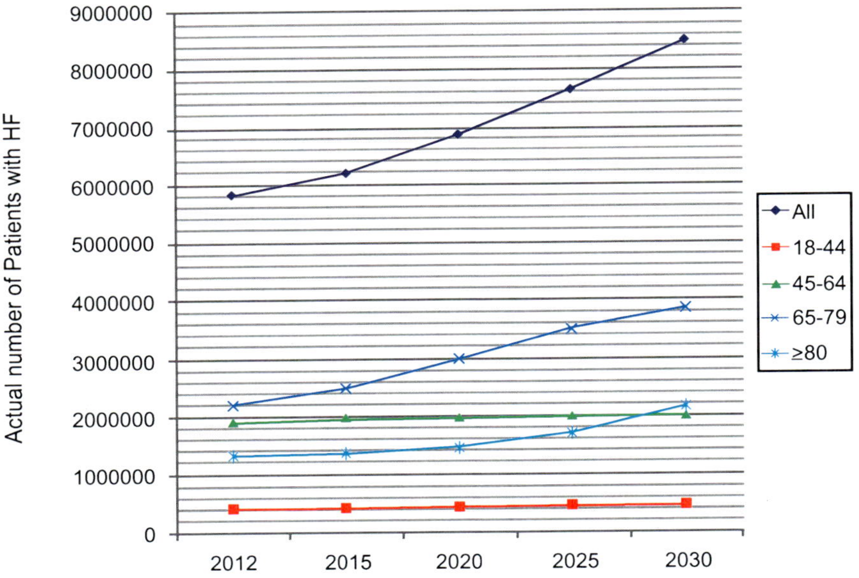

Fig. (5). Projected US prevalence of heart failure from 2012 to 2030 for different age groups [18].

Table 2. Prevalence, incidence, mortality rates, hospital discharges and total cost for heart failure by population groups.

Population group	**Prevalence, 2012, age ≥20 y**	**Incidence (new cases), age ≥55 y**	**Mortality, 2011, all ages***	**Hospital discharges, 2010, all ages**	**Cost, 2012**[†]
Both sexes	5 700 000 (2.2%)	870 000	58 309	1 023 000	30.7 billion
Males	2 700 000 (2.3%)	415 000	24 609 (42.2%)[‡]	501 000	. . .
Females	3 000 000 (2.2%)	455 000	33 700 (57.8%)[‡]	522 000	. . .
NH white males	2.2%	365 000[§]	21 802	. . .	. . .
NH white females	2.2%	395 000[§]	30 036	. . .	. . .
NH black males	2.8%	50 000[§]	2 371	. . .	. . .
NH black females	3.2%	60 000[§]	3 143	. . .	. . .
Hispanic males	2.1%	. . .	*	. . .	. . .
Hispanic females	2.1%	. . .	*	. . .	. . .

(Table 2) contd.....

Population group	Prevalence, 2012, age ≥20 y	Incidence (new cases), age ≥55 y	Mortality, 2011, all ages*	Hospital discharges, 2010, all ages	Cost, 2012†
Asian or Pacific islander	...	...	727	...	...
American Indian or Alaska native	...	...	230	...	...

Heart failure includes people who answered "yes" to the question of ever having congestive heart failure.
Ellipses (...) indicate data not available; NH: non-Hispanic.
*Mortality data for the white, black, Asian or Pacific Islander, and American Indian or Alaska Native populations include deaths among people of Hispanic and non-Hispanic origin. Death rates for Hispanic, American Indian or Alaska Native, and Asian and Pacific Islander people should be interpreted with caution because of inconsistencies in reporting Hispanic origin or race on the death certificate compared with censuses, surveys, and birth certificates. Studies have shown underreporting on death certificates of American Indian or Alaska Native, Asian and Pacific Islander, and Hispanic decedents, as well as undercounts of these groups in censuses.
†Cost data are from Heidenreich *et al.* Forecasting the impact of heart failure in the United States. Circ Heart Fail. 2013;6:606-619.
‡These percentages represent the portion of total mortality attributable to heart failure that is for males *vs* females.
§Estimates include Hispanics and non-Hispanics. Estimates for whites include other nonblack races; Chinese, Filipino, Hawaiian, Japanese, and Other Asian or Pacific Islander.
Sources:
Prevalence: National Health and Nutrition Examination Survey 2009 to 2012 (National Center for Health Statistics) and National Heart, Lung, and Blood Institute. Percentages are age adjusted for Americans ≥20 years of age. Age-specific percentages are extrapolated to the 2012 US population estimates. These data are based on self-reports.
Incidence: Atherosclerosis Risk in Communities Study Community Surveillance, 2005 to 2011 from National Heart, Lung, and Blood Institute.
Mortality: Centers for Disease Control and Prevention/National Center for Health Statistics, 2011 Mortality Multiple Cause-of-Death–United States.

Table 3. Projections of the US population with heart failure from 2010 to 2030 [18].

Year	18 – 44 y	45 – 64 y	65 – 79 y	≥80 y	All
2012	396 578	1 907 141	2 192 233	1 317 310	5 813 262
2015	402 926	1 949 669	2 483 853	3 354 158	6 190 606
2020	417 600	1 974 585	3 004 002	1 463 436	6 859 623
2025	434 635	1 969 852	3 526 347	1 713 840	7 644 674
2030	450 275	2 000 896	3 857 729	2 180 528	8 489 428

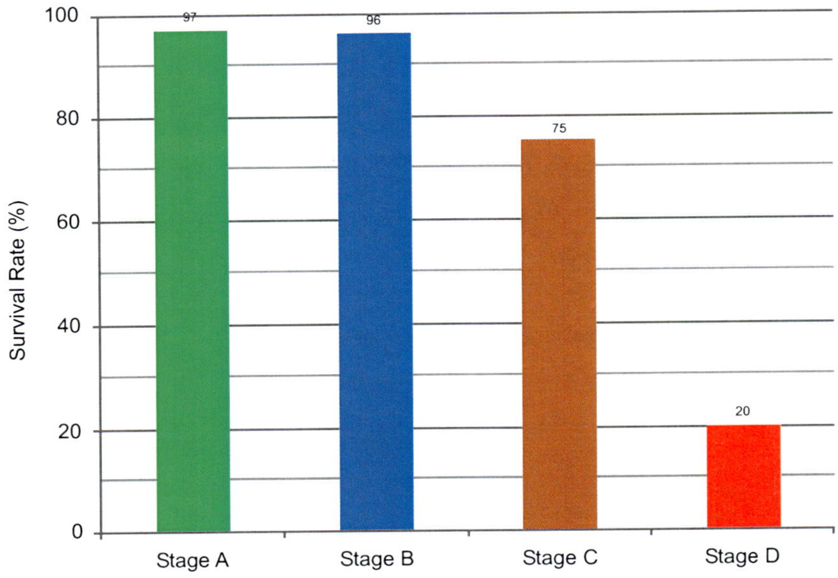

Fig. (6). 5-year survival rates by heart failure stage. A, B, C, and D heart failure was 97%, 96%, 75%, and 20% [20].

Mortality

In the United States HF is mentioned on the death certificate in 1 in 9 deaths. Approximately 7% of all cardiovascular deaths are due to HF. Although survival has improved with the implementation of life-saving therapies, the absolute numbers still remain high with approximately 50% of HF patients dying within 5 years of diagnosis [17, 19]. Data from the ARIC study suggest a 30-day mortality rate post-discharge of 10.4%; the numbers for 1-year and 5-year case fatality rates after hospitalization are 22% and 42.3% respectively [13]. In the Olmsted County, Minnesota population cohort study the 5-year survival rates for stage A, B, C, and D HF was 97%, 96%, 75%, and 20%, respectively (Fig. **6**) [20]. Thirty day post-admission mortality rates have decreased from 12.6% to 10.8% from 1993 to 2005, mainly due to lower in-hospital death rates. Post-discharge mortality actually rose from 4.3% to 6.4% during the same time period [21]. These temporal trends in HF survival are primarily observed in patients with HF-rEF and are not recorded in those with HF-pEF. The prevalence of HF-pEF has been changing as a consequence of alterations in population demographics and in the prevalence and treatment of HF risk factors. Owan and colleagues studied all over 6,000 patients hospitalized with decompensated HF at Mayo Clinic Hospitals in Olmsted County, Minnesota, from 1987 through 2001 [22]. Of these, 53% had HF-rEF and 47% had HF-pEF. The proportion of patients with the diagnosis of HF-pEF rose over time and was significantly higher among community patients than among referral patients (55% *vs.* 45%). The prevalence rates of hypertension, atrial fibrillation, and diabetes among HF patients increased significantly over time. Survival was slightly higher among patients with preserved EF. Interestingly, an improvement of survival was observed over time for those with reduced EF but not for those with preserved EF.

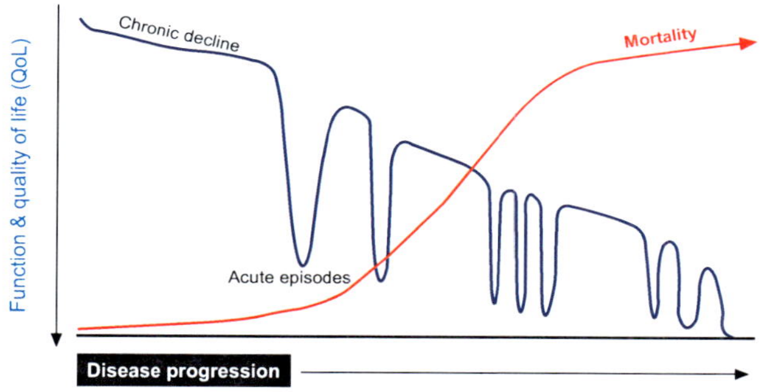

Fig. (7). The progressive nature of chronic HF and the change in natural history of the syndrome with episodes of acute decompensation. Increasing frequency of acute events with disease progression leads to high rates of hospitalization and increased risk of mortality. With each acute event, myocardial injury may contribute to progressive LV dysfunction.
HF: heart failure; LV: left ventricular.

Hospitalizations

Hospitalization represents a crucial event in the natural history of HF (Fig. **7**), resulting in frequent re-hospitalizations and worse outcomes as compared with patients that do not need hospice care [23]. Patients with HF are hospitalized over a million times annually in the United States. Actually, HF is the primary diagnosis in >1.2 million hospitalizations annually (Fig. **8**) [10]. Among patients with HF, hospitalizations are common after HF diagnosis, with 4 out of 5 patients hospitalized at least once and almost half hospitalized more than 3 times. 50% of these are non-cardiovascular hospitalizations, especially in patients with HF-pEF. HF patients that have been hospitalized remain at high risk for repeated hospitalizations and demonstrate a 1-month readmission rate of 25% [24]. 75% of all HF hospitalizations are linked to exacerbation of symptoms in patients with known HF. 50% of hospitalized HF patients have to be re-admitted to the hospital within 6 months. Obviously, preventing HF re-hospitalization is an important parameter for better patient outcomes.

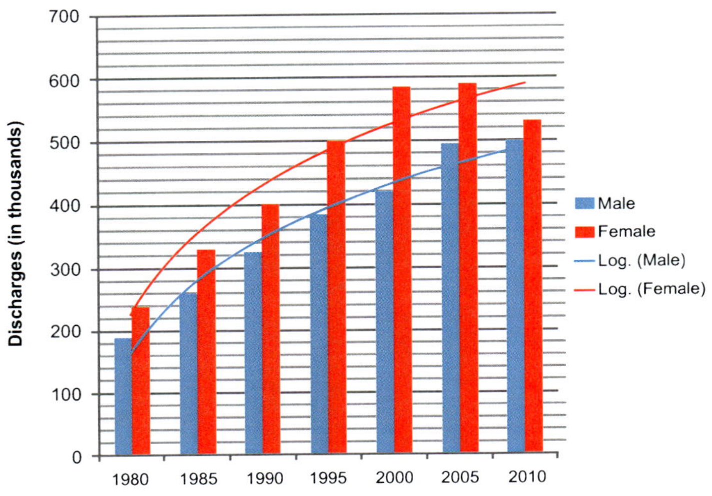

Fig. (8). Hospital discharges for heart failure by sex (United States: 1980–2010). Hospital discharges include people discharged alive, dead, and status unknown. Source: National Hospital Discharge Survey / National Center for Health Statistics and National Heart, Lung, and Blood Institute [10].

ECONOMIC COST

Heart failure importantly contributes to both the burden and the cost of national healthcare expenditures, since more elderly patients in the developed countries are hospitalized for HF than for any other medical condition. With the aging of the population, the impact of HF could rise substantially. In the United States the total cost for HF care exceeds \$30 billion annually (\$30.7 billions in 2012, Table **2**), taking into account: i) the cost of healthcare services, ii) the cost of medications, and iii) the cost for lost productivity [18]. Over half of these costs are spent on hospitalizations, with the mean cost of HF-related hospitalizations approaching

$25.000 per patient and being higher when HF is a secondary rather than the primary diagnosis (Fig. **9**) [25]. Obviously, preventing HF hospitalization and re-hospitalization is important to curb health care costs. In 2013, physician office visits for HF cost $1.8 billion. Projections show that by 2030, the total cost of HF will increase almost 127% to $69.7 billion from 2012. This equals ≈$244 for every US adult [18]. Direct costs (cost of medical care) are expected to increase more rapidly than indirect costs due to lost productivity and early mortality (Fig. **10**). Table **4** provides detailed 15-year projections of the total cost of care for HF stratified by different age groups of the US Population.

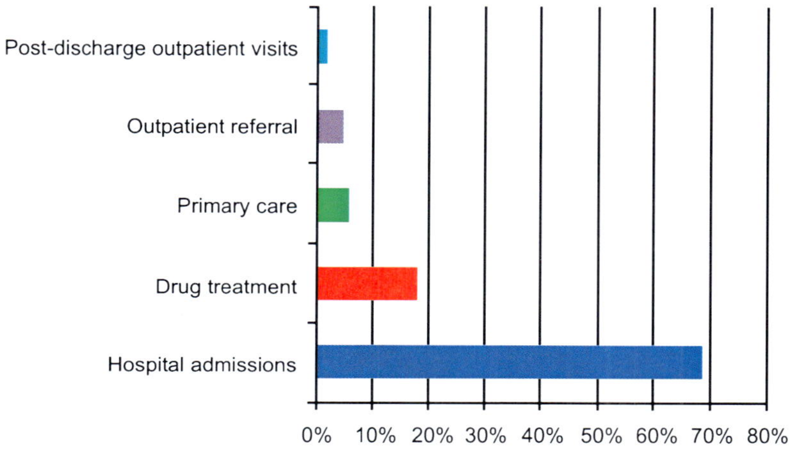

Fig. (9). Economic cost of heart failure (HF). Hospitalization accounts for most HF-associated costs [25].

Table 4. Projections of total cost of care ($ Billions) for heart failure for different age groups of the US Population* [18].

Year	18 – 44 y	45 – 64 y	65 – 79 y	≥80 y	All
2012	0.33	3.67	8.46	8.42	20.9
Direct	0.52	1.92	2.05	0.93	5.42
Indirect: Morbidity	0.66	2.53	0.98	0.18	4.35
Indirect: Mortality	1.51	8.12	11.5	9.53	30.7
Total					

(Table 4) contd.....

Year	18 – 44 y	45 – 64 y	65 – 79 y	≥80 y	All
2020					
Direct	0.43	4.58	14.2	11.8	31.1
Indirect: Morbidity	0.66	2.20	3.11	1.12	7.09
Indirect: Mortality	0.79	2.89	1.49	0.22	5.39
Total	1.88	9.67	18.8	13.2	43.6
2030					
Direct	0.59	5.86	23.3	23.4	53.1
Indirect: Morbidity	0.91	2.54	4.48	1.87	9.80
Indirect: Mortality	0.98	3.32	2.16	0.37	6.84
Total	2.48	11.7	29.9	25.6	69.7

*Excludes heart failure care costs that have been attributed to comorbid conditions.

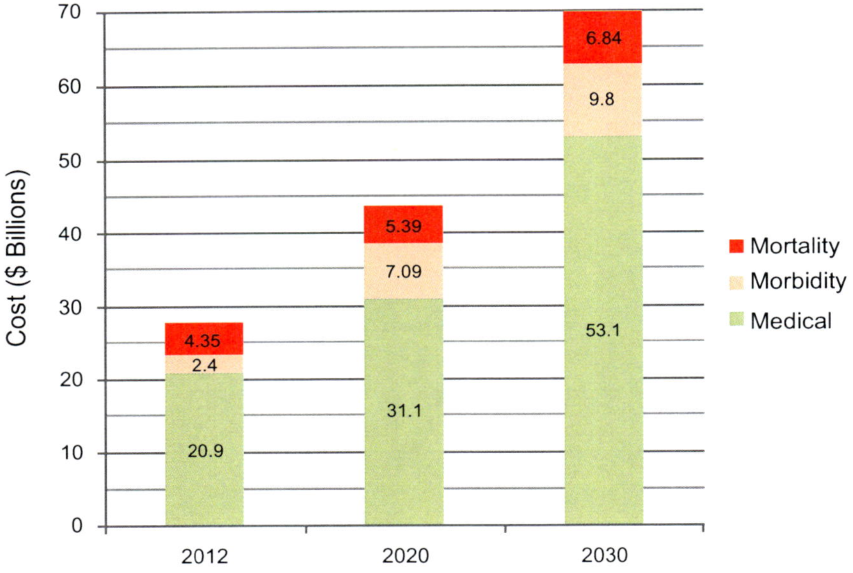

Fig. (10). Projected increase in direct and indirect costs attributable to heart failure from 2012 to 2030. Direct costs (cost of medical care) are expected to increase at a faster rate than indirect costs because of lost productivity and early mortality [18].

HEALTH POLICIES

Prevention of Heart Failure (HF)

Main health policy goals should include health improvement of the general population, HF prevention measures and reducing use of the limited healthcare resources. Prevention is an applicable strategy through optimal treatment of predisposing conditions such as coronary artery disease, hypertension, and diabetes mellitus [26]. Very similarly, prevention strategies need to be applied widely across different ethnic and racial groups as well [18]. Further research on HF prevention by sex is also awaited. In addition, a shift in the care model aiming to lower hospitalization rate could have a significant impact on the overall HF-related costs.

Early Diagnosis

Early diagnosis of non-acute new-onset HF in primary care is challenging but crucial because prompt initiation of evidence-based treatment can prevent or slow down further progression. In a cross-sectional diagnostic accuracy study with external validation, Kelder and colleagues evaluated the diagnostic value of physical examination and additional testing in primary care patients with suspected HF [3]. All patients underwent standardized diagnostic work-up including chest x-ray, spirometry, electrocardiography (ECG), N-terminal B-type natriuretic peptide (NT-proBNP) measurement, and echocardiography in specially equipped outpatient diagnostic HF clinics. The diagnosis of HF was established by an outcome panel using the initial clinical findings and 6-month follow-up evidence, blinded to biomarker data. The combination of three items from history (age, coronary artery disease, and loop diuretic use) plus six from physical examination (pulse rate and regularity, displaced apex beat, rales, heart murmur, and increased jugular vein pressure) showed independent diagnostic value, whereas NT-proBNP was identified as the supplementary test with the strongest diagnostic performance. For daily practice, a diagnostic rule was derived to quantify the probability of HF in patients with new symptoms suggestive of HF that may help to improve clinical decision making.

Heart Failure (HF) Clinics

Specialized multidisciplinary clinics have been found to reduce HF mortality serving as a cost effective way of delivering ambulatory care to HF patients. Wijeysundera and colleagues performed a cost-effectiveness analysis, with a 12-year time frame, from the perspective of the Ontario Ministry of Health and

Long-term Care, comparing a standard care cohort, consisting of all HF patients admitted to hospital in 2005, to a hypothetical cohort treated in HF clinics [27]. HF clinics were associated with a 29% decline in all-cause mortality but a 12% increase in hospitalizations. Projected life-expectancy of HF clinic patients was 3.91 years, compared to 3.21 years for standard care patients. The cost of care in the HF clinic was $52 per 30 patient-days, whereas the 12-year cumulative cost per patient in the HF clinic group was $66,532 *versus* $53,638 in the standard care group. The incremental cost-effectiveness ratio (ICER, a statistic used in cost-effectiveness analysis to summarize the cost-effectiveness of a health care intervention, defined as the difference in cost between two possible interventions divided by the difference in their effect) was $18,259 per life-year gained [27].

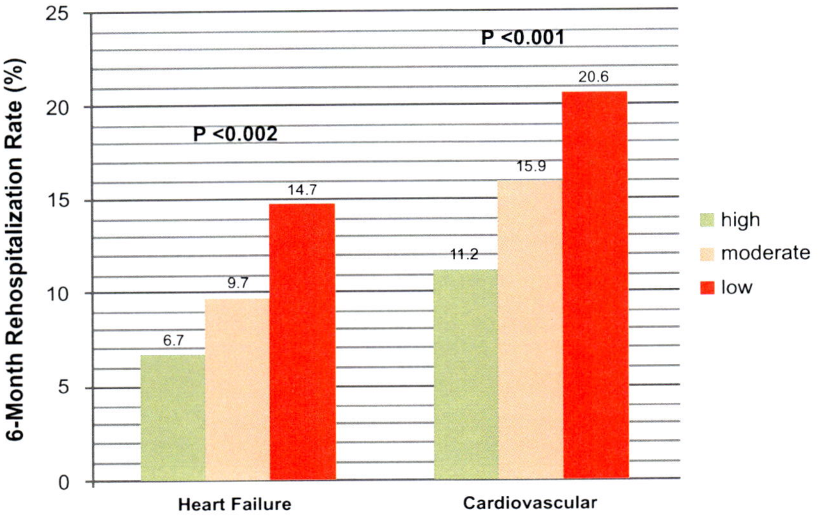

Fig. (11). Adherence to heart failure (HF) guidelines predicts HF hospitalizations. [Reprinted from ref [28] with kind permission from Oxford University Press].

Adherence to Heart Failure (HF) Guidelines

Adherence to HF guidelines has been constantly associated with improved outcome and should be the main target of every HF clinic and every health-care provider. The impact on outcome of the implementation of European guidelines for the treatment of chronic HF was recently evaluated in a study by Komajda and colleagues [28]. The investigators demonstrated that adherence of physicians to treatment guidelines is related to lower hospitalization rate in actual practice and underscored the importance to develop further quality improvement programs in this condition (Fig. **11**).

Patient Selection

Selecting HF patients carefully for certain interventions, especially those of very high cost (cardiac resynchronization therapy, implantable defibrillator, valve repair, *etc*) is important. Well-chosen patients usually have a shorter in-hospital length of stay, impose a lower cost burden, and may even generate a long-term profit in the society. Each hospital medical review board should select the patients likely to have the best outcomes. On the other hand, those patients at too high level of risk for advanced therapies may benefit more from disease management and palliative care. Rather than use an expensive, fully implantable LV assist device (LVAD) for high-risk patients in cardiogenic shock, it might be preferable to select a temporary device, providing time to reassess these patients and subsequently evaluate their neurologic and psychological status [29].

Nutritional Care

Malnutrition is a common finding especially in advanced HF patients and is associated with an increased risk of re-hospitalization and all-cause mortality. To achieve optimal long-term outcomes in these patients, an interdisciplinary approach that incorporates a nutrition-support team is vital, both in the in-hospital and in the out-patient period.

Post-operative Discharge Planning

HF patients who undergo hemodynamic interventions carry an increased risk of infection and prolonged hospitalization. Long hospitalizations can lead to a substantial deficit in even the most profitable HF programs. Ideally, one nurse should focus on post-operation discharge planning - examining each patient daily and preparing them for discharge. In order to decrease the length of stay, some HF centers have developed partnerships with long-term acute-care facilities that have personnel specifically trained in advanced HF therapies [29].

Educational Programs

Patient education is very important and documentation of learning goals and results should be provided at discharge, a task that can be undertaken by experienced nurses. Very similarly, group-based multi-professional educational programs for family members increase knowledge about HF and, therefore, should also be provided at clinics [30]. This information should preferably be repeated frequently during post-discharge period to maintain knowledge level.

Telemonitoring

Telemonitoring is a novel diagnostic tool that has been reported to be beneficial for HF patients. Physiological data (such as body weight, heart rate, arterial blood pressure, electrocardiogram, and other data by portable devices) are recorded and transmitting remotely (*via* a telephone line, a mobile phone, or a computer) to a server where they can be stored, reviewed, and analyzed [31]. Currently available trial results, although ambiguous, tend to be in favor of telemonitoring regarding reduced hospitalization rates. Importantly, improvement of the quality of life has been observed in all studies, whereas telemonitoring is also highly acceptable by chronic HF patients.

CONCLUDING REMARKS

The complex clinical syndrome, termed as "heart failure" is an important healthcare issue due to its high prevalence, mortality and morbidity rates, and economic costs. 2-3% of the general population worldwide has HF with prevalence increasing with age. Among those ≥80 years of age, almost 12% of both men and women have HF. Mortality is high, with 50% of patients not surviving 5 years after the initial diagnosis. The cost of HF care is extremely high, mostly driven by the frequent hospitalizations for HF, and poses a significant concern for the healthcare systems. Both prevalence and cost will increase markedly in the near future because of the aging of the population and the implementation of life-prolonging therapies in HF patients. Understanding the epidemiology and pathophysiology of the syndrome, identifying the predictors with the higher clinical significance, and cost-effectively implementing the available diagnostic modalities are essential parameters in order to devise effective preventive interventions and take advantage of novel therapeutic approaches to curb this epidemic.

CONFLICT OF INTEREST

The authors confirm that they have no conflict of interest to declare for this publication.

ACKNOWLEDGEMENTS

Declared none.

REFERENCES

[1] Yancy CW, Jessup M, Bozkurt B, *et al.* 2013 ACCF/AHA guideline for the management of heart failure: a report of the American College of Cardiology Foundation/American Heart Association Task Force on practice guidelines. Circulation 2013; 128(16): e240-327. [http://dx.doi.org/10.1161/CIR.0b013e31829e8807] [PMID: 23741058]

[2] McMurray JJ, Adamopoulos S, Anker SD, *et al.* ESC guidelines for the diagnosis and treatment of acute and chronic heart failure 2012: the task force for the diagnosis and treatment of acute and chronic heart failure 2012 of the European society of cardiology. Developed in collaboration with the heart failure association (HFA) of the ESC. Eur Heart J 2012; 33(14): 1787-847. [http://dx.doi.org/10.1093/eurheartj/ehs104] [PMID: 22611136]

[3] Kelder JC, Cramer MJ, van Wijngaarden J, *et al.* The diagnostic value of physical examination and additional testing in primary care patients with suspected heart failure. Circulation 2011; 124(25): 2865-73. [http://dx.doi.org/10.1161/CIRCULATIONAHA.111.019216] [PMID: 22104551]

[4] Fonarow GC, Stough WG, Abraham WT, *et al.* Characteristics, treatments, and outcomes of patients with preserved systolic function hospitalized for heart failure: a report from the OPTIMIZE-HF Registry. J Am Coll Cardiol 2007; 50(8): 768-77. [http://dx.doi.org/10.1016/j.jacc.2007.04.064] [PMID: 17707182]

[5] Borlaug BA, Paulus WJ. Heart failure with preserved ejection fraction: pathophysiology, diagnosis, and treatment. Eur Heart J 2011; 32(6): 670-9. [http://dx.doi.org/10.1093/eurheartj/ehq426] [PMID: 21138935]

[6] Paulus WJ, Tschöpe C, Sanderson JE, *et al.* How to diagnose diastolic heart failure: a consensus statement on the diagnosis of heart failure with normal left ventricular ejection fraction by the Heart Failure and Echocardiography Associations of the European Society of Cardiology. Eur Heart J 2007; 28(20): 2539-50. [http://dx.doi.org/10.1093/eurheartj/ehm037] [PMID: 17428822]

[7] Hunt SA, Baker DW, Chin MH, *et al.* ACC/AHA Guidelines for the Evaluation and Management of Chronic Heart Failure in the Adult: Executive Summary A Report of the American College of Cardiology/American Heart Association Task Force on Practice Guidelines (Committee to Revise the

1995 Guidelines for the Evaluation and Management of Heart Failure): Developed in Collaboration With the International Society for Heart and Lung Transplantation; Endorsed by the Heart Failure Society of America. Circulation 2001; 104(24): 2996-3007.
[http://dx.doi.org/10.1161/hc4901.102568] [PMID: 11739319]

[8] Djoussé L, Driver JA, Gaziano JM. Relation between modifiable lifestyle factors and lifetime risk of heart failure. JAMA 2009; 302(4): 394-400.
[http://dx.doi.org/10.1001/jama.2009.1062] [PMID: 19622818]

[9] Lloyd-Jones DM, Larson MG, Leip EP, *et al.* Lifetime risk for developing congestive heart failure: the Framingham Heart Study. Circulation 2002; 106(24): 3068-72.
[http://dx.doi.org/10.1161/01.CIR.0000039105.49749.6F] [PMID: 12473553]

[10] Mozaffarian D, Benjamin EJ, Go AS, *et al.* Heart disease and stroke statistics--2015 update: a report from the American Heart Association. Circulation 2015; 131(4): e29-e322.
[http://dx.doi.org/10.1161/CIR.0000000000000152] [PMID: 25520374]

[11] Curtis LH, Whellan DJ, Hammill BG, *et al.* Incidence and prevalence of heart failure in elderly persons, 1994-2003. Arch Intern Med 2008; 168(4): 418-24.
[http://dx.doi.org/10.1001/archinternmed.2007.80] [PMID: 18299498]

[12] Bahrami H, Kronmal R, Bluemke DA, *et al.* Differences in the incidence of congestive heart failure by ethnicity: the multi-ethnic study of atherosclerosis. Arch Intern Med 2008; 168(19): 2138-45.
[http://dx.doi.org/10.1001/archinte.168.19.2138] [PMID: 18955644]

[13] Loehr LR, Rosamond WD, Chang PP, Folsom AR, Chambless LE. Heart failure incidence and survival (from the Atherosclerosis Risk in Communities study). Am J Cardiol 2008; 101(7): 1016-22.
[http://dx.doi.org/10.1016/j.amjcard.2007.11.061] [PMID: 18359324]

[14] Liu L, Eisen HJ. Epidemiology of heart failure and scope of the problem. Cardiol Clin 2014; 32(1): 1-8, vii.
[http://dx.doi.org/10.1016/j.ccl.2013.09.009] [PMID: 24286574]

[15] Redfield MM, Jacobsen SJ, Burnett JC Jr, Mahoney DW, Bailey KR, Rodeheffer RJ. Burden of systolic and diastolic ventricular dysfunction in the community: appreciating the scope of the heart failure epidemic. JAMA 2003; 289(2): 194-202.
[http://dx.doi.org/10.1001/jama.289.2.194] [PMID: 12517230]

[16] Jong P, Yusuf S, Rousseau MF, Ahn SA, Bangdiwala SI. Effect of enalapril on 12-year survival and life expectancy in patients with left ventricular systolic dysfunction: a follow-up study. Lancet 2003; 361(9372): 1843-8.
[http://dx.doi.org/10.1016/S0140-6736(03)13501-5] [PMID: 12788569]

[17] Roger VL, Weston SA, Redfield MM, *et al.* Trends in heart failure incidence and survival in a community-based population. JAMA 2004; 292(3): 344-50.
[http://dx.doi.org/10.1001/jama.292.3.344] [PMID: 15265849]

[18] Heidenreich PA, Albert NM, Allen LA, *et al.* Forecasting the impact of heart failure in the United States: a policy statement from the American Heart Association. Circ Heart Fail 2013; 6(3): 606-19.
[http://dx.doi.org/10.1161/HHF.0b013e318291329a] [PMID: 23616602]

[19] Levy D, Kenchaiah S, Larson MG, *et al.* Long-term trends in the incidence of and survival with heart

failure. N Engl J Med 2002; 347(18): 1397-402.
[http://dx.doi.org/10.1056/NEJMoa020265] [PMID: 12409541]

[20] Ammar KA, Jacobsen SJ, Mahoney DW, *et al.* Prevalence and prognostic significance of heart failure stages: application of the American College of Cardiology/American Heart Association heart failure staging criteria in the community. Circulation 2007; 115(12): 1563-70.
[http://dx.doi.org/10.1161/CIRCULATIONAHA.106.666818] [PMID: 17353436]

[21] Bueno H, Ross JS, Wang Y, *et al.* Trends in length of stay and short-term outcomes among Medicare patients hospitalized for heart failure, 1993-2006. JAMA 2010; 303(21): 2141-7.
[http://dx.doi.org/10.1001/jama.2010.748] [PMID: 20516414]

[22] Owan TE, Hodge DO, Herges RM, Jacobsen SJ, Roger VL, Redfield MM. Trends in prevalence and outcome of heart failure with preserved ejection fraction. N Engl J Med 2006; 355(3): 251-9.
[http://dx.doi.org/10.1056/NEJMoa052256] [PMID: 16855265]

[23] Giamouzis G, Kalogeropoulos A, Georgiopoulou V, *et al.* Hospitalization epidemic in patients with heart failure: risk factors, risk prediction, knowledge gaps, and future directions. J Card Fail 2011; 17(1): 54-75.
[http://dx.doi.org/10.1016/j.cardfail.2010.08.010] [PMID: 21187265]

[24] Krumholz HM, Merrill AR, Schone EM, *et al.* Patterns of hospital performance in acute myocardial infarction and heart failure 30-day mortality and readmission. Circ Cardiovasc Qual Outcomes 2009; 2(5): 407-13.
[http://dx.doi.org/10.1161/CIRCOUTCOMES.109.883256] [PMID: 20031870]

[25] Stewart S, Jenkins A, Buchan S, McGuire A, Capewell S, McMurray JJ. The current cost of heart failure to the National Health Service in the UK. Eur J Heart Fail 2002; 4(3): 361-71.
[http://dx.doi.org/10.1016/S1388-9842(01)00198-2] [PMID: 12034163]

[26] Triposkiadis F, Giamouzis G, Butler J. The importance of managing diabetes correctly to prevent heart failure. Expert Rev Cardiovasc Ther 2011; 9(3): 257-9.
[http://dx.doi.org/10.1586/erc.11.6] [PMID: 21438801]

[27] Wijeysundera HC, Machado M, Wang X, *et al.* Cost-effectiveness of specialized multidisciplinary heart failure clinics in Ontario, Canada. Value Health 2010; 13(8): 915-21.

[28] Komajda M, Lapuerta P, Hermans N, *et al.* Adherence to guidelines is a predictor of outcome in chronic heart failure: the MAHLER survey. Eur Heart J 2005; 26(16): 1653-9.
[http://dx.doi.org/10.1093/eurheartj/ehi251] [PMID: 15827061]

[29] Bogaev RC. Cost considerations in the treatment of heart failure. Tex Heart Inst J 2010; 37(5): 557-8.
[PMID: 20978567]

[30] Löfvenmark C, Karlsson MR, Edner M, Billing E, Mattiasson AC. A group-based multi-professional education programme for family members of patients with chronic heart failure: effects on knowledge and patients' health care utilization. Patient Educ Couns 2011; 85(2): e162-8.
[http://dx.doi.org/10.1016/j.pec.2010.09.026] [PMID: 21050694]

[31] Giamouzis G, Mastrogiannis D, Koutrakis K, *et al.* Telemonitoring in chronic heart failure: a systematic review. Cardiol Res Pract 2012. 410820
[http://dx.doi.org/10.1155/2012/410820]

CHAPTER 2

Basics of Cardiac Physiology

Isaac Aidonidis*, **Rodopi Stamatiou, Sotirios Zarogiannis, Chrissi Hatzoglou, Konstantinos Gourgoulianis** and **Paschalis-Adam Molyvdas**

Department of Physiology, School of Medicine, Faculty of Health Sciences, University of Thessaly, Larissa, Greece

Abstract: Despite painstaking investigations on the pathogenetic mechanisms of heart failure, there still remains a long distance to completely understand the complexity of the events dominating its progression. In this direction, many efforts have been made by recruiting both basic physiology and imaging techniques in order to overcome gaps that are present in diagnostic and therapeutical interventions in heart failure. Intact heart muscle physiology and circulation are the cornerstone for a comprehensive insight into the mechanistic understanding of the relationship between contractility, coronary blood flow, and myocardial perfusion. The latter seems to be a major cause of cardiac muscle damage leading to progression into systolic heart failure. Therefore, it is a matter of urgency to re-evaluate and extend the spectrum of imaging techniques for achieving a better assessment of myocardial perfusion based on fundamental concepts of cardiac cellular and subcellular physiology.

Keywords: Actin, Calcium kinetics, Cardiac physiology, Diastolic dysfunction, Endothelin, Excitation-contraction coupling, Myocardial contractility, Myocardial perfusion, Myosin, Phospholamban, Relaxation, Ryanodine receptor, Tropomyosin, Troponin.

INTRODUCTION

This chapter emphasizes the physiologic mechanisms governing cardiac muscle systole and diastole in order to facilitate understanding of possible dysfunctions

* **Corresponding author Isaac Aidonidis:** Department of Physiology (Cardiovascular Research Section), School of Medicine, Faculty of Health Sciences, University of Thessaly, Larissa, Greece; Tel: +30 2410 68 5560; Fax: +30 2410 68 5546; E-mail: iaido@med.uth.gr.

Panagiotis Georgoulias (Ed.)

that may eventually intermingle in pump incompetence of failing heart. More specifically, the role of intracellular calcium (Ca^{+2}) kinetics for an adequately ejected blood volume and an isovolumic relaxation phase will be presented in detail.

Molecular processes taking place in contractility of physiologic cardiac myocytes that could be affected in the setting of heart failure would be the major objective of this chapter. The topic upon cardiac contractility and coronary flow physiology will synoptically focus on the mechanisms addressing regulation of myocardial perfusion.

CARDIAC MECHANIC FUNCTION

Excitation - Contraction Coupling

Major players in excitation-contraction coupling (ECC) are free Ca^{+2} concentration in the myoplasm, and integrity of the components of the cross-bridge complex (contractile apparatus). This system incorporates the contractile proteins (actin and myosin) and the regulatory proteins (troponin and tropomyosin). Contraction is possible to occur only when adenosine triphosphate (ATP) and Ca^{+2} are present. Availability of adequately high cytosolic Ca^{+2} concentrations is gained by Ca^{+2} entering the cell *via* the voltage-gated L-type Ca channels after depolarization of the cell membrane, which activates in cardiac muscle the mechanism of Ca-induced Ca^{+2} release from the sarcoplasmic reticulum (SR) [1].

Normally, the actin and myosin filaments do not interact (non-contracted state). This happens only when Ca^{+2} binds to the regulatory domain of troponin C, an action that abrogates inhibition of actin-myosin interaction through troponin I. Muscle shortening (systole) occurs by interaction of myosin heads with binding sites on the actin filament, resulting to increased overlapping of actin and myosin, an effect that brings the Z lines together during contraction.

When the intracellular Ca^{+2} concentration is reduced during electrical repolarization, predominantly *via* the reverse-mode activation of Na/Ca exchanger (NCX) and by re-entering of Ca^{+2} into the SR *via* the SR Ca-ATPase (SERCA), diastole starts. This process is significantly slower than the contraction event. By interventions aiming at enhancing cardiac muscle contractility of a failing myocardium, the mechanisms governing deranged myofilament Ca^{+2} sensitivity and altered Ca^{+2} fluxes still remain investigational.

Removal of cytosolic Ca^{+2} is necessary to allow relaxation and diastole of the heart. SERCA seems to be responsible for removing 70% of the activator Ca^{+2} from the cytosol, followed by activation of the forward-operated NCX that removes almost the rest of Ca^{+2} content. After a contraction phase, slowed or inhibited Ca^{+2} extrusion from the cytoplasm (*e.g.*, due to failed sarcolemmal Ca-ATPase or reverse-mode NCX activation by high [Na]i) may impede relaxation and increase appearance of Ca-triggered after depolarizations and cardiac arrhythmias. Moreover, sustained increase of intercellular Ca^{+2} during diastole may augment cardiac oxygen demand and compress small intramural coronary vessels, particularly in subendocardium, thus reducing coronary blood flow [2].

Pathophysiologic Alterations in Heart Failure

Defective ECC could be responsible for many contractility abnormalities encountered in congestive heart failure. It has been suggested that the mechanism of Ca-induced Ca release (ECC gain) is impaired in the failing heart, possibly due to a widening of the space between the T tubular membrane and the SR [3]. It must be pointed out that in order to have a normal ECC, several signalling pathways have to function properly. The checkpoints of these pathways enable therapeutic interventions in both arrhythmia management and hemodynamic improvement of the failing heart.

Certain types of cardiac G-protein-coupled receptors (GPCRs), including the beta-adrenergic and the angiotensin II type 1 receptors, are abundantly expressed in myocyte membranes and represent possible targets of drug action, directly modulating cardiac contractility and function [4, 5]. Lymperopoulos *et al.* highlighted in a review article the molecular pathways governing the pathophysiology of cardiac inotropic function in heart failure [6]. They focused on multiple genetic variations in several genes responsible for encoding abnormal intracellular proteins that could derange these molecular pathways in the failing heart and finally the translation of specific stimuli, such as hormones or drugs into the contractile response. Specifically, they pointed out that inhibition of all signaling pathways indiscriminately, typically resulting from a non-selective GPCR blockade to endogenous agonists (*e.g.* catecholamines), cannot always be beneficial for heart failure therapy because, despite blockade of beta-adrenoceptors, circulating plasma catecholamine levels remained elevated in heart failure patients. Lymperopoulos *et al.* found that this is due to the fact that sympatholytic agents did not effectively target the alpha2-adrenoceptor-mediated catecholamine inhibition, explaining their failure of efficient sympatholytic activity. This has been attributed to a substantial alpha2-adrenoceptor dysregulation during heart failure in the adrenal gland, triggered by increased expression and activity of GPCR kinase 2 [7]. Accordingly, novel heart failure therapies have to be based on updated knowledge on cardiac GPCR signaling, including the beta-adrenoceptors and the renin-angiotensin-aldosterone system [8]. In this sense, GPCR signalling is a matter deserving further investigation in order to elucidate difficulties by selective targeting of GPCR-induced signalling pathways preferentially on the intracellular interface of the receptor [9]. Substantial experimental investigations have been made on various molecular topics on the pathophysiology of myocardial contractility and relaxation. Accordingly, heart failure may arise from deranged Ca^{+2} storing and/or Ca^{+2} releasing mechanisms in the SR that are partially associated with lower phospholamban levels, or defective regulation of the ryanodine receptor 2 (RyR2) in the failing heart, respectively [10, 11].

For years, beta-adrenoceptor signalling pathways modulation has been the most preferential pharmacological option in heart failure patients. Long-term blockade of these receptors can reverse their down-regulation and have positive effects by increasing signalling mediated by inhibitory G proteins and GPCR kinase 2, thereby ameliorating abnormalities by the production of ECC proteins. However, there are different effects of beta-blockers (beta1 or beta2), since these receptors can interact with signalling pathways that act as cardioprotective factors against apoptosis or necrosis of the cardiomyocytes. Furthermore, several genetic factors exist that are involved in the effectiveness of such drugs. Other therapeutic approaches include blunting the activity of GPCR kinase 2 or up-regulating the expression of the gene encoding adenyl cyclase 6 [7, 12].

Another research field has been the blockade of various pro-inflammatory cytokines such as endothelin, or tumor necrosis factor. However, anticytokine drugs yielded disappointing results due to the complexity of the interactions between these cytokines and other signalling pathways. Pharmacologic targets in abnormal ECC may be also the natriuretic peptides [atrial natriuretic peptide (ANP) and brain natriuretic peptide (BNP)], which are cardioprotective. The endogenous circulating concentrations of ANP and BNP are often increased in heart failure and serve as diagnostic markers of disease progression. Apart from direct alterations in the levels of these peptides, suppression of hydrolysis of cyclic guanosine monophosphate (GMP) through phosphodiesterase 5 (PDE5) antagonists, such as sildenafil, can affect their action.

Myocardial Contractility and Relaxation

Contraction of cardiac muscle must be followed by relaxation, which mainly results from re-uptake of Ca^{+2} into the SR, as well as from the extrusion of Ca^{+2} predominantly *via* the forward-operated NCX (Fig. **1**).

Once the propagated impulse depolarizes the ventricular cells, the voltage-gated L-type Ca channels open and Ca^{+2} flows into the cell. Intracellular Ca^{+2} interacts with the RyR2 causing molecular conformational changes that may result in Ca^{+2} release from the SR. Sufficient Ca^{+2} released from the SR (Ca-induced Ca release, CICR) may critically increase cytosolic Ca^{+2} concentrations to values able to trigger contraction. Importantly, the increasing cytosolic Ca^{+2}*per se* triggers a negative feedback pathway causing Ca-induced inactivation of the L-type channels, thereby reducing further Ca^{+2} influx and maintaining Ca^{+2} homeostasis.

In detail, after completion of contraction and unbinding from the actin-myosin complex, cytosolic Ca^{+2} has to be drastically reduced and this happens mainly *via* the phospholamban-modulated Ca uptake pump, allowing Ca^{+2} ions to re-enter into the SR (initiation of relaxation). Under basal conditions, phospholamban exerts inhibition on SERCA, whereas disinhibiting of SERCA happens when phospholamban is phosphorylated through activation of protein kinase A and Ca/calmodulin–dependent kinase II. Abrogation of phospholamban inhibition may increase SERCA-mediated uptake of Ca^{+2}, speeding relaxation.

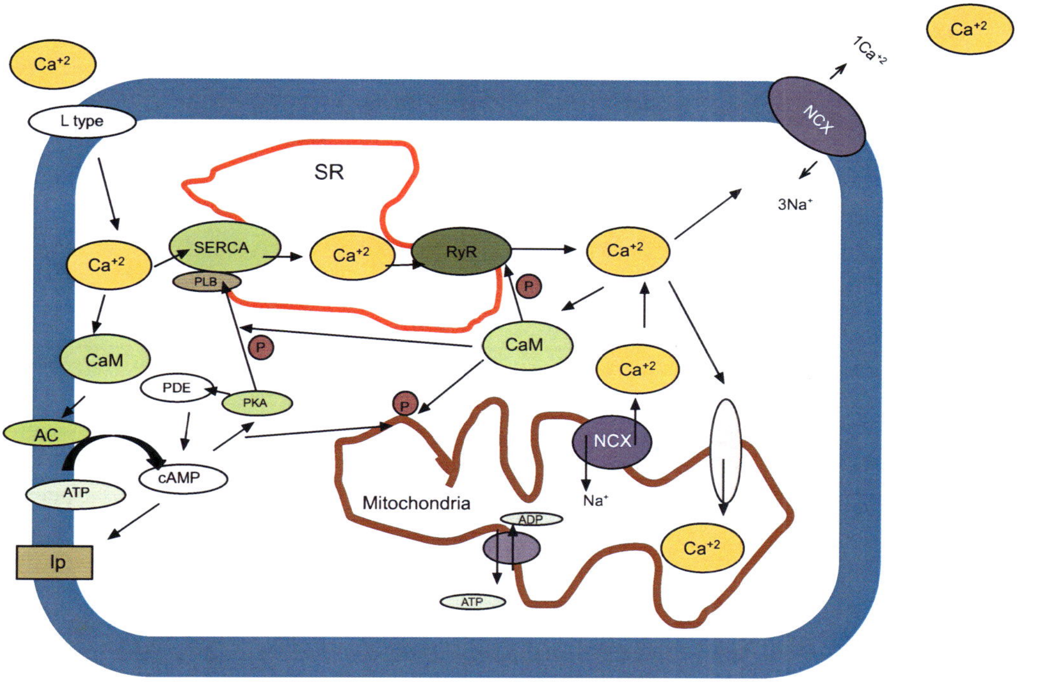

Fig. (1). This illustration depicts the pathways of Ca^{+2} kinetics in the cytoplasm. Crucial roles of PLB and RyR activation and deactivation dependence from phosphorylation in the SR are shown.
AC: adenylyl cyclase; ADP: adenosine diphosphate; ATP: adenosine triphosphate; cAMP: cyclic adenosine monophosphate; CaM: calmodulin; NCX: Na/Ca exchanger; P: phosphorylation; PDE: phosphodiesterase; PKA: protein kinase A; PLB: phospholamban; RyR: ryanodine receptor; SERCA: SR Ca-ATPase; SR: sarcoplasmic reticulum.

It is reasonable to assume that an interaction between the Ca^{+2} uptake pump and the Ca^{+2} release channel may modulate Ca^{+2} accumulation in the cytosol of cardiomyocytes. Disorders of this intracellular Ca^{+2} cycling may increase SR-Ca and generate spontaneous Ca^{+2} transients leading to propagated Ca^{+2} waves, triggering arrhythmias or impairing contractile activity of cardiac muscle [13]. The densities of Ca^{+2} release channels, beta-adrenergic receptor, Ca^{+2} pump ATPase molecules, and phospholamban decrease in systolic heart failure [1, 14].

Hemodynamic Determinants of Physiologic Left Ventricular Function

Left ventricular (LV) ejection and filling constitute the two principal hemodynamic heart functions. Three important determinants of LV ejection (systole) are the end-diastolic fibre length, the myocardial contractility and the aortic impedance (afterload). LV compliance and its reciprocal, the myocardial stiffness, represent two determinants of LV filling during diastole (end-diastolic volume-pressure relationship).

Notably, clinically asymptomatic chronic derangements in LV wall relaxation (heart failure with preserved ejection fraction) often precede the development of decreasing compliance promoting hypertrophy, dilation, and transition into overt systolic failure. Left atrial stiffness may play a crucial role for the course of LV relaxation abnormalities, thereby deteriorating hypertrophy and accelerating progression to systolic pump failure. The absence of an adequate decrease in LV pressure (end-systolic pressure) during isovolumic relaxation represents also an indicator of non compliant ventricle with impaired elasticity.

Increased LV end-systolic pressure may hinder normal ventricular diastolic filling due to prematurely reached end-diastolic pressure that overcomes left atrial pressure, thereby forcing the mitral valve to close earlier. This may result in diminished ejection volume due to retention of blood in left atrium, resulting in a stronger atrial contraction. All these changes may primarily arise from decreased compliance as the principal cause for diastolic dysfunction, increasing LV pressures and left atrial stretch. The perpetuation of a vicious cycle may lastly lead to LV hypertrophy and congestive heart failure.

Increases in LV contractility is affected by beta1-adrenergic agonists and PDE inhibitors *via* elevated cyclic AMP (cAMP) levels triggered by adenylate cyclase (AC) activity (Fig. **1**). The mechanism is that cAMP-dependent protein kinases catalyse the phosphorylation of plasma membrane Ca^{+2} channels, thus increasing the probability of channel opening and resulting in a positive inotropic effect. Because beta1-adrenoceptor desensitization in chronic heart failure leads to blunted functional effects of sympathetic stimulation, Ca^{+2} sensitizing drugs (*e.g.*, levosimendan), selectively targeting on the contractile proteins, may be used to enhance Ca^{+2} binding to troponin C, improving cardiac performance [14].

Pressure or volume overload as causes of heart failure may lead to qualitatively different molecular changes, indicating different signal transduction pathways participating in the development of the disease.

CORONARY BLOOD FLOW

Myocardial perfusion with oxygenated blood is mediated through the coronary arteries during diastole, since contraction of cardiac muscle during the systolic phase may compress intramural vessels or increase their resistance by deforming their cavity. Obviously, subendocardial regions, where tissue pressure is higher, may show a larger impediment of perfusion than epicardial regions during cardiac systole. As a consequence of changes in diastolic intervals, heart rate may modulate myocardial perfusion by spending different times in diastole and by altering the myocardial supply-demand ratio in oxygen. Accordingly, an increase in heart rate raises oxygen consumption of cardiac muscle. Increased end-diastolic filling pressure or end-systolic pressure, at the early stages of heart failure (diastolic dysfunction), might expect to have potent influences on normal subendocardial circulation during the diastolic interval. An additional factor is the decreasing compliance of cardiac muscle, principally being the primary cause initializing diastolic dysfunction.

The association of impaired contractility and coronary flow is very important as it constitutes a vicious cycle by which abnormal contractility further reduces cardiac muscle perfusion and vice versa. After reperfusion of ischemically damaged myocardium, delayed re-normalization of contractility (stunning) may negatively influence coronary flow which in turn deteriorates impaired diastolic relaxation. One of the major players in this phenomenon is a sustained cytosolic Ca^{+2} overload that occurs during the repolarization phase of cellular action potential, frequently extending beyond the end of repolarization (diastole).

Long-lasting working of the myocardial wall against an abnormally high intraventricular pressure may lead to reduced subendocardial and intramural coronary flow that accelerates ischemic myocardial damage, hypertrophy, and fibrotic degeneration of cardiac tissue. Ischemia-induced vasoconstriction *per se* may potentially contribute, together with abnormal regional contractility, to the so-called no-reflow phenomenon after coronary reperfusion. Specifically, release of endothelin, as well as endothelial damage and swelling or persistent critical closing due to low coronary perfusion pressure are possible determinants of no-reflow phenomenon. No-reflow phenomenon in turn might be a causing factor of stunned myocardium accompanied by delayed recovery from contractile dysfunction after reperfusion of ischemic heart.

Vascular smooth muscle cell contraction (VSMC) is primarily dependent on the opening of membrane voltage-gated L-type Ca channels and intracellular Ca release from the endoplasmic reticulum stores mediated through alpha-adrenergic mechanisms (Fig. **2**). Although the dilatory responses of coronary arteries to exercise are faster than the constrictor ones, the alpha-adrenergic effect on the coronary flow not only exists during exercise or ischemia, but it seems important for preventing circulatory steal from the subendocardium, thereby equalizing transmural myocardial perfusion [1]. In congestive heart failure, the coronary artery endothelium reduces the alpha-adrenergic response to norepinephrine. Therefore, it may play a protective role against vasoconstrictor hormones. Probably, this could explain the finding that patients with nonischemic heart failure show dilated coronary arteries in the angiographic examination.

Myocardial ischemia promotes vasodilation *via* adenosine formation and opening of ATP-sensitive potassium (K^+) channels. ATP levels holding the K^+ channel closed are reduced due to ischemia-related ATP breakdown; as a consequence, release of K^+ from the cytosol to the extracellular space shortens the plateau phase of repolarization, thereby decreasing Ca^{+2} entry and producing vasodilation.

In spite of substantial knowledge gained about the perfusion of subendocardium, evidently being the most vulnerable region during an ischemic episode, further investigation on early diagnostic procedures is needed to protect irreversible damage. Collectively, better technologies have to be developed in evaluating subendocardial perfusion that could incorporate the presently available methods, such as perfusion scintigraphy and positron emission tomography (PET). PET measures coronary blood flow in humans by monitoring the uptake of $^{13}N\text{-}NH_3$, while thallium-201 (^{201}TI) enables recognition of poorly contracting myocardial segments without, however, revealing absolute blood flow measurements [15].

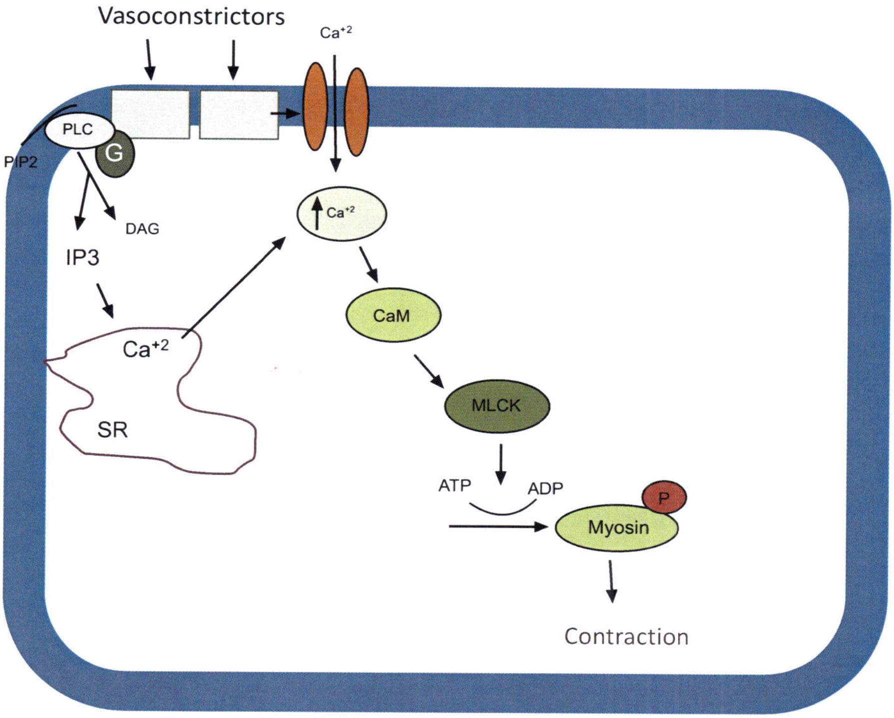

Fig. (2). Mechanisms of VSMC contraction. Intracellular Ca^{+2} is increased *via* the voltage-sensitive L-type Ca^{+2} channels, as well as through stimulation of alpha1-adrenoceptors in the cell membrane (vasoconstrictors). By the latter, Ca^{+2} concentration is increased *via* a IP3-receptor activation mechanism resulting in Ca^{+2} release from the SR. Ca^{+2} binds with CaM and activates the MLCK which then activates myosin *via* phosphorylation. Active myosin is able to interact with actin, producing contraction of the muscle. CaM: calmodulin; DAG: diacylglycerol; IP3: inositol trisphosphate; MLCK: myosin light chain kinase; P: phosphorylation; PIP2: phosphatidylinositol biphosphate; PLC: phospholipase C; SR: sarcoplasmic reticulum; VSMC: vascular smooth muscle cell.

CONTRACTION - PERFUSION MATCHING AND DIAGNOSTIC IMAGING PROCEDURES

Imaging of myocardial viability after re-opening of an occluded coronary artery is essential for choosing the correct therapeutic regimen in clinical settings. Cardiac PET may provide substantial information of regional myocardial perfusion and metabolism by documenting the efficacy of reperfusion therapy after thrombolysis, percutaneous transluminal coronary angioplasty (PTCA), or coronary artery bypass graft surgery (CABG) [15]. Main target is to quantify the degree of restoration of myocardial perfusion after recanalizing of an occluded coronary artery. Many factors, however, may influence the reliability of the measurement method in assessing regional perfusion of ischemically damaged myocardium. Common problems could be stunned myocardium, no-reflow phenomenon, abnormal vascular wall contractility and permeability, and metabolic disorders (*e.g.* oxidative stress). All these situations are able to produce derangements in contraction-perfusion matching, thereby limiting the global reliability of the imaging techniques used.

Discoordinated contractility in failing heart, as well as depletion of ATP and ATP-dependent functionality of several electrogenic ion pumps, including the Na^{+}/K^{+} ATPase pump, may particularly influence the active transport of certain radionuclides from the capillaries into the myocardiocytes of failing hearts. For example, ^{201}Tl exits the vessel faster than ^{99m}Tc (sestamibi or tetrofosmin), but its uptake into the myocyte is partly dependent on the Na^{+}/K^{+} ATPase pump [15]. In cases of decreased ATP levels in the myocardium (*i.e.* ischemia, stunning), whereby the active transport of radionuclides is reduced or even blocked, lipophilic (*e.g.* ^{99m}Tc-labelled) agents are preferred.

Patterns of regional distribution and redistribution of certain radiotracers make possible the non-invasive assessment of myocardial perfusion after coronary artery occlusion and reperfusion. Perfusion imaging techniques enable the estimation of the amount of apparent myocardial salvage before thrombolysis (area at risk for infarction) and after therapy, guiding the decision towards revascularization of the occluded infarct artery. According to this concept of myocardial perfusion imaging, one can quantitatively estimate the percentage of the initial risk area that has been salvaged by thrombolytic therapy using ^{99m}Tc-labelled radiotracers. The effectiveness of many pharmacologic and nonpharmacologic interventions can be determined using this method to visualize successful patency of the occluded artery. On the other hand, some pharmacologic interventions, such as potassium channel openers or other vasodilators, might limit accuracy of imaging methods in determining effectiveness of coronary reperfusion.

CONCLUDING REMARKS

Basic knowledge of physiologic cardiac muscle function, comprising the influence of intracellular and extracellular mechanisms regulating Ca^{+2} mobilization and binding/unbinding times to the ECC organelles, may represent absolute necessary elements for understanding heart failure development, progression, and therapy. Scattered myocardial ischemia, due to perfusion defects and fibrosis, has to be early diagnosed in order to limit uncontrolled progression of the disease. In this context, certain radiolabelled agents used to estimate regional myocardial perfusion cannot assess myocardial viability accurately [15]. The latter is strongly associated with metabolic changes related to the duration of the preceded ischemic period as well as to reperfusion injury.

In addition, the no-reflow phenomenon and stunning occurring in reperfused heart may also hamper assessment of myocardial viability. On the other hand, PET seems generally better for the evaluation of myocardial perfusion and metabolism and for the quantification of viable myocardium compared to other methods, since it is partially independent from macrovascular patency of the occluded artery. Furthermore, remote ischemic preconditioning and postconditioning, increasingly implemented to reduce reperfusion injury in clinical practice, could be fields challenging the applicability and diagnostic relevance of various noninvasive imaging techniques in an effort to estimate myocardial viability after flow restoration of an occluded coronary artery. Collectively, cardiac imaging techniques could have a significant role among various invasive and noninvasive procedures for detecting no-reflow phenomenon and assessing myocardial perfusion after PTCA or bypass surgery.

CONFLICT OF INTEREST

The authors confirm that they have no conflict of interest to declare for this publication.

ACKNOWLEDGEMENTS

The authors wish to thank C. Malavaki, MSc, PhD for the preparation of figures.

REFERENCES

[1] Spaan JA, Piek JJ, Siebes M. Coronary circulation and hemodynamics. In: Sperelakis N, Kurachi Y, Terzic A, Cohen MV, Eds. Heart Physiology and Pathophysiology. San Diego: Academic Press 2001; pp. 19-44. [http://dx.doi.org/10.1016/B978-012656975-9/50004-3]

[2] Opie LH. Myocardial contraction and relaxation. In: Opie LH, Ed. The Heart Physiology, From Cell to Circulation. Philadelphia: Lippincott-Raven Publishers 1998; pp. 209-31.

[3] Katz AM. Mechanism and control of the cardiac contractile process. In: Katz AM, Ed. Physiology of the Heart. Philadelphia: Lippincott Williams & Wilkins 2010; pp. 151-66.

[4] Capote LA, Mendez Perez R, Lymperopoulos A. GPCR signaling and cardiac function. Eur J Pharmacol 2015; 763(Pt B): 143-58. [http://dx.doi.org/10.1016/j.ejphar.2015.05.019]

[5] Salazar NC, Chen J, Rockman HA. Cardiac GPCRs: GPCR signaling in healthy and failing hearts. Biochim Biophys Acta 2007; 1768(4): 1006-18. [http://dx.doi.org/10.1016/j.bbamem.2007.02.010] [PMID: 17376402]

[6] Lymperopoulos A, Garcia D, Walklett K. Pharmacogenetics of cardiac inotropy. Pharmacogenomics 2014; 15(14): 1807-21. [http://dx.doi.org/10.2217/pgs.14.120] [PMID: 25493572]

[7] Lymperopoulos A, Rengo G, Funakoshi H, Eckhart AD, Koch WJ. Adrenal GRK2 upregulation mediates sympathetic overdrive in heart failure. Nat Med 2007; 13(3): 315-23. [http://dx.doi.org/10.1038/nm1553] [PMID: 17322894]

[8] Siryk-Bathgate A, Dabul S, Lymperopoulos A. Current and future G protein-coupled receptor signaling targets for heart failure therapy. Drug Des Devel Ther 2013; 7: 1209-22. [PMID: 24143078]

[9] Rengo G, Lymperopoulos A, Koch WJ. Future g protein-coupled receptor targets for treatment of heart failure. Curr Treat Options Cardiovasc Med 2009; 11(4): 328-38. [http://dx.doi.org/10.1007/s11936-009-0033-5] [PMID: 19627665]

[10] Brittsan AG, Kranias EG. Phospholamban and cardiac contractile function. J Mol Cell Cardiol 2000; 32(12): 2131-9. [http://dx.doi.org/10.1006/jmcc.2000.1270] [PMID: 11112989]

[11] Marks AR. Ryanodine receptors/calcium release channels in heart failure and sudden cardiac death. J Mol Cell Cardiol 2001; 33(4): 615-24. [http://dx.doi.org/10.1006/jmcc.2000.1343] [PMID: 11273716]

[12] Christian TF. Contraction-perfusion matching in reperfused acute myocardial infarction. In: Sechtem U, Ed. Imaging and intervention in Cardiology Dordecht. Nienaber, CA: Kluwer Academic Publishers 1996; pp. 13-27. [http://dx.doi.org/10.1007/978-94-009-0115-5_2]

[13] Schmidt TA, Larsen JS, Kjeldsen K. Myocardial Na/K-ATPase concentration and heart failure. In: Dhalla NS, Singal PK, Takeda N, Beamish RE, Eds. Pathophysiology of Heart Failure. Boston: Kluwer Academic Publishers 1996; pp. 353-65.

[http://dx.doi.org/10.1007/978-1-4613-1235-2_22]

[14] Antzelevitch C, Burashnikov A, Di Diego J. Mechanisms of Cardiac Arrhythmia. In: Gussak I, Antzelevitch C, Eds. Electrical Diseases of the Heart. London: Springer-Verlag 2013; pp. 65-132. [http://dx.doi.org/10.1007/978-1-4471-4881-4_6]

[15] Mudd JO, Kass DA. Tackling heart failure in the twenty-first century. Nature 2008; 451(7181): 919-28. [http://dx.doi.org/10.1038/nature06798] [PMID: 18288181]

CHAPTER 3

Aetiology and Pathophysiology: Cellular and Molecular Alterations of Heart Failure

Filippos Triposkiadis*, **Gregory Giamouzis** and **John Skoularigis**

Department of Cardiology, University Hospital of Larissa, Larissa, Greece

Abstract: Heart failure is a worldwide health challenge representing the most common admission diagnosis in patients aged ≥65 years. It is associated with worse prognosis even compared to that of most malignancies, despite therapeutic improvements. Research efforts are underway to combat this complex disease by increasing our understanding of the underlying molecular mechanisms associated with the structural and functional abnormalities. Here we review the molecular changes associated with the fundamental derangements observed in heart failure such as the depressed myocardial contractility and relaxation, increased cardiac fibrosis, increased cardiomyocyte stiffness and profound cytoskeletal changes.

Keywords: Calcium kinetics, Cardiomyocyte physiology, Contraction, Coupling mechanisms, Diastolic function, Excitation, Heart failure, Myocardial contractility, Myocardial perfusion, Myofibroblasts, Phospholamban, Relaxation.

INTRODUCTION

In developed countries, heart failure (HF) prevalence is 1–2% in adults and rises to ≥10% among individuals aged ≥70 years [1]. Although about 50% of HF patients show a preserved left ventricular (LV) ejection fraction (HF-pEF), and the remainder display reduced ejection fraction (HF-rEF), it has not been delineated yet whether HF-pEF and HF-rEF are distinct or overlapping phenotypes within the HF spectrum [2 - 4]. Increased LV mass is a common characteristic of most forms of HF. However, the patterns of LV remodeling in

* **Corresponding author Filippos Triposkiadis:** Department of Cardiology, University Hospital of Larissa, Larissa, Greece; Tel: +30 2413 50 2821; Fax: +30 2410 67 0248; E-mail: ftriposk@med.uth.gr.

Panagiotis Georgoulias (Ed.)

HF-pEF and HF-rEF differ, with LV chamber dilation being a defining characteristic of HF-rEF, and increased wall thickness with normal or near normal size of ventricular chamber, increased ratio of wall thickness to chamber dimension, and increased ratio of ventricular mass to chamber volume being reported in most but not all studies in HF-pEF [3, 5, 6].

Exercise intolerance, impaired LV filling dynamics, disordered relaxation and neurohumoral activation are observed not only in HF-rEF but also in HF-pEF patients [7]. Moreover, although the normal LV ejection fraction indicates that the hemodynamic compression pump performance is adequately compensated in HF-pEF, strain imaging detects impaired myocardial systolic function contributing to the pathophysiology of the syndrome [8]. Regardless of the LV ejection fraction, the severity of HF, patients' prognosis and the grade of impaired exercise tolerance are strictly linked to the degree of diastolic filling impairments [9]. Finally, chronic catecholamine excess has a fundamental role in HF pathophysiology [10]. Sympathetic nervous system upregulation is organ specific and directly proportional to disease severity. Patients with mild to moderate HF exhibit preferential stimulation of the sympathetic nervous system in the cardiac tissue, whereas the upregulation of sympathetic neurotransmission in the kidney and other organs becomes apparent only in severe HF. Other neurohormonal factors in HF pathophysiology include the renin-angiotensin-aldosterone system, natriuretic peptides, and vasopressin [10].

CARDIOMYOCYTE CONTRACTION AND RELAXATION

Histopathological studies have shown that the cardiomyocyte is narrow and elongated in HF-rEF, with reduced myofibrillar density, whereas the myocyte diameter and resting tension are both increased in HF-pEF, particularly among diabetics [11 - 13]. Abnormalities in calcium-handling proteins and disordered metabolic pathways are present.

Cardiomyocyte function is based on the coordinated calcium currents both intracellularly and out of the cell, and the adequate provision of ATP to energy-utilizing enzymes (Fig. **1**). Normally, depolarization of the plasma membrane and the transverse tubules stimulates the entry of small amounts of calcium into the cardiomyocyte, *via* L-type ion-specific channels located in the sarcoplasmic reticulum (SR) membrane of the cell [14]. Calcium influx leads to the opening of the adjacent calcium release channels, termed type 2 ryanodine receptors (RyR2), which are large tetrameric polypeptide complexes. The activation of L-type calcium channels and RyR2 is regulated by the sympathetic nervous system through the β1-adrenoreceptors on cardiomyocytes [10]. The release of much greater amounts of calcium from the SR *via* the RyR2 causes a significant rise of calcium into the cytoplasm. The binding of calcium on troponin C is a crucial step for the activation of the cross bridges between actin and myosin filaments in the sarcomeres, resulting in cardiac contraction [15]. Catecholamine - induced RyR2 hyper-activation is linked to ventricular arrhythmias in HF patients due to disordered cardiomyocyte calcium handling.

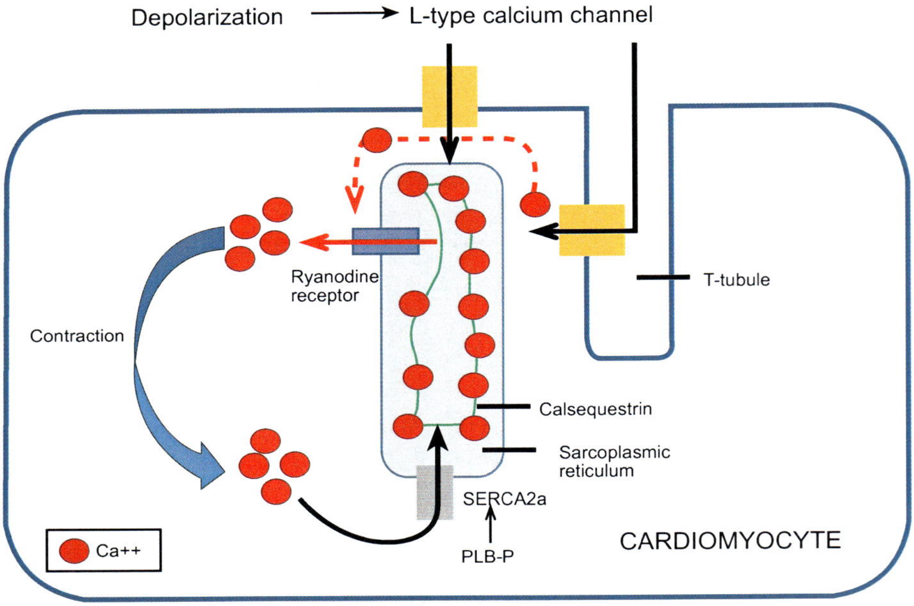

Fig. (1). After depolarization, calcium enters the cardiomyocyte *via* L-type calcium channels and activates the ryanodine receptors on the SR, leading to release of calcium stored within the SR by calsequestrin and increasing intracellular calcium availability, which initiates contraction. Subsequently, calcium is pumped back into the SR by SERCA2a, the calcium uptake pump which is ATP-dependent. An enhanced rate of calcium uptake into the SR increases the myocyte relaxation rate. PLB phosphorylation reverses the SERCA2a pump inhibition, enhancing calcium uptake either in response to increased cytosolic calcium or to β-adrenergic agonists or both.

ATP: adenosine triphosphate; P: phosphorylated; PLB: phospholamban; SERCA2a: sarcoplasmic-endoplasmic reticulum ATPase 2a; SR: sarcoplasmic reticulum.

Myocardial β1-adrenoreceptors have also an important role in cardiomyocyte relaxation rate through the indirect stimulation of sarcoplasmic-endoplasmic reticulum calcium ATPase (SERCA) [10]. SERCA2a is responsible for the calcium ions (Ca^{+2}) movement back into the SR from the cytoplasm, ending contraction and inducing cardiomyocyte relaxation. Phospholamban (PLB) is a cardiac SR – located phosphoprotein reversibly regulating SERCA2a activity and cardiomyocyte contractility [16]. Particularly, dephosphorylated PLB negatively regulates SERCA2a activity and PLB phosphorylation, at either serine 16 [Ser(16)] by protein kinase A (PKA) or threonine 17 [Thr(17)] by Ca^{+2}-calmodulin-dependent protein kinase (CaMKII), reverses this effect. Based on these biochemical processes, PLB is considered as a fundamental regulator of SR Ca^{+2} uptake, Ca^{+2} load, contractility, and relaxation [17]. Further, PLB phosphorylation has an important role in cardiac β1-adrenergic pathways. Although CaMKII-dependent Thr(17) phosphorylation contributes to these processes, its role is auxiliary to the PKA-mediated rise in cytosolic Ca^{+2}, necessary to stimulate CaMKII. Moreover, the effects of PLB and the consequences of its phosphorylation on cardiac physiology are also regulated by additional factors, the anti-apoptotic [hematopoietic lineage cell-specific protein-1 (HCLS-1)] – associated protein X-1 (HAX-1) and Gm or the anchoring unit of protein phosphatase 1 [18]. PLB activity modulation through this multimeric complex becomes predominant under pathological states, linked to aberrant Ca^{+2}-cycling. Particularly, CaMKII-dependent PLB phosphorylation has been related to positive effects not only in acidosis but also in ischemia/reperfusion [19]. However, the protective effects of rising SR Ca^{+2} uptake based on PLB phosphorylation may be lost or even reversed, when these actions take place in combination with changes in SR Ca^{+2} leak. Principal feature both in clinical and experimental HF is depressed SR Ca^{+2} uptake, linked to low SERCA2a levels and dephosphorylation of PLB, resulting in low SR Ca^{+2} load and disordered cardiac contraction. Therefore, manipulations of SERCA2a and/or PLB levels or activity to restore impaired SR Ca^{+2} uptake constitute a potential treatment strategy for HF therapeutic management.

Other mechanisms of cardiomyocyte dysfunction in HF-rEF include reduction in the expression and regulation of additional proteins involved in calcium cycling into and out of the SR, depressed β-adrenergic signalling, oxidative stress targeting calcium-handling proteins, and decreased recoil of elastic elements compressed during systolic phase [20 - 23]. Similar abnormalities are suspected in HF-pEF, though evidence remains limited given the lack of live tissue for human myocardial testing [24]. In a study of biopsy samples from HF-pEF and HF-rEF patients, the expression of calcium-handling proteins and phosphorylation of myofilament proteins were not significantly different between the two groups. However, β1-adrenergic receptor expression was slightly reduced in HF-pEF, whereas G-protein receptor kinase 2 and 5 expression, which can restrain stimulatory adrenergic signaling, was far more increased in HF-rEF [25].

MYOCARDIAL STIFFNESS

High myocardial diastolic stiffness has usually been attributed to fibrosis and excessive myocardial collagen deposition. However, stiff cardiomyocytes have also been identified as important contributors to high myocardial diastolic stiffness, especially in HF-pEF [12, 13, 26].

Cardiac Fibrosis

Cardiac fibrosis refers to net extracellular matrix (ECM) accumulation in the myocardium and is a principal finding in most cardiac pathologic conditions [27]. ECM constitutes a living protein network that is important for the integrity of myocardial structure, and permits the transmission of electrical currents and mechanical forces between the myocytes during cardiac cycle [28]. When LV remodelling takes place due to hemodynamic overload, increased collagen production (the main ECM component) leads to occupation of the space between myocytes and vessels by this component. Progressively, this pathophysiologic process results in fibrosis (reparative fibrosis), which has a compensatory role at early stages, but it may finally affect tissue stiffness and compromise ventricular function [28]. The development of replacement fibrosis at areas of previous myocardial necrosis preserves the integrity of myocardial structure, but there are adverse functional consequences due to the subsequent scar tissue formation. In general, progressive collagen accumulation affects diastolic function and impairs systolic mechanics.

Due to the negligible regenerative capacity of the adult mammalian myocardium, the most extensive fibrotic LV remodelling is observed in diseases linked to acute cardiomyocyte death [29]. After acute myocardial infarction, sudden death of a significant number of cardiomyocytes is accompanied by an inflammatory process, resulting in the replacement of necrotic myocardial regions with a collagen-based scar, as previously mentioned [30]. Other pathophysiologic states, without completed infarction, lead to more subtle interstitial and perivascular collagen deposition. Aging is related to progressive fibrosis that may lead to diastolic dysfunction and HF in elderly patients. Pressure overload, caused by hypertension or aortic stenosis, induces extensive cardiac fibrosis that is related to enhanced stiffness and diastolic dysfunction at early stages; a chronic pressure load may eventually contribute to the development of ventricular dilation and combined diastolic and systolic HF [27]. Further, volume overload in patients with heart valve regurgitation can lead to cardiac fibrosis, characterized by the presence of non-collagenous matrix in disproportionately larger amounts [31].

Myofibroblasts are mesenchymal cells within connective tissue that are responsible for the development of fibrotic tissue. These cells contain α-smooth muscle actin (α-SMA), which is a highly contractile protein [32]. α-SMA is assembled into stress fibers that can induce remodelling of the neighbouring ECM, because myofibroblasts are connected to ECM through focal adhesions that are specialized cell membrane structures [33]. Notably, β2 adrenoreceptors constitute the predominant adrenoreceptor type on cardiac fibroblasts, possibly exerting important actions regarding HF pathophysiology [32]. Chronic catecholamine excess is also associated with both atrial and ventricular arrhythmias in HF patients due to cardiac fibrosis and remodelling.

A complex interaction between various growth factors/cytokines and hormones is responsible *in vivo* for the initiation and progression of the fibrotic responses. Particularly, angiotensin II (Ang-II), endothelin-1 (ET-1), transforming growth factor-β (TGF-β), and platelet-derived growth factor (PDGF) seem to co-operate in order to activate resident interstitial fibroblasts. Moreover, they promote myofibroblasts' persistence and work together to induce the expression of different ECM components, including collagen type I [34]. Aldosterone also promotes cardiac fibrosis based on the activation of mineralocorticoid receptors on cardiac myofibroblasts [34]. The origin of myofibroblasts remains under investigation; various mechanisms may be involved including growth factor–dependent differentiation of resident mesenchymal cells, recruitment of pericyte-like progenitor cells, or epithelial–mesenchymal transition [35].

Recent evidence has suggested that the cellular microenvironment also has a crucial role in promoting pathological responses triggered by these growth factors/cytokines and hormones. For example, increased mechanical loading/tension and enhanced pro-adhesive signalling that is promoted by matricellular proteins, such as CCN2 (previously termed connective tissue growth factor), seem to represent significant cellular parameters [34]. On the other hand, the natriuretic peptides [atrial natriuretic peptide (ANP), B-type natriuretic peptide (BNP), and C-type natriuretic peptide (CNP)] promote adaptive mechanisms in HF and oppose the effects mediated by the sympathetic nervous system upregulation and renin-angiotensin-aldosterone system activation [2, 3].

Matricellular proteins include various structurally unrelated extracellular macromolecules that interact with cell surface receptors, growth factors, proteases, other bioactive factors, and polypeptides of the matrix, without demonstrating a direct structural effect [36]. Initially, the matricellular family included thrombospondin (TSP)-1, SPARC (secreted protein acidic and rich in cysteine), and tenascin-C; however, subsequent studies have led to the inclusion of various additional molecules, such as TSP-2 and -4, tenascin-X, osteopontin (OPN), periostin, and the members of the CCN family. A minimal expression of most matricellular proteins is observed in normal hearts of young adults, but these molecules are significantly upregulated post myocardial injury. Several members of the matricellular family crucially affect various cardiac disorders promoting angiogenesis, inflammation, tissue repair, and fibrosis. These effects are mediated through changes of biochemical processes in cardiomyocytes and interstitial cells and are based on regulation of matrix organization and metabolism [36]. Myocardial infarction induced - matricellular proteins seem to contribute to molecular signaling during cardiac repair, regulating cell migration, proliferation and adhesion [37]. In the pressure-overloaded myocardium, cytokine and growth factors signalling is regulated by matricellular proteins located in the interstitium. Based on these regulatory mechanisms, matricellular proteins modulate the susceptibility of cardiomyocytes to apoptosis and hypertrophic growth, affect matrix assembly and metabolism, and change the fibrogenic potential of inflammatory cells and fibroblasts [38]. In the elderly, up-regulation of some matricellular proteins may tend to preserve the integrity of cardiac structure, whereas other members of matricellular family may contribute to the pathophysiology of age-related fibrosis [39]. Since the functional and structural characteristics of the heart are associated with the complex interactions between myocardial cells and the matrix, systolic and diastolic ventricular disorders are closely linked to the consequences of matricellular proteins regulatory effects regarding cardiac physiology.

Cardiomyocyte Stiffness

Cardiomyocyte stiffness is predominantly modulated by titin, a giant cytoskeletal protein with a molecular mass of up to ≈3800 kDa. In humans, titin is encoded by a single gene containing 363 exons [40, 41]. It should be noted, however, that titin has various roles beyond viscoelastic force generation, including [42 - 44]:

a. Centering the thick filaments in the sarcomere and permitting optimum active force development.
b. Taking part in the assembly of the sarcomeres.
c. Participation in mechano-chemical signaling interactions through its binding partners.
d. Contribution to the length-dependent stimulation of the contractile apparatus, which underlies the Frank–Starling law.

Titin extends from the Z-disk (NH2 terminus) to the M-band (COOH terminus) of the half sarcomere (Fig. **2**). Through alternative splicing, particularly in the I-band region of the molecule (≈230 exons), 3 main isoforms are produced: N2B (≈3000 kDa) and N2BA (≈3200–3800 kDa) in cardiac tissue and N2A in skeletal muscles [45]. The N2B is the shorter and stiffer heart isoform, whereas N2BA is the longer and more compliant heart isoform [40]. Titin-isoform switching is observed in various HF types. Compliant N2BA variants were more abundant in end-stage HF, including subjects with ischemic cardiomyopathy, non-ischemic dilated cardiomyopathy, and other patients with HF-rEF, compared to non-failing donor hearts (45 – 50% *versus* ≈30%) [46 - 49]. The N2BA:N2B expression ratio has been found higher, unaltered or reduced in subjects with aortic stenosis compared to healthy control hearts [49 - 51]. Titin-isoform switching is not adequately investigated in patients with HF-pEF. According to an early report, a reduced N2BA:N2B ratio was demonstrated in a limited number of HF-pEF compared to HF-rEF patient hearts, whereas a follow-up study revealed an elevated ratio in advanced HF-pEF *versus* non-failing donor hearts [11, 49]. Therefore, titin-isoform shift is involved in the regulation of total myocardial passive stiffness in a number of HF patients, and titin-isoform transitions are linked to the different types of heart disease or the stages of cardiac impairment [41].

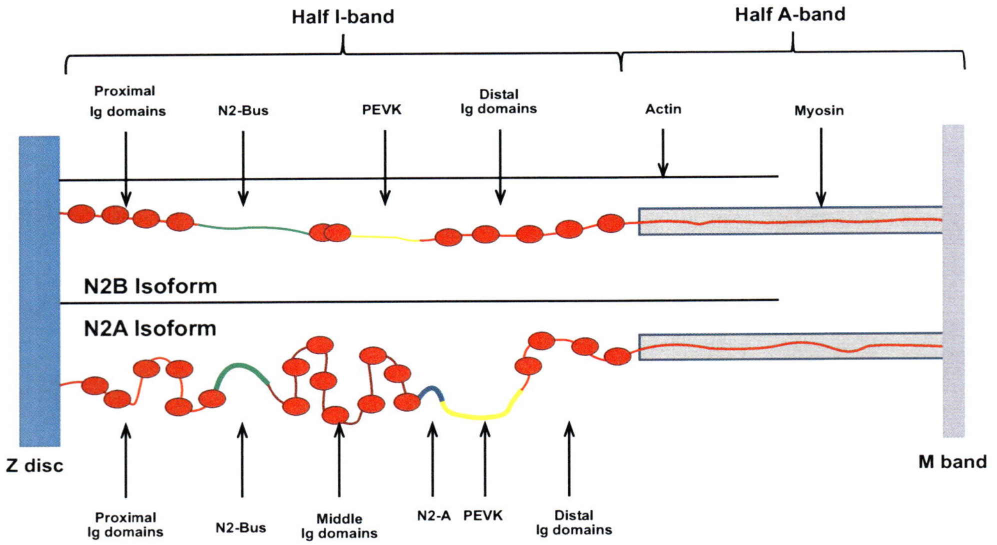

Fig. (2). Layout of titin-isoforms in the cardiac half-sarcomere.
Ig: immunoglobulin; N2-Bus: N2-B-unique sequence.

Besides isoform switches, titin adjusts cardiomyocyte stiffness through post-translational modifications such as phosphorylation or oxidation. PKA and protein kinase G phosphorylate titin at its N2B segment allowing β-adrenergic stimulation, nitric oxide and natriuretic peptides to lower cardiomyocyte stiffness [52, 53]. Protein kinase Cα phosphorylates titin at its proline-glutamate-valine-lysine region resulting in higher cardiomyocyte stiffness. This effect has been observed in cardiomyocytes isolated from normal myocardium but not in cells from an animal model [54, 55]. Titin can also be phosphorylated by extracellular signal-regulated kinase-2 and by calcium calmodulin-dependent kinase II [56, 57]. Both extracellular signal regulated kinase-2 and calcium calmodulin-dependent kinase II lower cardiomyocyte stiffness. Finally, the stiffness of cardiomyocytes increases in the presence of oxidative stress due to the formation within the titin molecule of disulphide bridges reducing the contour length of the N2B segment [58].

Increased Myocardial Stiffness: Increased Extracellular Matrix (ECM) Collagen or Increased Cardiomyocyte Stiffness?

In HF-pEF patients and animal models, the observed increase in cardiomyocyte stiffness is always accompanied by increased deposition of collagen; therefore, it remains unclear whether impaired elasticity of titin could be solely responsible for high myocardial diastolic stiffness and HF-pEF. The relative importance of cardiomyocyte stiffness was evaluated in studies of passive length-tension relations of skinned cardiac muscle strips obtained before and after KI/KCl administration which extracts thick and thin filaments and leaves titin unanchored [59, 60]. Therefore, the passive length-tension relation after KI/KCl corresponds to the elasticity of the extracellular matrix. By subtracting this relation from the one before KI/KCl administration, the elasticity attributable to titin can be calculated. In the normal myocardium, titin accounts for cardiac muscle elasticity at low and intermediate sarcomere lengths (Fig. **3**). Collagen starts to contribute at high sarcomere lengths and at the outer limit of the physiological range of sarcomere lengths (2.3 μm), the contributions of collagen and titin equalize [61]. When titin is stiffer than normal, equalization occurs beyond the outer limit, and the fit of interstitial collagen around cardiomyocytes becomes "loose" over the physiological range of sarcomere lengths. When there is excessive collagen deposition, equalization occurs at intermediate sarcomere length, and the fit of interstitial collagen becomes "tight." When both titin and extracellular matrix are stiffer, equalization occurs again at the outer limit of physiological sarcomere lengths, and the relative importance of titin and collagen resembles the normal situation [61].

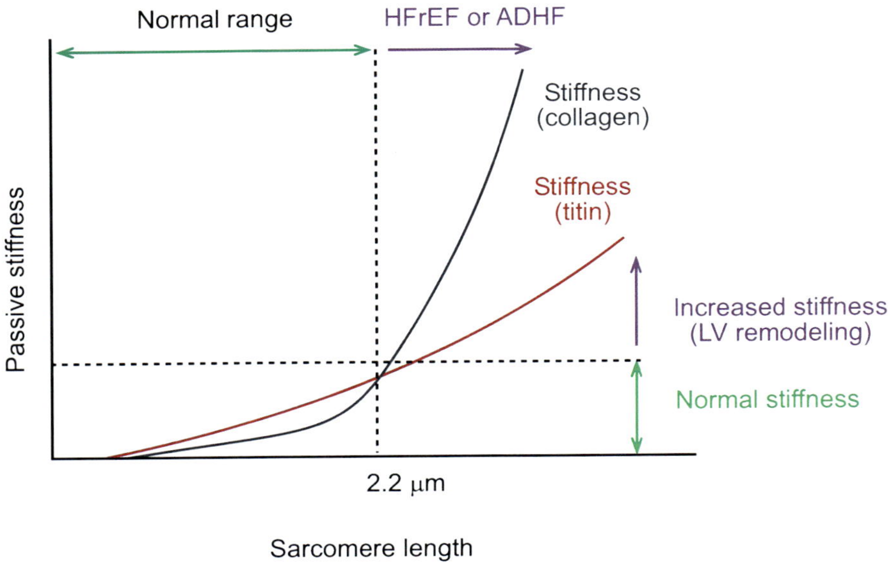

Fig. (3). Relative contributions of titin and collagen to overall myocardial passive stiffness at increasing sarcomere lengths. Overstretch occurs in HF-rEF and probably ADHF.
ADHF: acute decompensated heart failure; HF-rEF: heart failure with reduced LV ejection fraction; LV: left ventricular.

In a recent study, 70 patients underwent echocardiographic evaluation, plasma biomarkers measurements, and intraoperative LV epicardial anterior wall biopsy during coronary artery bypass grafting [62]. Subjects were categorized into 3 groups: referent control (n=17, no hypertension or diabetes mellitus), hypertension (HTN) without (–) HF-pEF (n=31), and HTN with (+) HF-pEF (n=22). Compared to both control and HTN(–) groups, patients with HTN(+) HF-pEF showed elevated LV end-diastolic pressure, left atrial volume, N-terminal propeptide of brain natriuretic peptide, total, collagen-dependent, and titin-dependent stiffness, insoluble collagen, increased titin phosphorylation on PEVK S11878(S26), decreased phosphorylation on N2B S4185(S469), and increased levels of inflammation markers. It was concluded that HTN without HF-pEF does not affect passive myocardial stiffness, whereas HTN(+) HF-pEF is associated with significantly increased passive myocardial stiffness; collagen-dependent and titin-dependent stiffness are elevated [62].

STRUCTURAL (SCAFFOLDING OR CYTOSKELETAL) PROTEINS

In sarcomeres, the contractile actin and myosin filaments are organized by a network of proteins with structural and signaling functions. This network forms the main cardiomyocyte scaffold, the sarcomeric cytoskeleton, which regulates cellular shape and mechanical integrity. Because of this scaffold, the transmission of tension is uniform along myofibrils. Moreover, the cytoskeleton permits the bidirectional signalling with the extracellular environment allowing myocardial cells to monitor and quickly respond to biomechanical stress.

The sarcomeric cytoskeleton can be divided into two main parts, the true cytoskeleton and the myofibril cytoskeleton [63]. True cytoskeleton proteins include actin, tubulin and desmin that firmly structure myofibrils. Three major structural constituents are observed in myofibril cytoskeleton [63]:

a. A pair of structures referred to as Z-disc which has a core consisting of actin filaments that come from adjacent sarcomeres and cross linked by α actinin molecules. Z-disc transversely delineates each side of the sarcomere and contributes to the mechanical linkage of thin filaments. It also uniforms force transmission and is involved in the connection of myofibrils to the sarcolemma and ECM.
b. Titin provides, as previously discussed, sarcomere flexibility and stability and significantly influences both passive shortening and mechanical signalling.
c. The M-band at the sarcomere centre contributes to the stable positioning of the thick filaments.

Sarcomeric proteins remodelling has been observed in impaired ventricular function [64]. Elevated levels of both local and circulating catecholamines result in cardiac hypertrophy by affecting directly the cardiomyocytes (β1-adrenoreceptors), or by promoting the paracrine release of other hormones, such as Ang-II and ET-1 [10]. Vasopressin effects are also linked to cardiac hypertrophy contributing to the progression of HF [10]. It seems that the progression from hypertrophy to HF includes two stages in sequence. Initially, a reversible accumulation of cytoskeletal proteins is observed in an effort to counteract the elevated myocardial strain, whereas the second stage is irreversible and involves the loss of contractile filaments and crucial sarcomeric proteins, including α-actinin, titin and myomesin. Various cardiac diseases have been related to remodelling of α-actinin and the Z-disk. In mouse myocytes, *Trypanosoma cruzi* affects α-actinin distributions; the periodic structure of these distributions is altered and α-actinin localizes to focal adhesion sites [65]. In the failing heart α-actinin-1 depositions are observed, and an electron dense material is accumulated around Z-lines in canines with arrhythmogenic cardiomyopathy [11, 66, 67]. Cardiac conditions such as dilated cardiomyopathy and hypertrophic cardiomyopathy have been also associated with mutations of the gene that encodes α-actinin-2. The remodelling of sarcomeric α-actinin was recently investigated in two HF models, synchronous HF (SHF) and dyssynchronous HF (DHF), as well as in a model of cardiac resynchronization therapy (CRT) [68 - 70]. α-Actinin spatial regularity was reduced in DHF cells in comparison to SHF cells. Furthermore, a partial restoration of α-actinin spatial regularity was observed after CRT. Longitudinal α-actinin depositions were found in SHF, DHF and CRT cells. These depositions spanned neighboring Z-disks and were characterized by a lower α-actinin density when compared to the Z-disk. The occurrence of depositions between SHF, DHF and CRT models was significantly different compared to controls. Further, a higher occurrence of depositions was found in CRT cells in comparison to SHF, but not DHF models. The accumulation of other sarcomeric proteins in the depositions was less significant *versus* α-actinin density. No differences were found regarding the gene responsible for α-actinin and the expression of this protein. The findings of this study implied that HF is related to two different forms of α-actinin remodelling; however, only one of these remodelling alterations was reversed through CRT performance [70].

FUTURE DIRECTIONS IN HEART FAILURE (HF) MEDICAL THERAPY BASED ON PATHOPHYSIOLOGICAL EVIDENCE

G Protein-Coupled Receptors Signaling (GPCRs) Targets

GPCRs represent fundamental components of the mechanisms regulating cardiac function and structure [71]. All adrenoreceptors in cardiac tissue mediate the signal of the sympathetic neurotransmitters, epinephrine and norepinephrine, through heterotrimeric G proteins (GPCRs) [72]. The structural and morphological characteristics of the heart are modulated by Ang-II receptors type-1, which are mainly expressed in endothelial cells or cardiac fibroblasts, and - to a lesser extent - in cardiomyocytes [73]. Further, heart rate is regulated by β-adrenoreceptors and muscarinic cholinergic receptors that are detected in several sites of the cardiac electrical conduction system [72]. Moreover, the functions of various GPCRs influence crucial neurohormonal regulatory components of the circulatory system, such as the renin-angiotensin-aldosterone system and the adrenal release of catecholamine and corticosteroids [74]. Notably, about a third of cardiovascular drugs currently used in clinical practice target directly GPCRs, located in the cell membrane of cardiomyocytes, endothelial cells and cardiac fibroblasts [71].

In fact, the positive effects of β-adrenoreceptor antagonists in HF patients are now well-established and include improvement of coronary blood flow, protection against catecholamine-induced cardiotoxic overstimulation, reversal of LV remodelling, better survival rates, and reduction of both the risk of hospitalization and the risk of life-threatening arrhythmias [74]. β-Adrenoceptor agonists (dobutamine, dopamine) and phosphodiesterase type-3 inhibitors (milrinone) are used in patients with decompensated acute HF because of their positive inotropic effects [74]. On the other hand, the antagonism of renin-angiotensin-aldosterone system has currently a pivotal role in the medical therapy of HF. Apart from angiotensin-converting enzyme inhibitors that affect negatively Ang-II synthesis, angiotensin receptor blockers act on Ang-II receptor type-1 ameliorating features of HF-related LV adverse remodelling, including myocardial stiffness, fibrosis, hypertrophy and dilatation [72].

During the last decades, research advances in the investigation of signaling pathways regulated by CPCRs have resulted in the identification of additional molecules, which may represent novel targets for HF therapeutic strategies [72]. Further, increasing evidence confirms that the activation of a single GPCR by the same endogenous ligand can lead to different, or even conflicting, cellular effects through a number of different signalling pathways [75]. More importantly, certain pathways linked to the stimulation of a single GPCR may have favourable effects regarding HF management. However, the agents currently administered for HF therapy cause an indiscriminate inhibition of all the signalling pathways mediated by the same GPCR. Therefore, the development of selective agents with the ability to target certain pathways intracellularly may improve essentially HF therapy in the future [75].

β-Adrenoreceptor Signalling

In general, the activation of β1-adrenoreceptors and, to a lesser extent, β2-adrenoreceptors is associated with a positive inotropic effect, which is opposite to that induced by β3-adrenoreceptors [74]. Under normal physiologic conditions, β3-adrenoreceptors are mainly inactive, but their activation tends to compensate adrenergic hyperstimulation by decreasing cardiac contractility [72]. Other effects of the stimulation of β1- and β2-adrenoreceptors in cardiac tissue include a rise of cardiac frequency and rate of relaxation (positive chronotropic effect and lusitropic effect, respectively), acceleration of impulse conduction *via* the atrioventricular node (positive dromotropic effect), and higher pacemaker activity from the sinoatrial node [74].

Particularly, the stimulation of β1- and β2-adrenoreceptors leads to the activation of stimulatory G proteins. However, β2-adrenoreceptors stimulation in the heart can also result in the activation of inhibitory G proteins. Interestingly, β2-adrenoreceptor phosphorylation by PKA may be responsible for this switching of signalling from stimulatory to inhibitory G proteins [76]. This fundamental difference between β1- and β2-adrenoreceptors may have important implications for HF management. Selective stimulation and overexpression of β2-adrenoreceptors have been associated with anti-apoptotic and cardioprotective effects [74]. On the other hand, β1-adrenoreceptors hyperstimulation or overexpression has been linked to detrimental effects in the myocardium [74]. Furthermore, in the failing human heart, β1-adrenoreceptors were found to be selectively downregulated. This reduction in the number of functional β1-adrenoreceptors results in a stoichiometric shift in favor of β2-adrenoreceptors [74]. Based on the above-mentioned cardioprotective properties of β2-adrenoreceptors, this shift could have positive consequences for the failing heart. However, β2-adrenoreceptor signalling is also impaired in HF. According to the results of a recent study, β2-adrenoreceptor signalling in HF differs from that observed in the normal heart, resembling the pre-apoptotic pattern linked to β1-adrenoreceptors [77].

Chronic β-blocker therapy progressively improves LV performance by reducing cardiac workload and increasing oxygen and energy supply [72]. Given the possible cardioprotective properties of β2-adrenoreceptor signalling, HF patients may benefit more from β-adrenoreceptor antagonists selectively blocking β1-adrenoreceptor signalling (such as metoprolol), or the administration of a β-adrenoreceptor antagonist combined with a β2-adrenoreceptor selective agonist [78].

α-Adrenoreceptor Signalling

α1-Adrenoreceptors are expressed in the human heart, but their involvement in cardiac physiology remains under investigation. In the pathophysiology of HF, the activation of α1-adrenoreceptors has been associated with the promotion of cardiac survival and the preservation of cardiac inotropy [72]. However, their compensatory actions seem to be limited to situations of cardiac hypertrophy. Indeed, α1-adrenoreceptors stimulation has been linked to the activation of hypertrophic mechanisms in cardiomyocytes [79]. Therefore, the inhibition of certain molecules involved in cardiac a1-adrenoreceptor signalling, or the antagonism of these receptors have been suggested as novel targets in HF management [80, 81].

Chronically increased norepinephrine release associated with enhanced sympathetic nervous system activity in the heart, and increased circulating catecholamines due to elevated adrenal catecholamine secretion, are recognized as the hallmark abnormalities of chronic HF [82]. Notably, $\alpha 2_A$- and $\alpha 2_C$-adrenoreceptors represent the only presynaptic adrenoreceptors that can inhibit norepinephrine release from sympathetic nerve terminals in the heart [83]. Given their crucial role regarding the control of norepinephrine actions, the dysfunction of these receptors is associated with adverse clinical outcomes in HF patients [72]. Thus, α2-adrenoreceptor agonism has been proposed for the management of chronic HF patients; this strategy aims to control sympathetic nervous system outflow in the heart and decrease the circulating catecholamine levels [84, 85].

Unfortunately, research efforts targeting α2-adrenoreceptor in order to cause catecholamine inhibition did not lead to satisfactory results [86]. Lymperopoulos *et al.* reported that the enhanced expression and activity of G protein-coupled receptor kinase-2 (GRK-2) in the adrenal gland were linked to a significant dysregulation of α2-adrenoreceptor in different experimental models of HF [86]. More importantly, adrenal gland-specific inhibition of GRK-2 had several positive consequences [86]. The dysregulation of α2-adrenoreceptor was reversed leading to a reduction of catecholamine levels. Moreover, α2-adrenoreceptor signalling and function in the heart were improved and the sympatholytic efficacy of the α2-adrenoreceptor agonist moxonidine was increased. Thus, adrenal GRK-2 may represent another target in the medical therapy of HF [86].

Angiotensin II (Ang-II) Receptor Type 1 Signalling

Ang-II receptor type 1 is a G protein-coupled receptor, but it can also signal *via* β arrestins (βarrs) [73]. Both in experimental and clinical models of HF, the activation of renin-angiotensin-aldosterone system is confirmed. Moreover, the antagonism of this system has been found to offer symptomatic relief to HF patients and provide a survival benefit [72]. Ang-II contributes to the adverse hemodynamic and LV remodelling responses in HF, acting through Ang-II receptor type 1. In the central nervous system, the activation of Ang-II receptors type 1 has been associated with the elevation of sympathetic nervous system activity that is a crucial pathophysiological characteristic of HF. Further, in the adrenal cortex, the stimulation of Ang-II receptors type 1 results in the production of aldosterone, which is the last component activated in the renin-angiotensin-aldosterone system. Recently, the antagonism of aldosterone has been suggested as a therapeutic option to restrain LV adverse remodelling and improve patient survival in advanced HF [87].

Endothelin Receptors

Endothelin is the most potent endogenous vasoconstrictor hormone, even compared to Ang-II. Its plasma levels correlate well with HF severity [88]. To date, promising strategies targeting the endothelin system have not provided any substantial benefit for HF management [88]. However, based on endothelin therapeutic value in pulmonary arterial hypertension patients, endothelin receptor antagonists may be useful in right-sided HF [72].

Adenosine Receptors

Adenosine binds to four GPCR subtypes, namely A1, A2a, A2b, and A3. The activation of the A1 receptor subtype is primarily involved in the cardioprotective effects of this purine nucleoside in ischemic preconditioning [89]. Interestingly, the administration of capadenoson, a partial A1 receptor agonist, resulted in LV functional improvement in a canine HF model, coupled with a preventive effect regarding adverse cardiac remodelling [90].

Adrenomedullin Receptor

Adrenomedullin receptor is also a GPCR, but its signalling capability requires the coupling of the receptor to one of the receptor activity-modifying proteins [91]. Adrenomedullin is released from the kidneys, adrenal medulla and other tissues. Increased adrenomedullin plasma concentrations have been reported in acute decompensated HF, whereas its levels were found to be independently predictive of 2-year survival in chronic HF [92]. Adrenomedullin receptor agonists seem promising agents for HF management, given the positive inotropic effect of adrenomedullin in the heart and its other beneficial actions, including hypertension and natriuresis [93].

Relaxin Receptors

In the cardiovascular system, two members of the relaxin hormone family, relaxin-1 and relaxin-2, have potent vasodilatory effects mediated by four types of relaxin family peptide receptors [72]. These receptors are all GPCRs. Further, the stimulation of relaxin family peptide receptor-1 and -2 has been linked to positive inotropic effects. Therefore, the development of recombinant relaxin peptides and peptide analogs may be of value, especially for acute HF treatment [72]. The administration of serelaxin, a recombinant human relaxin-2, in clinical trials has been associated with very promising results in the field of acute HF [94].

Corticotropin-Releasing Factor Receptors

Corticotropin-releasing factor family includes corticotropin-releasing hormone, urotensin-1 and urocortins. Their receptors belong to GPCRs group [72]. In particular, corticotropin-releasing factor receptor-2 is expressed in the heart and its activation is associated with cardiostimulatory effects. In a sheep HF model, the stimulation of corticotropin-releasing factor receptor-2 by urocortin-1 led to favourable results regarding cardiac function [95]. Similar beneficial effects were observed in humans after the activation of the same receptor by urocortin-2 or stresscopin, a corticotropin-releasing factor-like peptide that selectively stimulates this receptor [96, 97].

Vasopressin Receptors

Among the three types of vasopressin GPCRs, human cardiomyocytes express, to a limited extent, vasopressin receptor-1. Its activation leads to cardiac hypertrophy and vasoconstriction in vascular smooth muscle cells [72]. Therefore, vasopressin receptor antagonism may represent another therapeutic option regarding the control of the underlying mechanisms in HF; however, vasopressin receptor antagonists are currently approved for congestive HF treatment only in few countries [98].

Glucagon Peptide Hormone Receptors

Glucagon receptor and glucagon-like peptide receptor-1 are GPCRs that mediate the effects of glucagon and glucagon-like peptide-1, respectively [72]. In the heart, glucagon induces a positive inotropic mechanism, increasing cardiac output. It can be administered for the management of acute decompensations in HF patients treated with β-blockers [72]. On the other hand, the cardiac effects of glucagon-like peptide include cardiomyocyte proliferation, inhibition of apoptosis and positive inotropy [72]. Given these actions, glucagon-like peptide analogues have been investigated in previous HF studies, with encouraging results [99, 100].

Apelin Receptor

Apelin receptor shows significant sequence similarity compared to the Ang-II receptor type-1, without binding Ang-II [101]. Apelin is an endogenous peptide that exerts cardioprotective effects against ischemia/reperfusion injury [102]. Apelin receptor stimulation leads to hypotension and venodilation, increases cardiac contractility and induces diuresis and neovascularization [101].

Muscarinic Receptors

Muscarinic cholinergic receptors are also members of the GPCR family. Among their five types in mammals, muscarinic receptor type 2 mediates the classic cholinergic effect of bradycardia [74]. Cholinergic receptors seem to be expressed in atrial cardiomyocytes, but not in myocytes located at ventricular myocardium. Thus, they do not influence directly cardiac contractility.

Other Targets for Heart Failure (HF) Drug Development

Apart from the heterotrimeric G proteins mentioned above, there are also small G proteins that serve as a link between cell membrane and signalling pathways located intracellularly [72]. The Ras homolog gene family member A (RhoA) is a small G protein that stimulates a protein kinase, which is involved in the cardiac hypertrophic process [72]. Fasudil, a drug that inhibits this kinase, was reported to reverse LV remodelling in a mice model of myocardial infarction [103]. Furthermore, the exchange protein directly activated by cAMP (EPAC) is another promising target. This small G protein acts as an adapter molecule taking part in various protein–protein interactions in the cardiomyocytes [72]. Based on the available research findings, the inhibition of EPAC might be beneficial for cardiac arrhythmias, and potentially for HF management [104].

In the majority of GPCRs, continuous or repeated agonist stimulation is controlled by an agonist-promoted desensitization and downregulation that diminish receptor response [72]. The first stage of this regulatory process includes the phosphorylation of the receptor by GRKs. Then, βarrs bind to the GRK-phosphorylated receptor and its overstimulation is controlled. The inhibition of GRK-2 was found to induce positive inotropic and sympatholytic effects simultaneously; therefore, it represents an attractive option for chronic HF management in the future [72]. Similarly, selective targeting of βarrs, or other therapeutic manipulations of βarr signalling, seems to constitute very promising strategies for HF drug development [72].

Pharmacogenetic Approaches to the Treatment of Heart Failure (HF)

In the future, evidence obtained through pharmacogenetic studies might help the clinicians to make therapeutic decisions on an individualized basis. To date, the combination of the β1-adrenoreceptor Arg389Gly and $\alpha 2_C$-adrenoreceptor Ins/Del322-325 polymorphisms in black patients and the ABCB1 C3435T genotype in female patients treated with digoxin, are characterized by the greatest potential for future clinical applications [105].

Previous studies have identified several polymorphisms in genes responsible for the synthesis of proteins that are involved in cardiac contractility [105]. Polymorphisms in human β- and α-adrenoreceptor genes have been related to different HF phenotypes and seem to affect β-blocker therapy [105]. Moreover, these polymorphisms might also influence cardiac contractility. Increased cardiac contractility has been reported in the carriers of the Arg389 human β1-adrenoreceptor variant in comparison to Gly389 carriers [106]. In individuals of the European descent, the Arg389 β1-adrenoreceptor variant is more common, but the frequency of these variants is almost the same in African-Americans [107].

As previously stated, the effects of norepinephrine in cardiomyocytes are mediated by β1-adrenoreceptors and the Arg389 variant is related to increased function. On the other hand, norepinephrine release is negatively controlled through the presynaptic α2-adrenoreceptors; however, a polymorphic variant ($\alpha 2_C$Del322–325) shows reduced α2-adrenergic function [108]. The $\alpha 2_C$Del322–325 polymorphism is related to local norepinephrine concentration in the heart, but it does not influence directly cardiac contractility [105]. Small *et al.* investigated whether the combination of these variants would have HF-inducing properties, since the enhanced synaptic norepinephrine release is coupled with the increased β1-adrenergic function at the cardiomyocytes [108]. After genotyping at these loci in 159 HF patients and 189 control subjects, the researchers concluded that the β1Arg389 and $\alpha 2_C$Del322–325 variants exert a synergistic action leading to increased HF risk, especially in blacks.

Digoxin represents the only inotropic agent that is administered orally in HF patients. Due to the extremely narrow therapeutic index of this agent (recommended serum digoxin concentration between 0.7 – 0.9 ng/ml), genetic variations may result in alterations of serum digoxin levels with therapeutic significance. P-glycoprotein-1 (P-gp) is an ATP-dependent efflux protein with broad substrate specificity. This glycoprotein is encoded by ABCB1 gene in humans and digoxin is a substrate of P-gp. The common variation C3435T in ABCB1 has become the principal research area in most genetic studies investigating digoxin pharmacokinetics [105]. Almost all studies have confirmed that 3435T genotype is associated with higher serum digoxin concentration. However, there may be ethnic differences, since higher digoxin concentration was linked to 3435C genotype according to the results of two studies in Japan [105]. Moreover, it remains under investigation whether this genetic variation has clinically significant consequences regarding digoxin pharmacokinetics in HF patients [105]. Perhaps, the clinical relevance of ABCB1 C3435T polymorphism lies in the observed sex-specific differences on digoxin bioavailability. Neuvonen *et al.* investigated the association between ABCB1 genotype and post-mortem digoxin concentration [109]. The researchers revealed a relationship between 3435T allele frequency and post-mortem digoxin concentration with a more emphatic pattern for female subjects, implying the presence of a sex-related risk of digoxin intoxication. Notably, this finding may contribute to the interpretation of the higher mortality in females treated with digoxin *versus* placebo [110].

Pharmacogenetics of cardiac inotropy might change significantly aspects of HF management [105]. Current data indicates that polymorphisms of adrenoreceptors (mainly of β1-adrenoreceptors) may be involved in underlying mechanisms of HF pathophysiology. These genetic variants represent important parameters of cardiac inotropy and might be of therapeutic value for HF patients. Finally, another promising research area involves the pharmacokinetics of the inotropes (digoxin and levosimendan).

CONCLUDING REMARKS

HF represents a very important health problem worldwide, which may become crucial in the near future. Understanding of the underlying cellular and molecular alterations will hopefully lead to a more effective, safer, and personalized therapy, with new treatment modalities such as gene or cell therapy. Ethical and financial issues raised as these biological therapies progress to clinical application will be surpassed once safety requirements have been met and clinical benefits have been confirmed in subsequent studies.

CONFLICT OF INTEREST

The authors confirm that they have no conflict of interest to declare for this publication.

ACKNOWLEDGEMENTS

Declared none.

REFERENCES

[1] Mosterd A, Hoes AW. Clinical epidemiology of heart failure. Heart 2007; 93(9): 1137-46. [http://dx.doi.org/10.1136/hrt.2003.025270] [PMID: 17699180]

[2] De Keulenaer GW, Brutsaert DL. Systolic and diastolic heart failure are overlapping phenotypes within the heart failure spectrum. Circulation 2011; 123(18): 1996-2004. [http://dx.doi.org/10.1161/CIRCULATIONAHA.110.981431]

[3] Borlaug BA, Redfield MM. Diastolic and systolic heart failure are distinct phenotypes within the heart failure spectrum. Circulation 2011; 123(18): 2006-13.

[4] Owan TE, Hodge DO, Herges RM, Jacobsen SJ, Roger VL, Redfield MM. Trends in prevalence and outcome of heart failure with preserved ejection fraction. N Engl J Med 2006; 355(3): 251-9. [http://dx.doi.org/10.1056/NEJMoa052256] [PMID: 16855265]

[5] Maurer MS, El Khoury Rumbarger L, King DL. Ventricular volume and length in hypertensive diastolic heart failure. J Am Soc Echocardiogr 2005; 18(10): 1051-7. [http://dx.doi.org/10.1016/j.echo.2005.03.003] [PMID: 16198882]

[6] Maurer MS, Burkhoff D, Fried LP, Gottdiener J, King DL, Kitzman DW. Ventricular structure and function in hypertensive participants with heart failure and a normal ejection fraction: the Cardiovascular Health Study. J Am Coll Cardiol 2007; 49(9): 972-81. [http://dx.doi.org/10.1016/j.jacc.2006.10.061] [PMID: 17336721]

[7] Fukuta H, Ohte N, Brucks S, Carr JJ, Little WC. Contribution of right-sided heart enlargement to cardiomegaly on chest roentgenogram in diastolic and systolic heart failure. Am J Cardiol 2007; 99(1): 62-7. [http://dx.doi.org/10.1016/j.amjcard.2006.07.067] [PMID: 17196464]

[8] Kraigher-Krainer E, Shah AM, Gupta DK, *et al.* Impaired systolic function by strain imaging in heart failure with preserved ejection fraction. J Am Coll Cardiol 2014; 63(5): 447-56. [http://dx.doi.org/10.1016/j.jacc.2013.09.052] [PMID: 24184245]

[9] Brucks S, Little WC, Chao T, *et al.* Contribution of left ventricular diastolic dysfunction to heart failure regardless of ejection fraction. Am J Cardiol 2005; 95(5): 603-6.

[http://dx.doi.org/10.1016/j.amjcard.2004.11.006] [PMID: 15721099]

[10] Reed BN, Street SE, Jensen BC. Time and technology will tell: the pathophysiologic basis of neurohormonal modulation in heart failure. Heart Fail Clin 2014; 10(4): 543-57. [http://dx.doi.org/10.1016/j.hfc.2014.07.002] [PMID: 25217430]

[11] van Heerebeek L, Borbély A, Niessen HW, *et al.* Myocardial structure and function differ in systolic and diastolic heart failure. Circulation 2006; 113(16): 1966-73. [http://dx.doi.org/10.1161/CIRCULATIONAHA.105.587519] [PMID: 16618817]

[12] Borbély A, van der Velden J, Papp Z, *et al.* Cardiomyocyte stiffness in diastolic heart failure. Circulation 2005; 111(6): 774-81. [http://dx.doi.org/10.1161/01.CIR.0000155257.33485.6D] [PMID: 15699264]

[13] van Heerebeek L, Hamdani N, Handoko ML, *et al.* Diastolic stiffness of the failing diabetic heart: importance of fibrosis, advanced glycation end products, and myocyte resting tension. Circulation 2008; 117(1): 43-51. [http://dx.doi.org/10.1161/CIRCULATIONAHA.107.728550] [PMID: 18071071]

[14] Braunwald E. The war against heart failure: the Lancet lecture. Lancet 2015; 385(9970): 812-24. [http://dx.doi.org/10.1016/S0140-6736(14)61889-4] [PMID: 25467564]

[15] Gorski PA, Ceholski DK, Hajjar RJ. Altered myocardial calcium cycling and energetics in heart failure--a rational approach for disease treatment. Cell Metab 2015; 21(2): 183-94. [http://dx.doi.org/10.1016/j.cmet.2015.01.005] [PMID: 25651173]

[16] Mattiazzi A, Kranias EG. The role of CaMKII regulation of phospholamban activity in heart disease. Front Pharmacol 2014; 5: 5. [http://dx.doi.org/10.3389/fphar.2014.00005] [PMID: 24550830]

[17] Haghighi K, Bidwell P, Kranias EG. Phospholamban interactome in cardiac contractility and survival: A new vision of an old friend. J Mol Cell Cardiol 2014; 77: 160-7. [http://dx.doi.org/10.1016/j.yjmcc.2014.10.005] [PMID: 25451386]

[18] Kranias EG, Hajjar RJ. Modulation of cardiac contractility by the phospholamban/SERCA2a regulatome. Circ Res 2012; 110(12): 1646-60. [http://dx.doi.org/10.1161/CIRCRESAHA.111.259754] [PMID: 22679139]

[19] Vittone L, Mundina-Weilenmann C, Mattiazzi A. Phospholamban phosphorylation by CaMKII under pathophysiological conditions. Front Biosci 2008; 13: 5988-6005. [http://dx.doi.org/10.2741/3131] [PMID: 18508637]

[20] Kranias EG, Bers DM. Calcium and cardiomyopathies. Subcell Biochem 2007; 45: 523-37. [http://dx.doi.org/10.1007/978-1-4020-6191-2_20] [PMID: 18193651]

[21] Norman HS, Oujiri J, Larue SJ, Chapman CB, Margulies KB, Sweitzer NK. Decreased cardiac functional reserve in heart failure with preserved systolic function. J Card Fail 2011; 17(4): 301-8. [http://dx.doi.org/10.1016/j.cardfail.2010.11.004] [PMID: 21440868]

[22] Sag CM, Wagner S, Maier LS. Role of oxidants on calcium and sodium movement in healthy and diseased cardiac myocytes. Free Radic Biol Med 2013; 63: 338-49. [http://dx.doi.org/10.1016/j.freeradbiomed.2013.05.035] [PMID: 23732518]

[23] Helmes M, Lim CC, Liao R, Bharti A, Cui L, Sawyer DB. Titin determines the Frank-Starling relation in early diastole. J Gen Physiol 2003; 121(2): 97-110.
[http://dx.doi.org/10.1085/jgp.20028652] [PMID: 12566538]

[24] Sharma K, Kass DA. Heart failure with preserved ejection fraction: mechanisms, clinical features, and therapies. Circ Res 2014; 115(1): 79-96.
[http://dx.doi.org/10.1161/CIRCRESAHA.115.302922] [PMID: 24951759]

[25] Hamdani N, Paulus WJ, van Heerebeek L, *et al.* Distinct myocardial effects of beta-blocker therapy in heart failure with normal and reduced left ventricular ejection fraction. Eur Heart J 2009; 30(15): 1863-72.
[http://dx.doi.org/10.1093/eurheartj/ehp189] [PMID: 19487234]

[26] van Heerebeek L, Hamdani N, Falcão-Pires I, *et al.* Low myocardial protein kinase G activity in heart failure with preserved ejection fraction. Circulation 2012; 126(7): 830-9.
[http://dx.doi.org/10.1161/CIRCULATIONAHA.111.076075] [PMID: 22806632]

[27] Berk BC, Fujiwara K, Lehoux S. ECM remodeling in hypertensive heart disease. J Clin Invest 2007; 117(3): 568-75.
[http://dx.doi.org/10.1172/JCI31044] [PMID: 17332884]

[28] Segura AM, Frazier OH, Buja LM. Fibrosis and heart failure. Heart Fail Rev 2014; 19(2): 173-85.
[http://dx.doi.org/10.1007/s10741-012-9365-4] [PMID: 23124941]

[29] Kong P, Christia P, Frangogiannis NG. The pathogenesis of cardiac fibrosis. Cell Mol Life Sci 2014; 71(4): 549-74.
[http://dx.doi.org/10.1007/s00018-013-1349-6] [PMID: 23649149]

[30] Frangogiannis NG. Regulation of the inflammatory response in cardiac repair. Circ Res 2012; 110(1): 159-73.
[http://dx.doi.org/10.1161/CIRCRESAHA.111.243162] [PMID: 22223212]

[31] Borer JS, Truter S, Herrold EM, *et al.* Myocardial fibrosis in chronic aortic regurgitation: molecular and cellular responses to volume overload. Circulation 2002; 105(15): 1837-42.
[http://dx.doi.org/10.1161/01.CIR.0000014419.71706.85] [PMID: 11956128]

[32] Leask A. Getting to the heart of the matter: new insights into cardiac fibrosis. Circ Res 2015; 116(7): 1269-76.
[http://dx.doi.org/10.1161/CIRCRESAHA.116.305381] [PMID: 25814687]

[33] Gabbiani G. The myofibroblast in wound healing and fibrocontractive diseases. J Pathol 2003; 200(4): 500-3.
[http://dx.doi.org/10.1002/path.1427] [PMID: 12845617]

[34] Leask A. Potential therapeutic targets for cardiac fibrosis: TGFbeta, angiotensin, endothelin, CCN2, and PDGF, partners in fibroblast activation. Circ Res 2010; 106(11): 1675-80.
[http://dx.doi.org/10.1161/CIRCRESAHA.110.217737] [PMID: 20538689]

[35] Hinz B, Phan SH, Thannickal VJ, *et al.* Recent developments in myofibroblast biology: paradigms for connective tissue remodeling. Am J Pathol 2012; 180(4): 1340-55.
[http://dx.doi.org/10.1016/j.ajpath.2012.02.004] [PMID: 22387320]

[36] Frangogiannis NG. Matricellular proteins in cardiac adaptation and disease. Physiol Rev 2012; 92(2): 635-88.
[http://dx.doi.org/10.1152/physrev.00008.2011] [PMID: 22535894]

[37] Chatila K, Ren G, Xia Y, Huebener P, Bujak M, Frangogiannis NG. The role of the thrombospondins in healing myocardial infarcts. Cardiovasc Hematol Agents Med Chem 2007; 5(1): 21-7.
[http://dx.doi.org/10.2174/187152507779315813] [PMID: 17266545]

[38] Xia Y, Dobaczewski M, Gonzalez-Quesada C, *et al.* Endogenous thrombospondin 1 protects the pressure-overloaded myocardium by modulating fibroblast phenotype and matrix metabolism. Hypertension 2011; 58(5): 902-11.
[http://dx.doi.org/10.1161/HYPERTENSIONAHA.111.175323] [PMID: 21947471]

[39] de Castro Bras LE, Toba H, Baicu CF, *et al.* Age and SPARC change the extracellular matrix composition of the left ventricle. BioMed Res Int 2014.
[http://dx.doi.org/10.1155/2014/810562]

[40] LeWinter MM, Granzier HL. Cardiac titin and heart disease. J Cardiovasc Pharmacol 2014; 63(3): 207-12.
[http://dx.doi.org/10.1097/FJC.0000000000000007] [PMID: 24072177]

[41] Linke WA, Hamdani N. Gigantic business: titin properties and function through thick and thin. Circ Res 2014; 114(6): 1052-68.
[http://dx.doi.org/10.1161/CIRCRESAHA.114.301286] [PMID: 24625729]

[42] Gautel M. The sarcomeric cytoskeleton: who picks up the strain? Curr Opin Cell Biol 2011; 23(1): 39-46.
[http://dx.doi.org/10.1016/j.ceb.2010.12.001] [PMID: 21190822]

[43] Tskhovrebova L, Trinick J. Roles of titin in the structure and elasticity of the sarcomere. J Biomed Biotechnol 2010.

[44] Linke WA. Sense and stretchability: the role of titin and titin-associated proteins in myocardial stress-sensing and mechanical dysfunction. Cardiovasc Res 2008; 77(4): 637-48.
[PMID: 17475230]

[45] Freiburg A, Trombitas K, Hell W, *et al.* Series of exon-skipping events in the elastic spring region of titin as the structural basis for myofibrillar elastic diversity. Circ Res 2000; 86(11): 1114-21.
[http://dx.doi.org/10.1161/01.RES.86.11.1114] [PMID: 10850961]

[46] Neagoe C, Kulke M, del Monte F, *et al.* Titin isoform switch in ischemic human heart disease. Circulation 2002; 106(11): 1333-41.
[http://dx.doi.org/10.1161/01.CIR.0000029803.93022.93] [PMID: 12221049]

[47] Makarenko I, Opitz CA, Leake MC, *et al.* Passive stiffness changes caused by upregulation of compliant titin isoforms in human dilated cardiomyopathy hearts. Circ Res 2004; 95(7): 708-16.
[http://dx.doi.org/10.1161/01.RES.0000143901.37063.2f] [PMID: 15345656]

[48] Nagueh SF, Shah G, Wu Y, *et al.* Altered titin expression, myocardial stiffness, and left ventricular function in patients with dilated cardiomyopathy. Circulation 2004; 110(2): 155-62.
[http://dx.doi.org/10.1161/01.CIR.0000135591.37759.AF] [PMID: 15238456]

[49] Borbély A, Falcao-Pires I, van Heerebeek L, *et al.* Hypophosphorylation of the Stiff N2B titin isoform raises cardiomyocyte resting tension in failing human myocardium. Circ Res 2009; 104(6): 780-6. [http://dx.doi.org/10.1161/CIRCRESAHA.108.193326] [PMID: 19179657]

[50] Falcão-Pires I, Hamdani N, Borbély A, *et al.* Diabetes mellitus worsens diastolic left ventricular dysfunction in aortic stenosis through altered myocardial structure and cardiomyocyte stiffness. Circulation 2011; 124(10): 1151-9. [http://dx.doi.org/10.1161/CIRCULATIONAHA.111.025270] [PMID: 21844073]

[51] Williams L, Howell N, Pagano D, *et al.* Titin isoform expression in aortic stenosis. Clin Sci 2009; 117(6): 237-42. [http://dx.doi.org/10.1042/CS20080248] [PMID: 19154184]

[52] Fukuda N, Wu Y, Nair P, Granzier HL. Phosphorylation of titin modulates passive stiffness of cardiac muscle in a titin isoform-dependent manner. J Gen Physiol 2005; 125(3): 257-71. [http://dx.doi.org/10.1085/jgp.200409177] [PMID: 15738048]

[53] Krüger M, Kötter S, Grützner A, *et al.* Protein kinase G modulates human myocardial passive stiffness by phosphorylation of the titin springs. Circ Res 2009; 104(1): 87-94. [http://dx.doi.org/10.1161/CIRCRESAHA.108.184408] [PMID: 19023132]

[54] Hidalgo C, Hudson B, Bogomolovas J, *et al.* PKC phosphorylation of titin's PEVK element: a novel and conserved pathway for modulating myocardial stiffness. Circ Res 2009; 105(7): 631-8. [http://dx.doi.org/10.1161/CIRCRESAHA.109.198465]

[55] Hamdani N, Bishu KG, von Frieling-Salewsky M, Redfield MM, Linke WA. Deranged myofilament phosphorylation and function in experimental heart failure with preserved ejection fraction. Cardiovasc Res 2013; 97(3): 464-71. [http://dx.doi.org/10.1093/cvr/cvs353] [PMID: 23213108]

[56] Raskin A, Lange S, Banares K, *et al.* A novel mechanism involving four-and-a-half LIM domain protein-1 and extracellular signal-regulated kinase-2 regulates titin phosphorylation and mechanics. J Biol Chem 2012; 287(35): 29273-84. [http://dx.doi.org/10.1074/jbc.M112.372839] [PMID: 22778266]

[57] Hamdani N, Krysiak J, Kreusser MM, *et al.* Crucial role for Ca2(+)/calmodulin-dependent protein kinase-II in regulating diastolic stress of normal and failing hearts *via* titin phosphorylation. Circ Res 2013; 112(4): 664-74. [http://dx.doi.org/10.1161/CIRCRESAHA.111.300105] [PMID: 23283722]

[58] Grützner A, Garcia-Manyes S, Kötter S, Badilla CL, Fernandez JM, Linke WA. Modulation of titin-based stiffness by disulfide bonding in the cardiac titin N2-B unique sequence. Biophys J 2009; 97(3): 825-34. [http://dx.doi.org/10.1016/j.bpj.2009.05.037] [PMID: 19651040]

[59] Hudson B, Hidalgo C, Saripalli C, Granzier H. Hyperphosphorylation of mouse cardiac titin contributes to transverse aortic constriction-induced diastolic dysfunction. Circ Res 2011; 109(8): 858-66. [http://dx.doi.org/10.1161/CIRCRESAHA.111.246819] [PMID: 21835910]

[60] Chung CS, Hutchinson KR, Methawasin M, *et al.* Shortening of the elastic tandem immunoglobulin

segment of titin leads to diastolic dysfunction. Circulation 2013; 128(1): 19-28. [http://dx.doi.org/10.1161/CIRCULATIONAHA.112.001268] [PMID: 23709671]

[61] Hamdani N, Paulus WJ. Myocardial titin and collagen in cardiac diastolic dysfunction: partners in crime. Circulation 2013; 128(1): 5-8. [http://dx.doi.org/10.1161/CIRCULATIONAHA.113.003437] [PMID: 23709670]

[62] Zile MR, Baicu CF, Ikonomidis JS, *et al.* Myocardial stiffness in patients with heart failure and a preserved ejection fraction: contributions of collagen and titin. Circulation 2015; 131(14): 1247-59. [http://dx.doi.org/10.1161/CIRCULATIONAHA.114.013215] [PMID: 25637629]

[63] Sequeira V, Nijenkamp LL, Regan JA, van der Velden J. The physiological role of cardiac cytoskeleton and its alterations in heart failure. Biochim Biophys Acta 2014; 1838(2): 700-22. [http://dx.doi.org/10.1016/j.bbamem.2013.07.011] [PMID: 23860255]

[64] Hein S, Kostin S, Heling A, Maeno Y, Schaper J. The role of the cytoskeleton in heart failure. Cardiovasc Res 2000; 45(2): 273-8. [http://dx.doi.org/10.1016/S0008-6363(99)00268-0] [PMID: 10728347]

[65] Melo TG, Almeida DS, Meirelles MN, *et al.* Disarray of sarcomeric alpha-actinin in cardiomyocytes infected by Trypanosoma cruzi. Parasitology 2006; 133(Pt2): 171-8. [http://dx.doi.org/10.1017/S0031182006000011]

[66] Hein S, Block T, Zimmermann R, *et al.* Deposition of nonsarcomeric alpha-actinin in cardiomyocytes from patients with dilated cardiomyopathy or chronic pressure overload. Exp Clin Cardiol 2009; 14(3): e68-75. [PMID: 20098571]

[67] Oxford EM, Danko CG, Kornreich BG, *et al.* Ultrastructural changes in cardiac myocytes from Boxer dogs with arrhythmogenic right ventricular cardiomyopathy. J Vet Cardiol 2011; 13(2): 101-13.

[68] Mohapatra B, Jimenez S, Lin JH, *et al.* Mutations in the muscle LIM protein and alpha-actinin-2 genes in dilated cardiomyopathy and endocardial fibroelastosis. Mol Genet Metab 2003; 80(1-2): 207-15. [http://dx.doi.org/10.1016/S1096-7192(03)00142-2] [PMID: 14567970]

[69] Chiu C, Bagnall RD, Ingles J, *et al.* Mutations in alpha-actinin-2 cause hypertrophic cardiomyopathy: a genome-wide analysis. J Am Coll Cardiol 2010; 55(11): 1127-35. [http://dx.doi.org/10.1016/j.jacc.2009.11.016] [PMID: 20022194]

[70] Lichter JG, Carruth E, Mitchell C, *et al.* Remodeling of the sarcomeric cytoskeleton in cardiac ventricular myocytes during heart failure and after cardiac resynchronization therapy. J Mol Cell Cardiol 2014; 72: 186-95.

[71] Capote LA, Mendez Perez R, Lymperopoulos A. GPCR signaling and cardiac function. Eur J Pharmacol 2015; 763(Pt B): 143-8. [http://dx.doi.org/10.1016/j.ejphar.2015.05.019]

[72] Siryk-Bathgate A, Dabul S, Lymperopoulos A. Current and future G protein-coupled receptor signaling targets for heart failure therapy. Drug Des Devel Ther 2013; 7: 1209-22. [PMID: 24143078]

[73] Lymperopoulos A, Bathgate A. Arrestins in the cardiovascular system. Prog Mol Biol Transl Sci 2013; 118: 297-334.

[http://dx.doi.org/10.1016/B978-0-12-394440-5.00012-7] [PMID: 23764059]

[74] Lymperopoulos A, Rengo G, Koch WJ. Adrenergic nervous system in heart failure: pathophysiology and therapy. Circ Res 2013; 113(6): 739-53. [http://dx.doi.org/10.1161/CIRCRESAHA.113.300308] [PMID: 23989716]

[75] Rengo G, Lymperopoulos A, Koch WJ. Future g protein-coupled receptor targets for treatment of heart failure. Curr Treat Options Cardiovasc Med 2009; 11(4): 328-38. [http://dx.doi.org/10.1007/s11936-009-0033-5] [PMID: 19627665]

[76] Zhu WZ, Zheng M, Koch WJ, Lefkowitz RJ, Kobilka BK, Xiao RP. Dual modulation of cell survival and cell death by beta(2)-adrenergic signaling in adult mouse cardiac myocytes. Proc Natl Acad Sci USA 2001; 98(4): 1607-12. [http://dx.doi.org/10.1073/pnas.98.4.1607] [PMID: 11171998]

[77] Nikolaev VO, Moshkov A, Lyon AR, *et al.* Beta2-adrenergic receptor redistribution in heart failure changes cAMP compartmentation. Science 2010; 327(5973): 1653-7. [http://dx.doi.org/10.1126/science.1185988] [PMID: 20185685]

[78] Birks EJ, Tansley PD, Hardy J, *et al.* Left ventricular assist device and drug therapy for the reversal of heart failure. N Engl J Med 2006; 355(18): 1873-84. [http://dx.doi.org/10.1056/NEJMoa053063] [PMID: 17079761]

[79] Bers DM. Calcium cycling and signaling in cardiac myocytes. Annu Rev Physiol 2008; 70: 23-49. [http://dx.doi.org/10.1146/annurev.physiol.70.113006.100455] [PMID: 17988210]

[80] Esposito G, Prasad SV, Rapacciuolo A, Mao L, Koch WJ, Rockman HA. Cardiac overexpression of a G(q) inhibitor blocks induction of extracellular signal-regulated kinase and c-Jun NH(2)-terminal kinase activity in *in vivo* pressure overload. Circulation 2001; 103(10): 1453-8. [http://dx.doi.org/10.1161/01.CIR.103.10.1453] [PMID: 11245652]

[81] Hwang H, Robinson DA, Stevenson TK, *et al.* PKCβII modulation of myocyte contractile performance. J Mol Cell Cardiol 2012; 53(2): 176-86. [http://dx.doi.org/10.1016/j.yjmcc.2012.05.001] [PMID: 22587992]

[82] Rengo G, Lymperopoulos A, Zincarelli C, *et al.* Myocardial adeno-associated virus serotype 6-betaARKct gene therapy improves cardiac function and normalizes the neurohormonal axis in chronic heart failure. Circulation 2009; 119(1): 89-98. [http://dx.doi.org/10.1161/CIRCULATIONAHA.108.803999] [PMID: 19103992]

[83] Brede M, Wiesmann F, Jahns R, *et al.* Feedback inhibition of catecholamine release by two different alpha2-adrenoceptor subtypes prevents progression of heart failure. Circulation 2002; 106(19): 2491-6. [http://dx.doi.org/10.1161/01.CIR.0000036600.39600.66] [PMID: 12417548]

[84] Cohn JN, Pfeffer MA, Rouleau J, *et al.* Adverse mortality effect of central sympathetic inhibition with sustained-release moxonidine in patients with heart failure (MOXCON). Eur J Heart Fail 2003; 5(5): 659-67. [http://dx.doi.org/10.1016/S1388-9842(03)00163-6] [PMID: 14607206]

[85] Kao DP, Wagner BD, Robertson AD, Bristow MR, Lowes BD. A personalized BEST: characterization of latent clinical classes of nonischemic heart failure that predict outcomes and response to bucindolol. PLoS One 2012; 7(11): e48184.

[http://dx.doi.org/10.1371/journal.pone.0048184] [PMID: 23144856]

[86] Lymperopoulos A, Rengo G, Funakoshi H, Eckhart AD, Koch WJ. Adrenal GRK2 upregulation mediates sympathetic overdrive in heart failure. Nat Med 2007; 13(3): 315-23.
[http://dx.doi.org/10.1038/nm1553] [PMID: 17322894]

[87] Lang CC, Struthers AD. Targeting the renin-angiotensin-aldosterone system in heart failure. Nat Rev Cardiol 2013; 10(3): 125-34.
[http://dx.doi.org/10.1038/nrcardio.2012.196] [PMID: 23319100]

[88] Kaoukis A, Deftereos S, Raisakis K, *et al.* The role of endothelin system in cardiovascular disease and the potential therapeutic perspectives of its inhibition. Curr Top Med Chem 2013; 13(2): 95-114.
[http://dx.doi.org/10.2174/1568026611313020003] [PMID: 23470073]

[89] Mustafa SJ, Morrison RR, Teng B, Pelleg A. Adenosine receptors and the heart: role in regulation of coronary blood flow and cardiac electrophysiology. Handb Exp Pharmacol 2009; 193: 161-88.
[http://dx.doi.org/10.1007/978-3-540-89615-9_6]

[90] Sabbah HN, Gupta RC, Kohli S, *et al.* Chronic therapy with a partial adenosine A1-receptor agonist improves left ventricular function and remodeling in dogs with advanced heart failure. Circ Heart Fail 2013; 6(3): 563-71.
[http://dx.doi.org/10.1161/CIRCHEARTFAILURE.112.000208] [PMID: 23564604]

[91] Hong Y, Hay DL, Quirion R, Poyner DR. The pharmacology of adrenomedullin 2/intermedin. Br J Pharmacol 2012; 166(1): 110-20.
[http://dx.doi.org/10.1111/j.1476-5381.2011.01530.x] [PMID: 21658025]

[92] Nishikimi T, Kuwahara K, Nakagawa Y, Kangawa K, Nakao K. Adrenomedullin in cardiovascular disease: a useful biomarker, its pathological roles and therapeutic application. Curr Protein Pept Sci 2013; 14(4): 256-67.
[http://dx.doi.org/10.2174/13892037113149990045] [PMID: 23745694]

[93] Yoshizawa T, Sakurai T, Kamiyoshi A, *et al.* Novel regulation of cardiac metabolism and homeostasis by the adrenomedullin-receptor activity-modifying protein 2 system. Hypertension 2013; 61(2): 341-51.
[http://dx.doi.org/10.1161/HYPERTENSIONAHA.111.00647] [PMID: 23297372]

[94] Metra M, Cotter G, Davison BA, *et al.* Effect of serelaxin on cardiac, renal, and hepatic biomarkers in the Relaxin in Acute Heart Failure (RELAX-AHF) development program: correlation with outcomes. J Am Coll Cardiol 2013; 61(2): 196-206.
[http://dx.doi.org/10.1016/j.jacc.2012.11.005] [PMID: 23273292]

[95] Emeto TI, Moxon JV, Rush C, Woodward L, Golledge J. Relevance of urocortins to cardiovascular disease. J Mol Cell Cardiol 2011; 51(3): 299-307.
[http://dx.doi.org/10.1016/j.yjmcc.2011.06.002] [PMID: 21689660]

[96] Davis ME, Pemberton CJ, Yandle TG, *et al.* Urocortin 2 infusion in human heart failure. Eur Heart J 2007; 28(21): 2589-97.
[http://dx.doi.org/10.1093/eurheartj/ehm340] [PMID: 17720993]

[97] Gheorghiade M, Greene SJ, Ponikowski P, *et al.* Haemodynamic effects, safety, and pharmacokinetics of human stresscopin in heart failure with reduced ejection fraction. Eur J Heart Fail 2013; 15(6): 679-

89.
[http://dx.doi.org/10.1093/eurjhf/hft023] [PMID: 23471413]

[98] Kinugawa K, Imamura T, Komuro I. Experience of a vasopressin receptor antagonist, tolvaptan, under the unique indication in Japanese heart failure patients. Clin Pharmacol Ther 2013; 94(4): 449-51. [http://dx.doi.org/10.1038/clpt.2013.147] [PMID: 23872863]

[99] Brubaker PL. Minireview: update on incretin biology: focus on glucagon-like peptide-1. Endocrinology 2010; 151(5): 1984-9. [http://dx.doi.org/10.1210/en.2010-0115] [PMID: 20305008]

[100] Lorber D. GLP-1 receptor agonists: effects on cardiovascular risk reduction. Cardiovasc Ther 2013; 31(4): 238-49. [http://dx.doi.org/10.1111/1755-5922.12000] [PMID: 23865382]

[101] Galanth C, Hus-Citharel A, Li B, Llorens-Cortès C. Apelin in the control of body fluid homeostasis and cardiovascular functions. Curr Pharm Des 2012; 18(6): 789-98. [http://dx.doi.org/10.2174/138161212799277770] [PMID: 22236125]

[102] Yang Y, Lv SY, Lyu SK, Wu D, Chen Q. The protective effect of apelin on ischemia/reperfusion injury. Peptides 2015; 63: 43-6. [http://dx.doi.org/10.1016/j.peptides.2014.11.001] [PMID: 25447414]

[103] McKinsey TA, Kass DA. Small-molecule therapies for cardiac hypertrophy: moving beneath the cell surface. Nat Rev Drug Discov 2007; 6(8): 617-35. [http://dx.doi.org/10.1038/nrd2193] [PMID: 17643091]

[104] Pereira L, Cheng H, Lao DH, *et al.* Epac2 mediates cardiac β1-adrenergic-dependent sarcoplasmic reticulum Ca2+ leak and arrhythmia. Circulation 2013; 127(8): 913-22. [http://dx.doi.org/10.1161/CIRCULATIONAHA.12.148619] [PMID: 23363625]

[105] Lymperopoulos A, Garcia D, Walklett K. Pharmacogenetics of cardiac inotropy. Pharmacogenomics 2014; 15(14): 1807-21. [http://dx.doi.org/10.2217/pgs.14.120] [PMID: 25493572]

[106] Sandilands AJ, O'Shaughnessy KM, Brown MJ. Greater inotropic and cyclic AMP responses evoked by noradrenaline through Arg389 beta 1-adrenoceptors *versus* Gly389 beta 1-adrenoceptors in isolated human atrial myocardium. Br J Pharmacol 2003; 138(2): 386-92. [http://dx.doi.org/10.1038/sj.bjp.0705030] [PMID: 12540530]

[107] Johnson JA, Liggett SB. Cardiovascular pharmacogenomics of adrenergic receptor signaling: clinical implications and future directions. Clin Pharmacol Ther 2011; 89(3): 366-78. [http://dx.doi.org/10.1038/clpt.2010.315] [PMID: 21289619]

[108] Small KM, Wagoner LE, Levin AM, Kardia SL, Liggett SB. Synergistic polymorphisms of beta1- and alpha2C-adrenergic receptors and the risk of congestive heart failure. N Engl J Med 2002; 347(15): 1135-42. [http://dx.doi.org/10.1056/NEJMoa020803] [PMID: 12374873]

[109] Neuvonen AM, Palo JU, Sajantila A. Post-mortem ABCB1 genotyping reveals an elevated toxicity for female digoxin users. Int J Legal Med 2011; 125(2): 265-9. [http://dx.doi.org/10.1007/s00414-011-0550-0] [PMID: 21311904]

[110] Adams KF Jr, Patterson JH, Gattis WA, *et al.* Relationship of serum digoxin concentration to mortality and morbidity in women in the digitalis investigation group trial: a retrospective analysis. J Am Coll Cardiol 2005; 46(3): 497-504.
[http://dx.doi.org/10.1016/j.jacc.2005.02.091] [PMID: 16053964]

CHAPTER 4

Gene Polymorphisms, Mutations and Epigenetics in Heart Failure

Daphne Koumbi[1,2], Constantina Sambani[1], George P. Patrinos[3] and **Panagoula Kollia[2,*]**

[1] *Laboratory of Health Physics, Radiobiology & Cytogenetics, NCSR "Democritus", Athens, Greece*

[2] *Department of Genetics & Biotechnology, Faculty of Biology, National & Kapodistrian University of Athens, Athens, Greece*

[3] *Department of Pharmacy, University of Patras, Patras, Greece*

Abstract: Heart Failure (HF) is a complex clinical syndrome characterized by compromised cardiac output that leads to inadequate blood supply failing to meet the requirements of the metabolizing tissues of the body. HF is a silent epidemic that affects ~2% of the general population in the western world and its prevalence is steadily increasing. Although survival has improved, high morbidity and mortality render HF the most devastating cardiovascular disorder with considerable financial burden on public health care. The phenotypic variability of HF syndrome reflects the complexity of the underlying genetic background of the disease, as well as the inter-individual susceptibility to external triggers. Although acquired clinical conditions account for the majority of HF development, a proportion of HF cases are due to inherited pathological states comprising myocardial disorders, mitochondrial diseases, metabolic disorders and congenital heart defect syndromes. Among those, inherited forms of cardiomyopathies constitute "naturally-occurring" disease models that provide the opportunity for an in depth investigation of the genotype–phenotype relationships. Advances in technology permitting high-throughput whole genome genotyping and sequencing, have provided invaluable insights into the genetic architecture, disease evolution and therapeutic response. However, despite the enormous wealth of genetic information derived from those studies and their contribution towards the identification

* **Corresponding author Panagoula Kollia:** Department of Genetics & Biotechnology, Faculty of Biology, National & Kapodistrian University of Athens, Athens, Greece; Tel: +30 210 727 4041; Fax: +30 210 727 4318; E-mail:pankollia@biol.uoa.gr

Panagiotis Georgoulias (Ed.)

of disease-specific genetic variants in complex diseases such as HF, a considerable amount of genetic information related to heritability is missing. In this chapter, we will review knowledge regarding the underlying complex genetic architecture of both acquired and inherited forms of HF, the role of epigenetics as a significant modifier mechanism in disease susceptibility and phenotypic heterogeneity, as well as advances in the field of pharmacogenetics of HF.

Keywords: Cardiomyopathies, Chromatin remodelling, Congenital heart defects, DNA methylation, Epigenetics, Genetics, Genetic testing, Heart failure, Histone, MicroRNAs, Pharmacogenetics, Single nucleotide polymorphisms.

INTRODUCTION

Heart failure (HF) is a complex clinical syndrome characterized by compromised cardiac output that leads to inadequate blood supply, failing to meet the requirements of the metabolizing tissues of the body. HF affects ~2% of the general population in the western world and its prevalence is increasing both in the developed and developing countries, mainly due to population aging, advances in clinical management of coronary artery disease (CAD) and growing incidence of clinical conditions that constitute important risk factors for HF (*e.g.* diabetes, hypertension). Although survival has improved, high morbidity is still a considerable issue and mortality rates remain approximately 50% within 5 years of diagnosis, thereby rendering HF the most devastating cardiovascular disorder with considerable financial burden on public health care. The clinical syndrome of HF may result from disorders mainly of the myocardium, and comorbid clinical conditions [CAD, hypertension, diabetes mellitus type 2 (T2DM)] are also underlying causes of this pathological state [1 - 5]. Although the majority of HF incidence is due to acquired forms of disorders, emerging data from the Framingham heart study project, shed light onto the genetic components of sporadic forms of HF in regard to the relative risks for offsprings of parents with HF (1.69 if one parent has HF and 1.92 if both parents are affected) [6]. Acquired forms of HF are characterized by a complex genetic architecture, interplaying between environmental and genetic factors, and numerous studies highlight the contribution of the genetic components to HF susceptibility, disease evolution and therapeutic outcome. In addition to sporadic/acquired forms of HF, a small but substantial proportion of HF cases are due to inherited clinical conditions comprising myocardial disorders, mitochondrial diseases, metabolic disorders and congenital heart defect syndromes. Mendelian-inherited myocardial disorders are due to myocardium impairment and comprise the following cardiomyopathies: hypertrophic cardiomyopathy (HCM), dilated cardiomyopathy (DCM), restrictive cardiomyopathy (RCM), arrhythmogenic right ventricular dysplasia/ cardiomyopathy (ARVD/ARVC) and left ventricular non-compaction (LVNC) [2, 5]. Inherited cardiomyopathies constitute "naturally-occurring" HF disease models and in this direction, more profound understanding of their genetic architecture may aid toward an in depth understanding of the cross-talk between inborn genetic composition and epigenetic modifiers. In recent years, with the application of high-throughput technologies, Genome Association-based Meta-analyses studies have enabled for the whole-genome screening of a large number of individuals and in this direction, substantial advances in the discovery of loci contributing to HF development have been achieved [7, 8]. Still, only a small fraction of the genetic information explaining the heritability of HF is known. In the future, larger-scale studies using higher-density reference panels will provide new biological insights into the complex nature of HF, with the ultimate goal to improve our understanding of the disease susceptibility and progression, as well as to identify novel targets for the treatment and prevention of this clinical condition.

GENETICS OF HEART FAILURE (HF) IN ACQUIRED DISORDERS

Genetic Defects and Inborn Genetic Variants in the Ca^{+2} Signaling Pathway - General Aspects

Cardiomyocytes express all three β-adrenergic receptor subtypes β1, β2 and β3, with β1 being the most prominent one. The latter mediates positive chronotropic, inotropic and lusitropic effects, thereby participating in the regulation of heart rate, muscular contraction and diastolic relaxation. β2 receptor is also involved in the enhancement of cardiac frequency and contractility, with a role in smooth muscle relaxation [9 - 12]. Following β-receptor coupling to stimulative regulative G-protein (Gs), increase in cAMP levels and ensuing activation of the protein kinase A (PKA) take place. The latter phosphorylates a number of proteins fundamental for cardiac function: L-type calcium channels (LTCC), phospholamban (PLN), troponin I and C, ryanodine receptors (RyR2) and cardiac sarcoplasmic reticulum Ca^{+2} - ATPase pump (SERCA2a) [13 - 17]. During sarcomere contraction, Ca^{+2} influx through the L-type channel occurs with ensuing release of Ca^{+2} from the sarcoplasmic reticulum (SR) through the RyR2. During cardiac relaxation, Ca^{+2} re-uptake into the SR occurs *via* SERCA2a. Ca^{+2} SERCA2a-mediated entry into SR is regulated by phospholamban (PLN), a 52 amino acid SR transmembrane phosphoprotein that acts as an inhibitor of SERCA2a activity. When phosphorylated, PLN dissociates from SERCA2a and accelerates ventricular relaxation [15]. Elevated cytosolic Ca^{+2} levels constitute a common final pathway in failing cardiomyocytes [18]. Given that intracellular Ca^{+2} handling is the central coordinator of cardiac contraction and relaxation, mutations affecting Ca^{+2} cycling proteins have been reported in several cardiomyopathies with high incidence of HF. In HF, β-receptor desensitization is a key event and β-receptor antagonist administration, pioneered in the 1970s, is a standard treatment in HF [19 - 23]. Increased G protein-coupled receptor kinase (GRK) activity appears to be a major factor contributing to β-receptor desensitization in failing hearts [24, 25]. During HF, the cardiac β1-receptor function is downregulated and the rest of the receptors are uncoupled from Gs, presumably *via* increased activity of the GRK2 and/or GRK5 [26, 27]. Normally, the β1-receptor system can handle short-term increases in cardiac function, yet prolonged activation causes damage. In this context, studies have shown that the level of disease severity is analogous to ~50% decrease in β1 mRNA and protein levels [28, 29]. Numerous studies have demonstrated upregulation of GRK activity and GRK2 mRNA in patients and animal models of HF and hypertrophy [30, 31]. Cardiac overexpression of β1-receptors in transgenic mouse models caused cardiomyocyte hypertrophy, followed by fibrosis and HF [32 - 34]. Given the cardinal role of PKA-mediated phosphorylation of downstream protein targets, several studies have focused on those calcium modulator molecules. Based on the aforementioned detection of an important genetic component even in sporadic forms of HF (the Framingham Offspring cohort study), with a multifactorial pattern of inheritance emerging, numerous transgenic mouse models mimicking pathological conditions with high propensity to HF occurrence have been developed [6].

Ryanodine Receptor (RyR2) Mutations

As mentioned above, Ca^{2+} influx from SR into the cytosol is mediated through the RyR2 calcium channel [35]. RyR2 mutations have been detected in catecholaminergic polymorphic ventricular tachycardia [36, 37], a rare inherited arrhythmic disorder characterized by normal heart structure and sudden cardiac death during physical or emotional stress. More rarely, RyR2 mutations have been encountered in ARVD [38].

Phospholamban (PLN) Mutations

As mentioned, PLN is a negative modulator of SERCA2a-facilitated calcium influx into SR. Upon PLN phosphorylation, SERCA2a is activated and allows for calcium entry into SR, thereby contributing to ventricular relaxation [15]. In accordance with this, experiments with PLN knockout mice suggest that PLN plays a role in the positive lusitropic and part of the positive inotropic β-receptor function [35, 39]. Rare human PLN mutations have been shown to be causative factors in familial DCM and HF [40, 41]. Based on results from PLN-mutant transgenic mouse model studies, constitutive SERCA2a inhibition occurred as a result of excessive PLN activity due to lack of PLN phosphorylation. The PLN Arg9Cys mutation abrogated PKA-mediated PLN phosphorylation, leading to delay of myocyte relaxation, lack of response to β-adrenergic stimulation, significant biventricular cardiac dilation and HF in the mutant mice [42]. In line with this, heterozygote SERCA2 null mice have been shown to exhibit compromised levels of calcium reuptake, leading to defects in systolic and diastolic function [43]. Another PLN null mutation (Leu39stop) has been detected in humans with DCM [41]. Striking enough, PLN-deficient mice exhibited increased calcium reuptake into the SR and enhanced basal contractility [39]. Accordingly, PLN ablation in mice null for the MLP gene - a gene encoding for MLP protein located in cardiac muscle with a role in calcium handling - has been shown to rescue DCM in the specific knock-out mice model [44]. However, in PLN-deficient myocytes, β-adrenergic activation was abrogated [45]. Taken these results together, either hindrance or excessive PLN activity has detrimental effects upon normal heart function.

Polymorphisms in the β- and α- Adrenergic Receptor Genes – General Aspects and Pharmacogenetics Implications

In a broad spectrum of clinical conditions, modulatory effects on disease susceptibility, progression and therapeutic response have been attributed to allelic variation. In this framework, inborn genetic variants (single nucleotide polymorphisms - SNPs) have been also implicated in the HF syndrome, being assigned a modulatory role in HF risk [46]. In the context of individualized therapeutic treatment and with the aim of alleviating drug complications and enhancing therapeutic outcome, investigation of the impact of inborn genetic variants (polymorphisms) on drug metabolism, efficacy and toxicity has been extensively carried out in an array of disorders and clinical conditions. These conditions include the cytochrome P450 enzyme CYP2D6 variants in tamoxifen therapy of breast cancer, the CYP2C9 polymorphic variants in warfarin administration for the prevention of thromboembolism and variants of C-reactive protein and interleukin-6 in stroke incidence following cardiothoracic surgery. Insufficient therapeutic regimes for the management of HF are main causes of increased mortality due to the HF. With the aim of exploiting existing information regarding the complex genetic pathways involved in HF (including the discovery of molecules with a clear-cut beneficial role in HF), the scientific community has shifted much of its interest in the field of pharmagogenetics, where efforts are being made to identify effective therapeutic molecules. The field of pharmacogenetics also explores a variety of chemical agents in terms of their role in the prevention of HF. In this framework, the protective effect of curcumin, a natural component of the spice turmeric, has been established in mouse models. Curcumin has been found to exert an inhibitory effect upon the activity of HATs, which are epigenetic modifiers of genes, such as the p300. Curcumin administration has managed to restore normal cardiac function either alone or in combination with angiotensin converting enzyme (ACE) inhibitors [47, 48]. Another study has shown that trichostatin A (TSA) administration, a histone deacetylase (HDAC) inhibitor, was able to attenuate pathological cardiac remodeling and cardiac hypertrophic growth in transgenic mice models [49, 50]. On the basis of the pronounced inter-individual variation regarding disease susceptibility, evolution and therapeutic response, considerable efforts are being made towards the era of individualized therapeutic approaches, by using accumulating knowledge regarding the drug-modifier activity of polymorphic genetic variants. Based on the patient's genetic profile, development of patient-tailored therapeutic strategies remains a challenge in the field. By applying three different methodological approaches, a number of genetic modifiers have been discovered. The first approach is the candidate-gene approach dealing with discovery of genetic variants involved in the pharmacogenetics cascades. The second approach is the Genome-Wide Association Studies (GWAS) by means of which whole-genome screening of SNPs is carried out. GWAS constitute a case-control approach setup, using a large group of individuals with a specific trait (cases) and a healthy control group. All individuals in each group are genotyped with the implementation of whole-genome SNP microarray platforms for the identification of genetic risk loci. The third approach is the Whole-Exome Sequencing methodology (WES) by means of which investigation for the detection of protein-coding genomic regions is performed.

β- Adrenergic Receptor Polymorphisms

SNPs have been found in all three β-receptor subtypes. More specifically, the SNP Arg389Gly in the β_1-receptor is important in G-protein binding with significant implications in β-blocker response. The Gly389 genetic variant has been shown to be accompanied by reduced cAMP levels, decreased inotropy and low sensitivity to beta-blocker administration [51]. By contrast, the Arg389 variant polymorphism, shown to display more consistent associations, have demonstrated that the Arg389 allele is associated with increased adenylyl cyclase (AC) enzyme signaling, and therefore with increased levels of cAMP, enhanced inotropy and increased susceptibility to beta-blockers [51 - 58]. Furthermore, individuals with the β_1-receptor Arg389 variant either in heterozygosity or homozygosity have been shown to display a satisfactory response to metoprolol and carvedilol β-blocker administration [59, 60]. In addition, studies have shown that the SNP Ser49Gly in the β_1-receptor gene exerts a more profound agonist-promoted down-regulation [61]. Moreover, clinical studies have shown that the coexistence of the Arg389Gly polymorphism in the β_1-receptor gene (ADRB1) and the Gln27Glu polymorphism in the adrenergic β_2-receptor gene (ADRB2) was associated with a two-fold increase in mortality relative to all other genotype combinations in carvedilol-administrated HF patients. By contrast, there was no difference in survival in metoprolol-administrated patients [62]. Both the Arg16Gly and the Gln27Glu polymorphisms have been associated with receptor down-regulation after agonist stimulation [63]. Finally, heterozygous carriers of the rare Ile164 polymorphic variant in β_2-receptor gene have been shown to exhibit lower chronotropic and inotropic response to the β_2 agonist terbutaline, reduced exercise capacity, and decreased survival in HF [64]. These findings underline the potential role of impaired β_1 and β_2 adrenergic receptor gene function as risk factor of HF incidence. To this direction, large cohort studies investigating more complete sets of such polymorphisms, including complete haplotypes, will be required to elucidate their role as modifiers of HF risk and biomarkers of therapeutic response.

α-Adrenergic Receptor Polymorphisms

The α2C Del322-325 polymorphic variant in the α2C-adrenergic receptor, whose mode of action is to inhibit the release of norepinephrine at the pre-junctional terminals, has been associated with higher HF risk [65]. Importantly, Del322-325 carriers were shown to be unresponsive to the administration of the β-blocker bucindolol, whereas wild-type α2C carriers had a 30% reduction in mortality [66].

Polymorphisms in G Protein-coupled Receptor Kinases (GRKs)

The allelic variant Gln41Leu in GRK5 has been shown to enhance desensitization, mimicking a beta-blocker mode of action [52, 67, 68]. In particular, the Leu41 variant appears to behave as an endogenous β-blocker agent. Clinical studies show improved transplant-free survival in patients homozygous or heterozygous for this particular genetic variant. In the light of these findings, the specific variant has been proposed to assume a gain-of-function protective property against the hyperactive adrenergic system in HF [69, 70].

Other Drug Response Modulating Genetic Variants

Polymorphisms in the Renin-Angiotensin-Aldosterone System (RAAS)

ACE is a component of the RAAS and catalyses the conversion of angiotensin I to angiotensin II, a potent vasoconstrictor. A common 287 bp insertion–deletion polymorphism (indels) located in intron 16 of the ACE gene, has been shown to account for almost half of the variation encountered in ACE enzyme levels [71]. More specifically, homozygous carriers for the two deletion alleles (D/D) were found to exhibit higher ACE enzyme levels as opposed to homozygous carriers of two insertion alleles (I/I) that showed lower ACE levels. Heterozygous carriers (I/D) exhibited intermediate ACE levels [72]. Based on the location of the specific genetic variants in non-coding regions, it has been postulated that another genetic variation in linkage disequilibrium with the ACE variant must account for the ACE serum levels. Interestingly enough, further studies discovered a strong association between the homozygous D/D genotype, evolution to DCM and to either ischaemic or non-ischaemic HF as well as with left ventricular hypertrophy (LVH) [73 - 86]. In addition, the D/D genotype was found to be more beneficial in terms of the patients' response to ACE inhibitors and beta-blocker therapeutic regimes [76, 77]. Further, a meta-analysis study corroborated the association between the D/D genotype and LVH but another one argued against any significant correlation between the specific ACE polymorphism and risk of HF [87, 88].

Polymorphisms in the P450 Cytochrome Family

The -344C/T polymorphism located in the promoter of the aldosterone synthase gene CYP11B2 was found to be associated with hypertension, maladaptive myocardial remodeling and higher HF risk, but with a better response to the administration of vasodilators such as hydralazine/isosorbide dinitrate [89, 90]. CYP2D6 encodes for a member of the P450 cytochrome family enzymes that are involved in Phase I drug metabolism. Polymorphic variants in this gene exert a modulatory effect upon β-blocker metabolism. Studies have shown that CYP2D6 variants confer distinct human pharmacokinetic phenotypes. More specifically, homozygous carriers of the loss-of-function polymorphism (deletion of both functional alleles) are poor metabolizers, exhibiting enhanced negative chronotropism and impaired drug clearance when administrated the β-blocker agent metoprolol [91 - 95]. The most important genetic variants involved in the pharmacogenetics of HF are summarized in Table **1**.

Table 1. Inborn genetic variants in heart failure syndrome.

Gene	Allelic variant	Mode of action
β1- adrenergic receptor gene (ADRB1)	Arg389Gly Ser49Gly	Arg389: enhanced inotropy, increased susceptibility to β-blockers 389Gly: decreased inotropy, low sensitivity to β-blocker Gly49: increased receptor down-regulation with agonist treatment
β2- adrenergic receptor gene (ADRB2)	Gln27Glu Arg16Gly Ile164	Glu27: decreased receptor down-regulation with agonist treatment Arg16: increased receptor down-regulation with agonist treatment lower chronotropic and inotropic response to the β2 agonist terbutaline, reduced exercise capacity, decreased survival in HF
α2C- adrenergic receptor gene (ADRA2C)	del322-325	unresponsive to the β-blocker bucindolol, decreased uptake, higher HF risk
G protein-coupled receptor kinase 5 (GRK5)	Gln41Leu	Leu41: endogenous β-blocker effect
Angiotensin I - converting enzyme (ACE)	D/D, D/I, I/I	D/D: higher ACE enzyme levels, responsive to ACE inhibitors and β-blockers D/I: intermediate ACE levels
Alderosterone synthase gene (CYP11B2)	-344C/T	hypertension, maladaptive myocardial remodeling, higher HF risk but with a better response to vasodilators
CYP2D6	CYP2D6*4 (gene deletion) CYP2D6*5 (splice-site variant)	poor metabolizers, enhanced negative chronotropism, impaired drug clearance

HF: heart failure.

Other Genomic Susceptibility Loci throughout the Genome

Using SNP microarray platforms with >2.4 million SNPs in >20,000 subjects, GWAS studies revealed an association between two genetic variants and HF risk occurrence [7]. The specific large-scale GWA-based meta-analysis identified an inborn allelic variant of USP3 gene and a genetic variant of the LRIG3 gene in individuals of European and African ancestry, respectively. The USP3 gene encodes for an ubiquitin-specific protease activated in cardiomyopathies and the LRIC3 gene is responsible for the production of a membrane protein involved in cardiac tissue development. A third variant in the CMTM7 gene (CKLF-like

MARVEL transmembrane domain containing 7) was associated with enhanced incidence of HF mortality [8]. The calculated odds ratios for all three polymorphic variants were around 1.5 (odds ratio: the likelihood that individuals who share a specific genotype will have the disease trait *versus* the likelihood that individuals who do not share a specific genotype will have the disease trait). In another set of GWAS studies using 50,000 SNPs spanning 2000 genes potentially implicated in the development of cardiovascular disorders, a close association between a SNP located in an non-coding region of the HSPB7 gene, encoding a heat shock protein, and HF was shown [96, 97]. Given the intronic location of the specific polymorphism and the fact that the HSPB7 gene was in linkage disequilibrium with the CLCNKA gene coding for the renal ClC-Ka voltage-gated chloride channel, further resequencing of the CLCNKA gene revealed a missense polymorphic variant, Arg83Gly. Importantly enough, the specific allelic variant exhibited a strong association with HF risk, with homozygous individuals showing ~55% increased risk of developing HF [98].

Genomic Susceptibility Loci in Comorbid Clinical Conditions with High Risk for Heart Failure (HF)

Implementation of GWAS has allowed the identification of SNPs with a significant component of genomic susceptibility loci in comorbid clinical conditions, with an elevated risk for acquired HF. In this framework, a considerable number of genetic variants throughout the genome have been implicated in the development of high risk disorders such as hypertension, CAD, T2DM and atherosclerotic heart disease. Hypertension is the most widespread cardiovascular disease with a high risk for HF development. The incidence of HF is greater with higher levels of blood pressure, older age, and longer duration of hypertension [99, 100]. Given that hypertension constitutes a significant public health issue and that blood pressure is a heritable trait influenced both by multiple biological pathways and environmental stimuli, efforts are being made in order to elucidate the genetic component underlying the propensity for HF development. GWAS have allowed the identification of numerous genomic loci closely associated with enhanced tendency for hypertension and ensuing HF incidence [101 - 103]. Moreover, heritability is known to account for 30–60% of the inter-individual variation encountered in the risk of CAD development, a clinical condition with the highest risk for HF development [104]. In this direction, and based on a significant number of GWA-based meta-analyses, identification of several genomic common variants have been shown to be associated with CAD risk [105 - 111]. T2DM is known to increase the likelihood of HF incidence in patients without structural cardiac defects [112]. GWAS and GWAS-based meta-analyses studies conducted in large groups of individuals, have identified a number of genomic variants predisposing to T2DM [113 - 115]. However, despite the enormous wealth of genetic information derived from GWAS studies and the significant contribution towards the identification of disease-specific genetic variants in complex diseases such as HF, a considerable amount of genetic information related to heritability is missing. Better management of population stratification, larger and well-defined phenotypic characterization of both case and control groups and a greater number of GWA-based meta-analysis studies are required.

GENETICS OF HEART FAILURE (HF) IN INHERITED DISORDERS

Inherited forms of cardiomyopathies comprise a small proportion of overall HF and their incidence is age- and population- dependent. The incidence of familial cardiomyopathies in children and adolescents is approximately 30-40% [116 - 118]. The phenotypic heterogeneity of the inherited forms of HF is a result of genetic heterogeneity due to allelic and locus heterogeneity. Allelic heterogeneity means that different variants within an individual gene can produce variable phenotypes. For instance, as it is discussed below, mutations in the gene encoding the sarcomeric protein cardiac troponin I (TNNT2) may cause the HCM, DCM, or RCM phenotype. Locus heterogeneity means that mutations in more than one type of gene (locus) are responsible for the clinical phenotype. Indeed, mutations in >50 genes cause a DCM phenotype and within these genes numerous variants exist. Variable expressivity and penetrance are also encountered in the inherited forms of the disease, suggesting that additional genetic, epigenetic and environmental factors function as modifiers in the final clinical manifestations. Digenic inheritance may also be encountered and in addition to that the proband with the disease may carry a *de novo* mutation. The proportion of cases caused by *de novo* mutations is unknown but estimated at 30%. *De novo* mutations pose an extra difficulty, given that in many instances it may not be possible to determine if a genetic variant is pathogenic or clinically irrelevant. Many mutations are known to be rare and frequently private and given that the index may be member of a small family, the potential pathogenicity of a missense genetic variant may be difficult to assess. It should be stressed that if no identification of a disease-causing mutation is achieved in an affected family member, longitudinal clinical evaluation for the disease is recommended for asymptomatic at-risk first degree relatives. Indeed, the use of genetic testing in everyday clinical practice has been challenging and identification of a pathogenic genetic variant is attained in approximately 30%-50% of familial HCM, DCM or ARVC cases [119 - 121]. Despite the difficulties encountered when screening for disease-causing genetic defects in cases of HF inherited forms, genetic testing and screening is extremely important because by identifying relatives at risk of developing the disease, early surveillance, risk stratification and therapeutic treatment can be implemented [28, 32, 33]. For this reason, genetic testing of at-risk family members is recommended in clinical guidelines and constitute standard of care practice [120, 122, 123]. Genetic testing also provides insight into the underlying genetic complexity of the disease.

Hypertrophic Cardiomyopathy (HCM)

HCM, a clinical condition characterized by left ventricular hypertrophy, affects 1 out of 500 people worldwide and is known to be the most common inherited cardiovascular disease. HCM is associated with high incidence of sudden death and increased likelihood of HF development (20% of patients will develop HF). HCM can occur at any age and is associated with enhanced frequency of HF during infancy. It is the most common cause of sudden cardiac death in adolescence and young adulthood. The disease exhibits a high degree of genetic heterogeneity. It is primarily a disorder of the sarcomere, with genetic variants located in 8 sarcomere genes in approximately 50-67% of clinical cases. In this framework, mutations have been located in genes encoding for protein components of the sarcomere (MYH7, MYBPC3, TNNT2, TNNI3) [124]. The MYH7 gene is responsible for the production of the cardiac beta (β)-myosin heavy chain, an essential component of the thick filament in sarcomeres. The MYH7 gene was the first HCM disease-causing gene discovered back in 1989. MYH7 mutations have been associated with early-onset phenotype and marked hypertrophy [125]. Together with MYBPC3, these two genes account for 80% of the disease-causing mutations in familial HCM cases. The MYBPC3 gene encodes the cardiac myosin binding protein C, which associates with the thick filament, thereby contributing to the structural support and assisting in the regulation of muscle contractions. As opposed to MYH7 mutations, MYBPC3 genetic variants have been correlated with later-onset disease manifestation [126, 127]. The TNNT2 and TNNI3 genes encode the cardiac troponin subunits T and I, respectively that form part of the troponin complex which in turn associates with the thin filament of sarcomeres. Production of altered or reduced amount of the aforementioned sarcomere proteins may lead to sarcomere impaired function, ultimately compromising myocardium normal contraction. Mutations in tropomyosin alpha-1 chain gene (TPM1) account for 2% of familial HCM cases. Tropomyosin is an important part of most actin filaments, thereby playing a pivotal role in cardiomyocyte contraction. More than 1,500 individual mutations have been identified. Mutations in any of the sarcomere genes are encountered not only in the 50%-67% of familial HCM cases, but also in 20%-30% of HCM cases without a family history [128, 129]. Importantly, occurrence of *de novo* mutations has been reported in 30% of HCM cases [130]. Some, if not all, of the sporadic forms of the disease may be caused by spontaneous mutations. The pattern of inheritance is autosomal dominant, with variable expressivity, penetrance and age of onset, ranging from asymptomatic left ventricular hypertrophy to arrhythmias and HF. The genotype in approximately 6% of affected individuals harbors either biallelic variants in any of the aforementioned sarcomere genes (compound heterozygosity) or heterozygous variants in more than one gene (double heterozygosity) [131 - 133]. The phenotypic heterogeneity characterizing HCM in terms of the severity of hypertrophy and the spectrum of clinical symptoms reflect the pronounced genetic heterogeneity. In this context, specific tropomyosin substitutions show only a mild degree of ventricular hypertrophy, although they carry a disproportionately high risk for sudden death. Adverse prognosis in situations of compound or double heterozygosity (5 to 10% of the patients) has been reported [132, 134]. Thus, a gene-dosage effect is encountered, with ≥ 2 genetic variants contributing to a more severe phenotype. In addition, studies show that the severity of the HCM phenotype is associated with detection of any sarcomere gene mutation compared to genotype-negative patients [135, 136].

Interestingly, despite the monogenic nature of familial HCM, a significant phenotypic variation is encountered even at the intrafamilial level, thereby pointing to the complex genetic architecture underlying the phenotypic clinical manifestations. Table **2** comprises the list of disease-causing genes in HCM.

Table 2. Disease-causing genes in hypertrophic cardiomyopathy [Data from OMIM (Online Mendelian Inheritance in Man Database)].

Genes	Protein name	OMIM
MYH7	Myosin-7	160760
MYBPC3	Myosin-binding protein C, cardiac type	115197
TNNT2	Troponin T, cardiac muscle	115195
TNNI3	Troponin I, cardiac muscle	191044
TPM1	Tropomyosin alpha-1 chain	115196
MYL2	Myosin regulatory light chain 2, ventricular/cardiac muscle isoform	160781
MYL3	Myosin light chain 3	160790
ACTC1	Actin, alpha cardiac muscle 1	102540
CSRP3	Cysteine and glycine-rich protein 3	600824
ACTN2	Alpha-actinin-2	102573
MYH6	Myosin-6	160710
TCAP	Telethonin	604488
TNNC1	Troponin C, slow skeletal and cardiac muscles	191040
PLN	Cardiac phospholamban	172405
MYOZ2	Myozenin-2	605602
NEXN	Nexilin	613121

Hypertrophic Cardiomyopathy (HCM) Phenotype and Related Phenocopies

Some clinical congenital heart defect diseases exhibit phenotypic similarities in terms of alterations in structure and function of the cardiovascular system. In this framework, HCM has been encountered in individuals with metabolic diseases such as Danon disease, caused by mutations in the LAMP2 gene that encodes a lysosomal-associated membrane protein. Danon disease is associated with striking LVH and ventricular arrhythmias related to accumulation of autophagic vacuoles, and rapid disease progression to end-stage HF. Fabry metabolic disease is another clinical condition resulting from deficient activity of the enzyme α-galactosidase (α-Gal) and progressive lysosomal deposition in cells throughout the body [137]. In middle age, most affected males develop cardiovascular and/or cerebrovascular disease. Pompe disease is an inborn glycogen storage disease (GSD II) associated with cardiac hypertrophy [138]. HCM is also encountered in the Noonan malformation syndrome characterized by gain-of-function mutations in PTPN11 gene that encodes for a protein interacting with the protein tyrosine kinase (PTK) - mitogen-activated protein kinase (MAPK) pathway [139]. Finally, the HCM is also part of the phenotypic manifestations seen in the neuromuscular disorder Friedreich ataxia (FRDA) caused by amplification of a triplet repeat within the FRDA gene that encodes for frataxin, a mitochondrial protein involved in iron metabolism [140].

Dilated Cardiomyopathy (DCM)

DCM is characterized by ventricular chamber enlargement and depressed myocardial contractile dysfunction associated with both systolic and diastolic dysfunction, often presenting with HF. It is the third most common cause of HF. DCM is one of the three traditional classes of cardiomyopathy, along with the HCM and RCM. The age-adjusted prevalence of DCM in the United States averages 36 cases per 100,000 population [141]. Following exclusion of all identifiable non-genetic causes, DCM is traditionally referred to as idiopathic dilated cardiomyopathy (IDCM). However, even in simplex cases, cases with a single occurrence of IDCM in a family, disease-causing mutations have been detected, thereby underlying the genetic basis of the disease [142]. More than 30% of the patients diagnosed with idiopathic DCM are finally found to have affected first-degree relatives. When two or more closely related family members are diagnosed with idiopathic (primary) DCM, diagnosis of familial DCM is established. Approximately 20%-50% of patients with idiopathic DCM have familial DCM [143, 144]. The mode of inheritance is mainly autosomal dominant (80%-90% of the cases), although other patterns of inheritance such as autosomal recessive, or X-linked inheritance have been reported. In patients ≥40 years of age, DCM penetrance levels up to almost 95%. Given that DCM exhibits a variable age of onset, (age-dependent penetrance) and the individual may be asymptomatic for years, the implementation of genetic testing is crucial both in cases of familial and idiopathic DCM.

Mutations in Dilated Cardiomyopathy (DCM)

Genetic defects in more than 80 genes encoding for sarcomere proteins, cytoskeleton proteins, nuclear envelope proteins, voltage-gated ion membrane channels and desmosomal proteins, have been reported in DCM [141, 143]. In addition to the genetic heterogeneity of the disease, significant allelic heterogeneity is also encountered.

Approximately in 40%-50% of familial DCM cases, causal gene mutations have been detected [143]. The disease exhibits significant allelic heterogeneity with ~25% of the familial cases harboring truncating mutations in the titin gene (TTN) [145]. TTN gene encodes for the giant protein titin spanning half the sarcomere. Importantly, idiopathic DCM cases show a TTN mutation frequency of 20%, thereby pointing to a genetic background of the disease [145]. Less frequently, mutations in MYH-7 myosin-7 gene (5%-10% frequency), a large LMNA deletion in the Lamin-A/C gene (6% frequency), SCN5A mutations in the sodium channel protein type 5 subunit alpha gene (4% frequency), TNNT2 mutations in the cardiac Troponin T (2.5% frequency) and a BAG3 whole-exon deletion in the BAG family molecular chaperone regulator 3 gene (2.5% frequency) have been also encountered, with many of the variants being private [146, 147]. LMNA mutations have been shown to be adverse prognostic factors with a high risk of sudden cardiac death [148 - 150]. SCN5A mutations have been associated with increased arrhythmogenicity and variants in the desmosomal genes DSP and PKP2 have been also detected in patients with DCM [151 - 153]. Table **3** comprises the list of disease-causing genes in DCM.

Dilated Cardiomyopathy (DCM) and Single Nucleotide Polymorphisms (SNPs)

A European consortium study on DCM identified three DCM-associated SNPs [154]. Two of these, rs10927875 and rs2234962, were replicated in independent samples. rs10927875 maps to a region on chromosome 1p36.13 which encompasses several genes, including the HSPB7 gene encoding for the heat shock protein beta. The second identified locus involves rs2234962, a non-synonymous SNP located within the coding sequence of BAG3 (BCL2-associated athanogene 3) on chromosome 10q26. A CNV harboring a 4.8-kb deletion in EYA4 gene has also been detected [155]. Rare variants in this gene were found to segregate in families. In another recent study, Norton *et al.* used GWAS and whole-exome sequencing and identified rare variants in BAG3 as a cause for familial DCM [147]. This is one of the rare examples of the same genetic locus showing an association between rare variants with large effect and rare familial monogenetic disease and common variants with small effects and sporadic common diseases. Finally, in another GWA study followed by exome sequencing, a pathogenic GATAD1 genetic variant encoding for the GATA zinc finger domain containing protein 1, was identified to cause DCM inherited in an autosomal recessive mode [156].

Table 3. Disease-causing genes in dilated cardiomyopathy [Data from OMIM (Online Mendelian Inheritance in Man Database)].

Genes	Protein name	OMIM
TTN	Titin	188840
LMNA	Lamin-A/C	150330
MYH7	Myosin-7	160760
MYH6	Myosin-6	160710
SCN5A	Sodium channel protein type 5 subunit alpha	600163
MYBPC3	Myosin-binding protein C, cardiac-type	600958
TNNT2	Troponin T, cardiac muscle	191045
BAG3	BAG family molecular chaperone regulator 3	603883
ANKRD1	Ankyrin repeat domain-containing protein 1	609599
RBM20	Probable RNA-binding protein 20	613171
TMPO	Lamina-associated polypeptide 2	188380
LDB3	LIM domain-binding protein 3	605906
TCAP	Telethonin	604488
VCL	Vinculin	193065
TPM1	Tropomyosin alpha-1 chain	191010
TNNI3	Troponin I, cardiac muscle	191044
TNNC1	Troponin C, slow skeletal and cardiac muscles	191040
ACTC1	Actin, alpha cardiac muscle 1	102540
ACTN2	Alpha-actinin-2	102573
CSRP3	Cysteine and glycine-rich protein 3	600824
DES	Desmin	125660
NEXN	Nexilin	613121
PSEN1	Presenilin-1	104311
PSEN2	Presenilin-2	600759
SGCD	Delta-sarcoglycan	601411
EYA4	Eyes absent homolog 4	603550
PLN	Cardiac phospholamban	172405
DSG2	Desmoglein-2	125671

Arrhythmogenic Right Ventricular Dysplasia/Cardiomyopathy (ARVD/ARVC)

ARVD/ARVC is mainly an inherited disorder characterized by structural and functional abnormalities in the right ventricle (RV) resulting in ventricular arrhythmias. Left ventricular dysfunction may also evolve with time. The prevalence is 1 in 1000 and constitutes an important cause of sudden cardiac death with a high risk of HF development (20% of the patients develop HF) [157 - 159]. It is more common in individuals of Greek and Italian origin. The median age at presentation is approximately 26 years of age. Familial cases account for up to 90% of cases, with the rest of the cases resulting from acquired etiology such as viral infection (myocarditis). The most common pattern of inheritance is autosomal dominance and a disease-causing gene has been found in approximately 40% of the patients. The penetrance is age-dependent, ranging from 20%-35% among family members. Digenic inheritance is also encountered. ARVD/ARVC is known as a disorder of the desmosome with the most common causal genes being the plakoglobin (JUP), desmoplakin (DSP), plakophilin-2 (PKP2), desmoglein-2 (DSG2), desmocollin-2 (DSC2), TGFB3, RYR2 and TMEM43. Four additional genes associated with ARVD/ARVC have been mapped but not identified (locus names ARVD3, ARVD4, ARVD6, and ARVD7 at 14q12-q22, 2q32.1-q32.3, 10p14-p12 and 10q22.3) [167, 168]. DSP, PKP2, DSG2, DSC2, and JUP encode for desmosomal proteins, with PKP2 exhibiting the highest mutation frequency (up to 50%) [160, 161]. ARVD/ARVC inheritance is characterized by compound and digenic heterozygosity, as well as significant level of reduced penetrance. Other frequent mutations occur in the DSG2 gene (3-20% frequency), DSP gene (1-16% frequency) and DSC2 gene (1-13% frequency). RYR2 plays an important role in calcium homeostasis by mediating its release from SR, thereby affecting cardiac muscle excitation-contraction coupling [38]. Genetic defects in RYR2 have shown that the resulting protein has impaired function, leading to excessive calcium influx into the cytosol and ultimately to arrhythmias. Production of an altered desmoplakin protein is proposed to be associated with desmosomal instability and mechanical stress in contracting cardiomyocytes [162, 163]. Similar to desmoplakin, plakophilin-2 (PKP2) desmosomal protein provides structural and functional integrity to adjacent cardiomyocytes. Lack of proper function as a result of mutations in the PKP2 gene has been speculated to contribute to arrhythmias. Mutations in the DSC2 gene lead to an altered desmocollin protein unable to bind plakoglobin. This impairment has been assumed to alter desmosome function. TMEM43 codes a novel transmembrane protein, speculated to be a target of PPARγ, known to be involved in PPARG fatty acid regulation storage and glucose metabolism. TGFB3 encodes transforming growth factor beta-3 which encodes cytokine-stimulating fibrosis and modulates cell adhesion. JUP gene encodes the cytoplasmic protein gamma catenin which is located within desmosomes and forms distinct complexes with cadherins and desmosomal cadherins. Genetic defects in JUP gene lead to structural alterations of JUP protein and this is assumed to interfere with regulatory mechanisms mediated by Wnt-signaling pathway involved in cell proliferation and migration. Genetic defects in RYR2, TMEM43, TGFB3 genes account for a small fraction of familial ARVD/ARVC cases. Emerging data from genotype-phenotype correlation studies has shown that the nature of the disease-causing gene as well as the occurrence of compound and digenic heterozygosity may have an impact upon the severity of clinical manifestations. In this regard, the presence of a heterozygous PKP2 mutation status was not found to suffice for development of the ARVD/ARVC phenotype. In a study of familial ARVD/ARVC cases, not all first-degree relatives of a proband with a PKP2 pathogenic variant met the clinical criteria for ARVD/ARVC [164]. In another set of familial ARVD/ARVC cases, compound and digenic heterozygosity with at least one mutation occurring in PKP2 were correlated with a more severe phenotype [165]. This led to the postulation of the insufficiency of only one pathogenic PKP2 variant as a causative genetic defect for the development ARVD/ARVC disorder. Furthermore, in a study including a substantial proportion of familial ARVD/ARVC cases, compound or digenic heterozygosity had a more detrimental effect upon the ensuing clinical phenotype as opposed to those individuals that were heterozygous for a single mutation [166]. By contrast, in another study conducted by Bauce *et al.*, the severity of the phenotype in individuals with ARVD/ARVC did not correlate with the presence or absence of compound or digenic heterozygosity [167]. Therefore, more research studies are needed in order to elucidate the exact impact of compound or digenic heterozygosity and PKP2 desmosomal mutations upon the clinical manifestations of the disease. Finally, mutations encountered both in HCM and DCM (*e.g.* TTN, MYH7, PKP2), have been also reported in ARVD/ARVC cases (phenotypic heterogeneity), thereby pointing to the activation of transcriptional, post-translational mechanisms and epigenetic gene expression modifications. Table **4** comprises the list of disease-causing genes in ARVD/ARVC.

Table 4. Disease-causing genes in arrhythmogenic right ventricular dysplasia/cardiomyopathy [Data from OMIM (Online Mendelian Inheritance in Man Database)].

Genes	Protein name	OMIM
PKP2	Plakophilin 2	602861
DSG2	Desmoglein 2	125671
DSP	Desmoplakin	125647
DSC2	Desmoglein 2	125645
RYR2	Ryanodine receptor 2	180902
TGFB3	Transforming growth factor, beta-3	190230
JUP	Junction plakoglobin	173325
TMEM43	Transmembrane protein 43	612048

Phenotypic Similarities in Other Congenital Heart Defect Syndromes and Diseases

The autosomal-recessive Naxos disease is a genetically related disorder characterized by ARVD/ARVC, palmoplantar keratosis and wooly hair. It is localized in the Greek island of Naxos. Genetic mutation occurs in JUP gene at 17q21 and penetrance is almost 100% [168]. The Carvajal syndrome is another genetically related disorder inherited in an autosomal recessive mode and characterized by ventricular dilated cardiomyopathy, palmoplantar keratoderma and woolly hair [169]. A homozygous nonsense DSP mutation has been reported to be responsible for the specific disorder.

Left Ventricular Non-Compaction Cardiomyopathy (LVNC)

LVNC is an uncommon, recently described, cardiomyopathy that is characterized by trabeculations in the left ventricle. Patients with LVNC may also have another type of heart muscle disease (HCM, DCM or RCM). The most serious complication of LVNC is HF and sudden cardiac arrest. In 20-40% of LVNC cases an underlying genetic cause is identified [170 - 172]. Although LVNC has been classified as a primary genetic cardiomyopathy, it is controversial whether LVNC should be considered as a distinct cardiomyopathy or rather a phenotypic variant of other primary cardiomyopathies [170, 171]. Familial disease accounts for 20%-70% of LVNC-diagnosed cases [172]. The mode of inheritance is predominantly autosomal dominant and the disease-causing gene is the alpha-dystrobrevin gene DTNA. The specific gene encodes for the dystrobrevin protein which is an integral component of the dystrophin-associated protein complex (DPC). Mutations in sarcomere protein genes (MYH7, MYBPC3, ACTC1, TPM1, TNNT2) have been also reported in approximately 20% of familial LVNC [173, 174].

Phenotypic Similarities in Other Congenital Heart Defect Syndromes and Diseases

LVNC can also occur as part of an X-linked disorder, Barth syndrome, characterized by mitochondrial cardiolipin deficiency [175]. It is caused by mutations in the TAZ gene on chromosome Xq28.

Restrictive Cardiomyopathy (RCM)

RCM is a rare myocardial disease, the least common of the 3 clinically recognized and described cardiomyopathies, characterized by diastolic dysfunction, specifically, restricted ventricular filling. RCM accounts for approximately 5% of all cases of primary heart muscle disease and is known to have a strong genetic cause. The pattern of the disease can be either idiopathic or familial. Mutations in familial RCM have been encountered in the genes encoding the sarcomere protein genes TNNI3, TNNT2, ACTC1, MYPN and MYL3 [176, 177]. Mutations in the DES gene encoding for the sarcomere protein desmin have been also reported [178]. In the majority of the cases there is no clear-cut correlation between the genetic variant and the specific RCM phenotype. Interestingly, a significant number of diagnosed RCM cases have been identified in family pedigrees, while HCM was diagnosed in the majority of affected individuals.

Mitochondrial Disorders and Cardiomyopathies

Cardiomyopathy is encountered in mitochondrial disorders with a frequency ranging from 17-40%. HCM is the most prevalent clinical manifestation (HCM 19%; RCM 3%; LVNC 3%). Myocardial tissue is highly affected by genetic defects altering normal oxidative phosphorylation and compromising adenosine triphosphate (ATP) production. However, phenotypic variation is characteristic of this spectrum of diseases when detrimental mutations occur in the mitochondrial genome. The phenotypic heterogeneity encountered, is due to the fact that a phenotypic threshold is required for the clinical condition to manifest. This threshold is due to mtDNA heteroplasmy, that is, the proportion of the mutant and normal mtDNA populations. Generally speaking, this threshold is approximately 60% for mutations in the mtDNA and 90% for mutations in the nuclear genome. Inheritance is matrilineal if the mutation occurs in the mitochondrial genome [179, 180]. MELAS disease (mitochondrial encephalopathy with lactic acidosis and stroke-like episodes) is associated with the m.3243A>G (MTTL1) mutation and cardiomyopathy is encountered at a frequency of 40% [181]. MERF disease (myoclonic epilepsy with ragged red fibrosis) is characterized by the m.8344A>G (MTTK) occurring within the mtDNA in the tRNA gene. 80% to 90% of the patients may develop HCM or DCM phenotype [182].

Metabolic Diseases and Cardiomyopathies

An array of inborn metabolic disorders exhibits a cardiomyopathy phenotype. Disorders of fatty acid metabolism, such as MCAD (medium-chain acyl-coenzyme A dehydrogenase) and LCAD (long-chain acyl CoA dehydrogenase), usually present with HCM phenotype [183, 184]. Glycogen storage disorders, such as Pompe disease, are associated with cardiac hypertrophy [138]. The majority of middle age individuals with mucopolysaccharidosis disorders, such as Fabry metabolic disease, develop cardiovascular disorders with HCM- or DCM-like phenotype.

Critical Congenital Heart Defect Syndromes (CCHD) and Cardiomyopathies

CCHD are the most common type of birth defect, accounting for more than 30% of all infant deaths. CCHD represent some of the most severe types of heart defects. CCHD that present as part of malformation syndromes are due to chromosomal aberrations, mutant gene disorders and environmental teratogens. Some of these genetic conditions that may present with cardiomyopathy are the followings:

a. Beckwith-Wiedemann syndrome, a clinical condition that is due to imprinting defects in genes (KCNQOT1, H19, CDKN1C, IGF2) located at 11p15. The specific syndrome often presents with cardiomyopathy [185].

b. Costello syndrome, a disorder caused by mutations in the HRAS gene, inherited in an autosomal dominant pattern. Patients often present with HCM [186].
c. Marfan syndrome, an autosomal dominant disorder caused by mutations in FBN1 gene [187].
d. Noonan syndrome inherited in an autosomal dominant pattern [139]. Gain-of-function mutations in PTPN11 gene that encode for a protein interacting with the PTK-MAPK pathway are the causing genetic defects responsible for the specific phenotype.

EPIGENETICS OF HEART FAILURE (HF)

Inherited clinical conditions of HF such as familial cardiomyopathies constitute excellent disease models for the elucidation of the underlying genetic background of HF development. The potential critical role of epigenomics in the clinical phenotype is supported by the high degree of phenotypic heterogeneity, due to the same or different mutations of the disease-causing gene. In this framework, recently, investigations of the mechanisms governing gene expression, protein synthesis as well as the participation of additional genetic modifiers in the final phenotypic profile of the HF syndrome have been undertaken both in humans suffering from cardiovascular diseases with enhanced incidence of HF as well as in transgenic mouse models.

Altered gene expression is a characteristic hallmark of HF. DNA methylation has already been proven in other devastating complex disorders such as cancer. The role of epigenomics in HF development has been under extensive study. However, this era of research needs further investigation. Initial reported results show that epigenomics could be a key determinant of the malfunctional re-programming of gene expression that occurs in cardiac hypertrophy [188]. Cardiac hypertrophy is known to be a condition characterized by dysfunctional cardiomyocyte remodeling in response to a variety of physiological and pathological stimuli (*e.g.* hypertension, valvular dysfunction). On a short time-scale, this constitutes an adjustment mechanism for the normal heart function. However, during prolonged periods of pathologically-induced hypertrophy, maladaptive cardiac remodeling takes place, resulting in cardiomyocyte death, ventricular dilation and HF [188]. Blockage of the signaling pathways mediating aberrant hypertrophy has been proposed as a way of reducing or ideally abolishing cardiac hypertrophy [188]. In this direction, agents that could negatively regulate those pathways could act as promising therapeutic agents for the management of cardiac hypertrophy and ultimately HF.

Chromatin Remodelling

The brahma-associated factor (BAF) complex is one of the four ATP-dependent chromatin remodelling complexes and brahma-related gene 1 (BRG1) is a key gene encoding for the ATPase subunit. During normal embryogenesis, BRG1, a fetal heart gene, through an interaction with the PRAP-1 DNA repair polymerase enzyme, participates in the inhibition of the myosin heavy chain switch, that is the shift from the myosin chain isoform (α-MHC or MYH6) to the MHC isoform (β-MHC or MYH7). PRAP-1 nuclear enzyme participates in transcription modulation by facilitating chromatin decondensation and PRAP-1 pharmacological repression has contributed to a decrease of cardiac hypertrophy [189, 190]. However, in the adult heart, BRG1 expression is repressed. Only under stress conditions and hypertrophic cardiomyopathy it is re-expressed with BRG1 expression levels being analogous to the aggressiveness of the clinical symptoms [191, 192].

DNA Methylation

DNA methylation is the most common epigenetic modification in the mammalian genome and has been shown to be a hallmark in HF [193, 194]. GWA studies have reported that in patients with end-stage cardiomyopathy, a differential methylation pattern emerged between up-regulated and down-regulated genes, with methylation pronouncedly being decreased in the promoter vicinity of up-regulated genes, whereas no considerable alteration took place in down-regulated genes [195].

Altered expression of the lymphocyte antigen 75 LY75 gene and the tyrosine kinase-type cell surface receptor ERBB3 gene has been exhibited in primary DCM patients. These two genes are known to be important modulators participating both in adaptive and maladaptive cardiac remodelling during HF [196]. In a study conducted by Watson *et al.*, hypoxia - induced DNA hypermethylation and increased DNA methyltransferase expression in cardiac fibroblasts, were reported to lead to aberrant ventricular remodelling and cardiac fibrosis [197]. Interestingly enough, expression of DNMT1 and DNMT3B methylating enzymes was shown to be regulated by hypoxia-inducible factor HIF-1 alpha, which may act as an effective therapeutic agent [197]. Studies have shown that in HF, attenuated expression of the platelet endothelial cell adhesion molecule 1 (PECAM-1) and the angiomotin- like protein 2 (AMOTL2) occurred, following hyper-methylation and hypo-methylation, respectively. By contrast, hyper-methylation within the Rho GTPase activating protein 24 gene (ARHGAP24) led to enhanced expression of ARHGAP24 in failing hearts [195]. Furthermore, DNA methylation inhibitors have been shown to reverse the hypertrophic promoting effects of norepinephrine in cardiac tissue [198]. Therefore, they may serve as therapeutic agents in cardiomyopathy.

Histone Modifications

Histone acetyltransferases (HATs) are enzymes that acetylate conserved lysine amino acids on histone proteins by transferring an acetyl group from acetyl CoA to form ε-N-acetyllysine. Histone acetylation leads to chromatin decondensation and to transcriptional gene activation and is accomplished by the HATs enzymes that acetylate the lysine amino acids located on histone tails. On the other hand, histone deacetylases (HDACs) are a class of enzymes that remove acetyl groups from an ε-N-acetyl lysine amino acid on a histone, thereby allowing for gene silencing. Dysregulation of the fine balance between HATs and HDACs activities may lead to aberrant gene expression and ultimately to HF development. In this direction, HDAC inhibitors have been suggested to restore the normal gene expression program in hypertrophic cardiomyocytes. In this framework, studies have shown that administration of class I HDAC inhibitors hindered cardiac hypertrophy, by enhancing acetylation of the sarcomeric proteins involved in myofilament calcium sensitivity in cardiac cells [199 - 202]. Identifying the molecular targets of HDAC inhibitors could provide important information for the development of new drugs for cardiac hypertrophy and HF. Surprisingly, another study revealed that estrogenic compounds derepressed the opposite effects of angiotensin II on the same parameters for HDAC4 and 5 (class II) [203]. In this context, estrogenic ERβ agonists have been proposed to act as HDAC modulators for prevention of cardiac hypertrophy [203].

Among the four known HDACs classes, class I HDACs are pro-hypertrophic whereas class IIa HDACs, found in abundance in cardiac tissues, are anti-hypertrophic [204 - 207]. Class IIa HDACs (HDAC4, -5, -7 and -9) have been shown to suppress MEF2 activity, leading to reduced cardiac hypertrophy [208]. Further studies have shown that activation of the transcriptional regulator CREB binding protein p300 can lead to cardiomyocyte hypertrophic growth and its mode of action is largely modulated by histone HAT activity. Inhibition of p300 repressed phenylephrine (PE)-induced hypertrophic cell growth [209]. p300 transgenic mouse models have developed HF, thereby underlying the role of p300 in maladaptive cardiac remodelling [210]. In addition to that, both HATs and HDACs have been shown to interact with sarcomeric proteins. In this context, binding of calcium/calmodulin-dependent kinase II (CaMKII) to HDAC4 has been shown to lead to cardiomyocyte hypertrophy, thereby indicating a central role for CaMKII- HDAC4 interactions in the development of cardiac hypertrophy [208]. Cao *et al.* reported that the TSA HDAC inhibitor reduces cardiac hypertrophy by suppressing autophagy [211]. Histone methylation is mediated by both histone methyltransferases and histone demethylases and as opposed to acetylation, histone methylation can act either by activating or by abrogating gene expression, depending on the target site and the degree of methylation. Genome-wide histone methylation studies in transgenic mice with cardiac hypertrophy have shown differential methylation of histone H3 on lysine 4 (H3K4) between normal and hypertrophic cardiomyocytes [212, 213].

RNA-Based Mechanisms

MicroRNAs

MicroRNAs are single-stranded, 22 nt-long non coding RNAs that act as regulators of gene expression. Initially, microRNAs are transcribed as primary miRNA (primiRNA). Following transport into the cytosol, the mRNA-inducing silencing complex RISC is formed and assumes action by forming partial hybrids with target mRNAs and acting as mRNA destabilizer and/or negative regulator of translation [214, 215]. Four miRNAs are highly expressed in the heart: miR-1, miR-133, miR-208, and miR-499 [216]. Gene expression-miRNAs patterns have shown differential expression in a set of miRNAs of cardiomyocytes from patients suffering from different forms of cardiovascular diseases (ischemic cardiomyopathy, idiopathic cardiomyopathy, aortic stenosis) [217, 218]. Alterations in the proportions of the two MHC isoforms, α- and β-MHC, known to participate in cardiomyocyte contractility, can lead to hypertrophy. During cardiac hypertrophy and HF development, β-MHC has been shown to be in excess [35]. Studies in transgenic mice with arrhythmia, fibrosis, and hypertrophic growth, have shown that increased levels of β- MHC are accompanied by miR-208a overexpression in cardiomyocytes and similar results have been obtained in humans with DCM [219]. Normally, miR-1 is highly expressed in the heart and downregulates calcium-calmodulin signaling [220]. In situations of pathological hypertrophy, miR-1 has been shown to be downregulated with direct modulatory effects upon the antiporter membrane protein sodium-calcium exchanger [221]. By contrast, miR-195 is upregulated during hypertrophy and HF [222]. miR-195 is speculated to be a modulator of several genes involved in the MAPK signaling pathway, thereby assuming a role in procedures of cell proliferation and apoptosis. A similar hypertrophic-promoting property has been reported for miR-499 that has been shown to enhance cardiomyogenesis *in vitro* and after infarction *in vivo* and to participate in maladaptive cardiac remodeling both in humans and mice [223, 224]. miR-23 and miR- 24 were recently shown to be upregulated in hypertrophic and ischemic cardiomyopathy, with a potential role in the regulation of MAPK and WNT signaling pathways [220]. Recently, published data reported that up-regulation of miR-25 in HF suppressed calcium kinetics in cardiomyocytes by interacting with mRNA that encodes SR calcium uptake pump SERCA2a [225]. Successful blockage of miR-25 action significantly halted established HF in a mouse model through the enhancement of SERCA2a activity that promotes intracellular calcium influx in heart muscle [225]. Further studies will be required in order to test the potential role of anti-miR-25 inhibitors as therapeutic agents in cardiac hypertrophy and HF. During normal cardiac function, miR-133 is highly expressed in adult cardiomyocytes and skeletal muscle. However, in situations of myocardial infarction and in pressure-overload cardiac hypertrophy models, miR-133 was found to be significantly down-regulated [226, 227]. Importantly, it was shown that miR-133 controls multiple components of the β_1-adrenergic receptor transduction pathway, serves as a potential cardioprotector in HF and could be a therapeutic target in the treatment of this syndrome [228]. Expression of miR-199b has been reported to be enhanced in mouse models with cardiac hypertrophy, as well as in humans with HF. Administration of antagomiR-199b has been reported to contribute to attenuation of cardiac hypertrophy and fibrosis [229]. Importantly, recent studies have shown that some miRNAs can be detected in the peripheral blood circulation and this could potentially render them effective diagnostic and prognostic biomarkers [230].

LncRNAs

LncRNAs are RNA molecules of >200 nucleotides in length, known to regulate the transcriptional and posttranscriptional gene expression [231]. LncRNAs have been found to protect the heart from hypertrophy through the BRG1-HDA--PARP pathway and MHRT-BRG1 feedback. LIPCAR lncRNA was discovered to be a novel biomarker of cardiac remodelling and a predictor of survival in HF patients [232]. Another LncRNA molecule, ANRIL, has been shown to achieve the shutdown of the genes INK4b, ARF, and INK4a that are involved in the CAD development [233].

CONCLUDING REMARKS

In recent years, novel genetic approaches based on GWA and NGS technologies have allowed for large-scale, high-throuput whole genome studies to be carried out, significantly broadening our knowledge regarding the genetic and phenotypic heterogeneity of acquired and inherited forms of HF. In this direction, the complex interplay between the underlying genetic background, epigenetic modifier factors and environmental triggers has become main field of current research. However, clear-cut genotype-phenotype associations have yet to be determined. The significant morbidity and mortality rates of HF syndrome in the Western world, urgently call for improvements in the era of genetic testing, screening, prognosis, therapy response and disease prevention. Although the role of the genetic component in HF is generally accepted, a significant amount of information in regard to heritability is missing. In this context, a lot of work remains to be done for the investigation of the inter-individual genetic predisposition in response to pathophysiological stressors and novel therapeutic agents. To this end and with the ultimate goal of translating research findings into the clinical practice with substantial public health benefits, improvements in the efficiency of the novel genomic technologies, applied onto larger cohorts of individuals with well-defined phenotypes and from diverse ethnic backgrounds, are urgently required. Parallel studies in the "epigenome" field will allow for a deeper understanding of the underlying mechanisms participating in phenotypic heterogeneity of HF syndrome, potentially allowing for the trial of novel therapeutic agents capable of restoring the 'normal' epigenetic landscape in HF syndrome.

CONFLICT OF INTEREST

The authors confirm that they have no conflict of interest to declare for this publication.

ACKNOWLEDGEMENTS

Declared none.

REFERENCES

[1] Hunt SA, Abraham WT, Chin MH, *et al.* 2009 focused update incorporated into the ACC/AHA 2005 guidelines for the diagnosis and management of heart failure in adults: a report of the American College of cardiology foundation/American Heart Association task force on practice guidelines: developed in collaboration with the international society for heart and lung transplantation. Circulation 2009; 119(14): e391-479.

[2] McMurray JJ, Adamopoulos S, Anker SD, *et al.* ESC guidelines for the diagnosis and treatment of acute and chronic heart failure 2012: The task force for the diagnosis and treatment of acute and chronic heart failure 2012 of the European society of cardiology. Developed in collaboration with the heart failure association (HFA) of the ESC. Eur J Heart Fail 2012; 14(8): 803-69. [http://dx.doi.org/10.1093/eurjhf/hfs105] [PMID: 22828712]

[3] Cowie MR, Fox KF, Wood DA, *et al.* Hospitalization of patients with heart failure: a population-based study. Eur Heart J 2002; 23(11): 877-85. [http://dx.doi.org/10.1053/euhj.2001.2973] [PMID: 12042009]

[4] Dickstein K, Cohen-Solal A, Filippatos G, *et al.* ESC Guidelines for the diagnosis and treatment of

acute and chronic heart failure 2008: the Task Force for the Diagnosis and Treatment of Acute and Chronic Heart Failure 2008 of the European Society of Cardiology. Developed in collaboration with the Heart Failure Association of the ESC (HFA) and endorsed by the European Society of Intensive Care Medicine (ESICM). Eur Heart J 2008; 29(19): 2388-442.
[http://dx.doi.org/10.1093/eurheartj/ehn309] [PMID: 18799522]

[5] Yancy CW, Jessup M, Bozkurt B, *et al.* 2013 ACCF/AHA guideline for the management of heart failure: a report of the American College of Cardiology Foundation/American Heart Association Task Force on Practice Guidelines. J Am Coll Cardiol 2013; 62(16): e147-239.
[http://dx.doi.org/10.1016/j.jacc.2013.05.019] [PMID: 23747642]

[6] Lee DS, Pencina MJ, Benjamin EJ, *et al.* Association of parental heart failure with risk of heart failure in offspring. N Engl J Med 2006; 355(2): 138-47.
[http://dx.doi.org/10.1056/NEJMoa052948] [PMID: 16837677]

[7] Smith NL, Felix JF, Morrison AC, *et al.* Association of genome-wide variation with the risk of incident heart failure in adults of European and African ancestry: a prospective meta-analysis from the cohorts for heart and aging research in genomic epidemiology (CHARGE) consortium. Circ Cardiovasc Genet 2010; 3(3): 256-66.
[http://dx.doi.org/10.1161/CIRCGENETICS.109.895763] [PMID: 20445134]

[8] Morrison AC, Felix JF, Cupples LA, *et al.* Genomic variation associated with mortality among adults of European and African ancestry with heart failure: the cohorts for heart and aging research in genomic epidemiology consortium. Circ Cardiovasc Genet 2010; 3(3): 248-55.
[http://dx.doi.org/10.1161/CIRCGENETICS.109.895995] [PMID: 20400778]

[9] Brodde OE. Beta-adrenoceptors in cardiac disease. Pharmacol Ther 1993; 60(3): 405-30.
[http://dx.doi.org/10.1016/0163-7258(93)90030-H] [PMID: 7915424]

[10] Brodde OE, Michel MC. Adrenergic and muscarinic receptors in the human heart. Pharmacol Rev 1999; 51(4): 651-90.
[PMID: 10581327]

[11] Chruscinski A, Brede ME, Meinel L, Lohse MJ, Kobilka BK, Hein L. Differential distribution of beta-adrenergic receptor subtypes in blood vessels of knockout mice lacking beta(1)- or beta(2)-adrenergic receptors. Mol Pharmacol 2001; 60(5): 955-62.
[PMID: 11641423]

[12] Lands AM, Arnold A, McAuliff JP, Luduena FP, Brown TG Jr. Differentiation of receptor systems activated by sympathomimetic amines. Nature 1967; 214(5088): 597-8.
[http://dx.doi.org/10.1038/214597a0] [PMID: 6036174]

[13] Zhao XL, Gutierrez LM, Chang CF, Hosey MM. The alpha 1-subunit of skeletal muscle L-type Ca channels is the key target for regulation by A-kinase and protein phosphatase-1C. Biochem Biophys Res Commun 1994; 198(1): 166-73.
[http://dx.doi.org/10.1006/bbrc.1994.1024] [PMID: 8292020]

[14] Gerhardstein BL, Puri TS, Chien AJ, Hosey MM. Identification of the sites phosphorylated by cyclic AMP-dependent protein kinase on the beta 2 subunit of L-type voltage-dependent calcium channels. Biochemistry 1999; 38(32): 10361-70.
[http://dx.doi.org/10.1021/bi990896o] [PMID: 10441130]

[15] Simmerman HK, Jones LR. Phospholamban: protein structure, mechanism of action, and role in cardiac function. Physiol Rev 1998; 78(4): 921-47.
[PMID: 9790566]

[16] Marx SO, Reiken S, Hisamatsu Y, *et al.* PKA phosphorylation dissociates FKBP12.6 from the calcium release channel (ryanodine receptor): defective regulation in failing hearts. Cell 2000; 101(4): 365-76.
[http://dx.doi.org/10.1016/S0092-8674(00)80847-8] [PMID: 10830164]

[17] Kunst G, Kress KR, Gruen M, Uttenweiler D, Gautel M, Fink RH. Myosin binding protein C, a phosphorylation-dependent force regulator in muscle that controls the attachment of myosin heads by its interaction with myosin S2. Circ Res 2000; 86(1): 51-8.
[http://dx.doi.org/10.1161/01.RES.86.1.51] [PMID: 10625305]

[18] Beuckelmann DJ, Näbauer M, Erdmann E. Intracellular calcium handling in isolated ventricular myocytes from patients with terminal heart failure. Circulation 1992; 85(3): 1046-55.
[http://dx.doi.org/10.1161/01.CIR.85.3.1046] [PMID: 1311223]

[19] Waagstein F, Hjalmarson A, Varnauskas E, Wallentin I. Effect of chronic beta-adrenergic receptor blockade in congestive cardiomyopathy. Br Heart J 1975; 37(10): 1022-36.
[http://dx.doi.org/10.1136/hrt.37.10.1022] [PMID: 1191416]

[20] Bristow MR. beta-adrenergic receptor blockade in chronic heart failure. Circulation 2000; 101(5): 558-69.
[http://dx.doi.org/10.1161/01.CIR.101.5.558] [PMID: 10662755]

[21] The Cardiac Insufficiency Bisoprolol Study II (CIBIS-II): a randomised trial. Lancet 1999; 353(9146): 9-13.
[http://dx.doi.org/10.1016/S0140-6736(98)11181-9] [PMID: 10023943]

[22] Effect of metoprolol CR/XL in chronic heart failure: metoprolol CR/XL Randomised Intervention Trial in Congestive Heart Failure (MERIT-HF). Lancet 1999; 353(9169): 2001-7.
[http://dx.doi.org/10.1016/S0140-6736(99)04440-2] [PMID: 10376614]

[23] Xamoterol in severe heart failure. Lancet 1990; 336(8706): 1-6.
[http://dx.doi.org/10.1016/0140-6736(90)91517-E] [PMID: 1694945]

[24] Lohse MJ. G-protein-coupled receptor kinases and the heart. Trends Cardiovasc Med 1995; 5(2): 63-8.
[http://dx.doi.org/10.1016/1050-1738(94)00034-4] [PMID: 21232239]

[25] Rockman HA, Koch WJ, Lefkowitz RJ. Seven-transmembrane-spanning receptors and heart function. Nature 2002; 415(6868): 206-12.
[http://dx.doi.org/10.1038/415206a] [PMID: 11805844]

[26] Ping P, Anzai T, Gao M, Hammond HK. Adenylyl cyclase and G protein receptor kinase expression during development of heart failure. Am J Physiol 1997; 273(2 Pt 2): H707-17.
[PMID: 9277487]

[27] Ungerer M, Parruti G, Böhm M, *et al.* Expression of beta-arrestins and beta-adrenergic receptor kinases in the failing human heart. Circ Res 1994; 74(2): 206-13.
[http://dx.doi.org/10.1161/01.RES.74.2.206] [PMID: 8293560]

[28] Kiuchi K, Shannon RP, Komamura K, *et al.* Myocardial beta-adrenergic receptor function during the development of pacing-induced heart failure. J Clin Invest 1993; 91(3): 907-14.

[http://dx.doi.org/10.1172/JCI116312] [PMID: 8383704]

[29] Engelhardt S, Böhm M, Erdmann E, Lohse MJ. Analysis of beta-adrenergic receptor mRNA levels in human ventricular biopsy specimens by quantitative polymerase chain reactions: progressive reduction of beta 1-adrenergic receptor mRNA in heart failure. J Am Coll Cardiol 1996; 27(1): 146-54. [http://dx.doi.org/10.1016/0735-1097(95)00425-4] [PMID: 8522688]

[30] Leineweber K, Brandt K, Wludyka B, *et al.* Ventricular hypertrophy plus neurohumoral activation is necessary to alter the cardiac beta-adrenoceptor system in experimental heart failure. Circ Res 2002; 91(11): 1056-62. [http://dx.doi.org/10.1161/01.RES.0000045088.59360.B7] [PMID: 12456492]

[31] Choi DJ, Koch WJ, Hunter JJ, Rockman HA. Mechanism of beta-adrenergic receptor desensitization in cardiac hypertrophy is increased beta-adrenergic receptor kinase. J Biol Chem 1997; 272(27): 17223-9. [http://dx.doi.org/10.1074/jbc.272.27.17223] [PMID: 9202046]

[32] Engelhardt S, Hein L, Wiesmann F, Lohse MJ. Progressive hypertrophy and heart failure in beta1-adrenergic receptor transgenic mice. Proc Natl Acad Sci USA 1999; 96(12): 7059-64. [http://dx.doi.org/10.1073/pnas.96.12.7059] [PMID: 10359838]

[33] Bisognano JD, Weinberger HD, Bohlmeyer TJ, *et al.* Myocardial-directed overexpression of the human beta(1)-adrenergic receptor in transgenic mice. J Mol Cell Cardiol 2000; 32(5): 817-30. [http://dx.doi.org/10.1006/jmcc.2000.1123] [PMID: 10775486]

[34] Ungerer M, Böhm M, Elce JS, Erdmann E, Lohse MJ. Altered expression of beta-adrenergic receptor kinase and beta 1-adrenergic receptors in the failing human heart. Circulation 1993; 87(2): 454-63. [http://dx.doi.org/10.1161/01.CIR.87.2.454] [PMID: 8381058]

[35] Bers DM. Cardiac excitation-contraction coupling. Nature 2002; 415(6868): 198-205. [http://dx.doi.org/10.1038/415198a] [PMID: 11805843]

[36] Laitinen PJ, Brown KM, Piippo K, *et al.* Mutations of the cardiac ryanodine receptor (RyR2) gene in familial polymorphic ventricular tachycardia. Circulation 2001; 103(4): 485-90. [http://dx.doi.org/10.1161/01.CIR.103.4.485] [PMID: 11157710]

[37] Priori SG, Napolitano C, Tiso N, *et al.* Mutations in the cardiac ryanodine receptor gene (hRyR2) underlie catecholaminergic polymorphic ventricular tachycardia. Circulation 2001; 103(2): 196-200. [http://dx.doi.org/10.1161/01.CIR.103.2.196] [PMID: 11208676]

[38] Tiso N, Stephan DA, Nava A, *et al.* Identification of mutations in the cardiac ryanodine receptor gene in families affected with arrhythmogenic right ventricular cardiomyopathy type 2 (ARVD2). Hum Mol Genet 2001; 10(3): 189-94. [http://dx.doi.org/10.1093/hmg/10.3.189] [PMID: 11159936]

[39] Luo W, Grupp IL, Harrer J, *et al.* Targeted ablation of the phospholamban gene is associated with markedly enhanced myocardial contractility and loss of beta-agonist stimulation. Circ Res 1994; 75(3): 401-9. [http://dx.doi.org/10.1161/01.RES.75.3.401] [PMID: 8062415]

[40] Schmitt JP, Kamisago M, Asahi M, *et al.* Dilated cardiomyopathy and heart failure caused by a mutation in phospholamban. Science 2003; 299(5611): 1410-3.

[http://dx.doi.org/10.1126/science.1081578] [PMID: 12610310]

[41] Haghighi K, Kolokathis F, Pater L, *et al.* Human phospholamban null results in lethal dilated cardiomyopathy revealing a critical difference between mouse and human. J Clin Invest 2003; 111(6): 869-76.
[http://dx.doi.org/10.1172/JCI17892] [PMID: 12639993]

[42] Anan R, Greve G, Thierfelder L, *et al.* Prognostic implications of novel beta cardiac myosin heavy chain gene mutations that cause familial hypertrophic cardiomyopathy. J Clin Invest 1994; 93(1): 280-5.
[http://dx.doi.org/10.1172/JCI116957] [PMID: 8282798]

[43] Periasamy M, Reed TD, Liu LH, *et al.* Impaired cardiac performance in heterozygous mice with a null mutation in the sarco(endo)plasmic reticulum Ca2+-ATPase isoform 2 (SERCA2) gene. J Biol Chem 1999; 274(4): 2556-62.
[http://dx.doi.org/10.1074/jbc.274.4.2556] [PMID: 9891028]

[44] Minamisawa S, Hoshijima M, Chu G, *et al.* Chronic phospholamban-sarcoplasmic reticulum calcium ATPase interaction is the critical calcium cycling defect in dilated cardiomyopathy. Cell 1999; 99(3): 313-22.
[http://dx.doi.org/10.1016/S0092-8674(00)81662-1] [PMID: 10555147]

[45] DeSantiago J, Maier LS, Bers DM. Phospholamban is required for CaMKII-dependent recovery of Ca transients and SR Ca reuptake during acidosis in cardiac myocytes. J Mol Cell Cardiol 2004; 36(1): 67-74.
[http://dx.doi.org/10.1016/j.yjmcc.2003.10.012] [PMID: 14734049]

[46] Dorn GW II. Adrenergic signaling polymorphisms and their impact on cardiovascular disease. Physiol Rev 2010; 90(3): 1013-62.
[http://dx.doi.org/10.1152/physrev.00001.2010] [PMID: 20664078]

[47] Morimoto T, Sunagawa Y, Kawamura T, *et al.* The dietary compound curcumin inhibits p300 histone acetyltransferase activity and prevents heart failure in rats. J Clin Invest 2008; 118(3): 868-78.
[PMID: 18292809]

[48] Sunagawa Y, Morimoto T, Wada H, *et al.* A natural p300-specific histone acetyltransferase inhibitor, curcumin, in addition to angiotensin-converting enzyme inhibitor, exerts beneficial effects on left ventricular systolic function after myocardial infarction in rats. Circ J 2011; 75(9): 2151-9.
[http://dx.doi.org/10.1253/circj.CJ-10-1072] [PMID: 21737953]

[49] Kook H, Lepore JJ, Gitler AD, *et al.* Cardiac hypertrophy and histone deacetylase-dependent transcriptional repression mediated by the atypical homeodomain protein Hop. J Clin Invest 2003; 112(6): 863-71.
[http://dx.doi.org/10.1172/JCI19137] [PMID: 12975471]

[50] Kee HJ, Sohn IS, Nam KI, *et al.* Inhibition of histone deacetylation blocks cardiac hypertrophy induced by angiotensin II infusion and aortic banding. Circulation 2006; 113(1): 51-9.
[http://dx.doi.org/10.1161/CIRCULATIONAHA.105.559724] [PMID: 16380549]

[51] Mason DA, Moore JD, Green SA, Liggett SB. A gain-of-function polymorphism in a G-protein coupling domain of the human beta1-adrenergic receptor. J Biol Chem 1999; 274(18): 12670-4.
[http://dx.doi.org/10.1074/jbc.274.18.12670] [PMID: 10212248]

[52] 1000 Genomes Project Consortium. A map of human genome variation from population-scale sequencing. Nature 2010; 467(7319): 1061-73.

[53] Joseph SS, Lynham JA, Grace AA, Colledge WH, Kaumann AJ. Markedly reduced effects of (-)-isoprenaline but not of (-)-CGP12177 and unchanged affinity of beta-blockers at Gly389-beta--adrenoceptors compared to Arg389-beta1-adrenoceptors. Br J Pharmacol 2004; 142(1): 51-6. [http://dx.doi.org/10.1038/sj.bjp.0705753] [PMID: 15037517]

[54] Rathz DA, Gregory KN, Fang Y, Brown KM, Liggett SB. Hierarchy of polymorphic variation and desensitization permutations relative to beta 1- and beta 2-adrenergic receptor signaling. J Biol Chem 2003; 278(12): 10784-9.
[http://dx.doi.org/10.1074/jbc.M206054200] [PMID: 12525504]

[55] Mialet Perez J, Rathz DA, Petrashevskaya NN, *et al.* Beta 1-adrenergic receptor polymorphisms confer differential function and predisposition to heart failure. Nat Med 2003; 9(10): 1300-5.
[http://dx.doi.org/10.1038/nm930] [PMID: 14502278]

[56] Liggett SB, Tepe NM, Lorenz JN, *et al.* Early and delayed consequences of beta(2)-adrenergic receptor overexpression in mouse hearts: critical role for expression level. Circulation 2000; 101(14): 1707-14.
[http://dx.doi.org/10.1161/01.CIR.101.14.1707] [PMID: 10758054]

[57] Bruck H, Leineweber K, Temme T, *et al.* The Arg389Gly beta1-adrenoceptor polymorphism and catecholamine effects on plasma-renin activity. J Am Coll Cardiol 2005; 46(11): 2111-5.
[http://dx.doi.org/10.1016/j.jacc.2005.08.041] [PMID: 16325050]

[58] Rochais F, Vilardaga JP, Nikolaev VO, Bünemann M, Lohse MJ, Engelhardt S. Real-time optical recording of beta1-adrenergic receptor activation reveals supersensitivity of the Arg389 variant to carvedilol. J Clin Invest 2007; 117(1): 229-35.
[http://dx.doi.org/10.1172/JCI30012] [PMID: 17200720]

[59] Terra SG, Hamilton KK, Pauly DF, *et al.* Beta1-adrenergic receptor polymorphisms and left ventricular remodeling changes in response to beta-blocker therapy. Pharmacogenet Genomics 2005; 15(4): 227-34.
[http://dx.doi.org/10.1097/01213011-200504000-00006] [PMID: 15864115]

[60] Chen L, Meyers D, Javorsky G, *et al.* Arg389Gly-beta1-adrenergic receptors determine improvement in left ventricular systolic function in nonischemic cardiomyopathy patients with heart failure after chronic treatment with carvedilol. Pharmacogenet Genomics 2007; 17(11): 941-9.
[http://dx.doi.org/10.1097/FPC.0b013e3282ef7354] [PMID: 18075464]

[61] von Homeyer P, Schwinn DA. Pharmacogenomics of β-adrenergic receptor physiology and response to β-blockade. Anesth Analg 2011; 113(6): 1305-18.
[http://dx.doi.org/10.1213/ANE.0b013e31822b887e] [PMID: 21965354]

[62] Petersen M, Andersen JT, Hjelvang BR, *et al.* Association of beta-adrenergic receptor polymorphisms and mortality in carvedilol-treated chronic heart-failure patients. Br J Clin Pharmacol 2011; 71(4): 556-65.
[http://dx.doi.org/10.1111/j.1365-2125.2010.03868.x] [PMID: 21395649]

[63] Green SA, Turki J, Innis M, Liggett SB. Amino-terminal polymorphisms of the human beta 2-

adrenergic receptor impart distinct agonist-promoted regulatory properties. Biochemistry 1994; 33(32): 9414-9.
[http://dx.doi.org/10.1021/bi00198a006] [PMID: 7915137]

[64] Small KM, McGraw DW, Liggett SB. Pharmacology and physiology of human adrenergic receptor polymorphisms. Annu Rev Pharmacol Toxicol 2003; 43: 381-411.
[http://dx.doi.org/10.1146/annurev.pharmtox.43.100901.135823] [PMID: 12540746]

[65] Lobmeyer MT, Gong Y, Terra SG, *et al.* Synergistic polymorphisms of beta1 and alpha2C-adrenergic receptors and the influence on left ventricular ejection fraction response to beta-blocker therapy in heart failure. Pharmacogenet Genomics 2007; 17(4): 277-82.
[http://dx.doi.org/10.1097/FPC.0b013e3280105245] [PMID: 17496726]

[66] Bristow MR, Murphy GA, Krause-Steinrauf H, *et al.* An alpha2C-adrenergic receptor polymorphism alters the norepinephrine-lowering effects and therapeutic response of the beta-blocker bucindolol in chronic heart failure. Circ Heart Fail 2010; 3(1): 21-8.
[http://dx.doi.org/10.1161/CIRCHEARTFAILURE.109.885962] [PMID: 19880803]

[67] Liggett SB, Cresci S, Kelly RJ, *et al.* A GRK5 polymorphism that inhibits beta-adrenergic receptor signaling is protective in heart failure. Nat Med 2008; 14(5): 510-7.
[http://dx.doi.org/10.1038/nm1750] [PMID: 18425130]

[68] Wang WC, Mihlbachler KA, Bleecker ER, Weiss ST, Liggett SB. A polymorphism of G-protein coupled receptor kinase5 alters agonist-promoted desensitization of beta2-adrenergic receptors. Pharmacogenet Genomics 2008; 18(8): 729-32.
[http://dx.doi.org/10.1097/FPC.0b013e32830967e9] [PMID: 18622265]

[69] Dorn GW II. Genetics of common forms of heart failure. Curr Opin Cardiol 2011; 26(3): 204-8.
[http://dx.doi.org/10.1097/HCO.0b013e328345d336] [PMID: 21464711]

[70] Cresci S, Kelly RJ, Cappola TP, *et al.* Clinical and genetic modifiers of long-term survival in heart failure. J Am Coll Cardiol 2009; 54(5): 432-44.
[http://dx.doi.org/10.1016/j.jacc.2009.05.009] [PMID: 19628119]

[71] Rigat B, Hubert C, Alhenc-Gelas F, Cambien F, Corvol P, Soubrier F. An insertion/deletion polymorphism in the angiotensin I-converting enzyme gene accounting for half the variance of serum enzyme levels. J Clin Invest 1990; 86(4): 1343-6.
[http://dx.doi.org/10.1172/JCI114844] [PMID: 1976655]

[72] Danser AH, Schalekamp MA, Bax WA, *et al.* Angiotensin-converting enzyme in the human heart. Effect of the deletion/insertion polymorphism. Circulation 1995; 92(6): 1387-8.
[http://dx.doi.org/10.1161/01.CIR.92.6.1387] [PMID: 7664416]

[73] Andersson B, Sylvén C. The DD genotype of the angiotensin-converting enzyme gene is associated with increased mortality in idiopathic heart failure. J Am Coll Cardiol 1996; 28(1): 162-7.
[http://dx.doi.org/10.1016/0735-1097(96)00098-8] [PMID: 8752809]

[74] Palmer BR, Pilbrow AP, Yandle TG, *et al.* Angiotensin-converting enzyme gene polymorphism interacts with left ventricular ejection fraction and brain natriuretic peptide levels to predict mortality after myocardial infarction. J Am Coll Cardiol 2003; 41(5): 729-36.
[http://dx.doi.org/10.1016/S0735-1097(02)02927-3] [PMID: 12628714]

[75] Huang W, Xie C, Zhou H, Yang T, Sun M. Association of the angiotensin-converting enzyme gene polymorphism with chronic heart failure in Chinese Han patients. Eur J Heart Fail 2004; 6(1): 23-7. [http://dx.doi.org/10.1016/j.ejheart.2003.09.004] [PMID: 15012915]

[76] McNamara DM, Holubkov R, Janosko K, *et al.* Pharmacogenetic interactions between beta-blocker therapy and the angiotensin-converting enzyme deletion polymorphism in patients with congestive heart failure. Circulation 2001; 103(12): 1644-8. [http://dx.doi.org/10.1161/01.CIR.103.12.1644] [PMID: 11273991]

[77] McNamara DM, Holubkov R, Postava L, *et al.* Pharmacogenetic interactions between angiotensin-converting enzyme inhibitor therapy and the angiotensin-converting enzyme deletion polymorphism in patients with congestive heart failure. J Am Coll Cardiol 2004; 44(10): 2019-26. [http://dx.doi.org/10.1016/j.jacc.2004.08.048] [PMID: 15542286]

[78] Marian AJ, Yu QT, Workman R, Greve G, Roberts R. Angiotensin-converting enzyme polymorphism in hypertrophic cardiomyopathy and sudden cardiac death. Lancet 1993; 342(8879): 1085-6. [http://dx.doi.org/10.1016/0140-6736(93)92064-Z] [PMID: 8105312]

[79] Tesson F, Dufour C, Moolman JC, *et al.* The influence of the angiotensin I converting enzyme genotype in familial hypertrophic cardiomyopathy varies with the disease gene mutation. J Mol Cell Cardiol 1997; 29(2): 831-8. [http://dx.doi.org/10.1006/jmcc.1996.0332] [PMID: 9140839]

[80] Lechin M, Quiñones MA, Omran A, *et al.* Angiotensin-I converting enzyme genotypes and left ventricular hypertrophy in patients with hypertrophic cardiomyopathy. Circulation 1995; 92(7): 1808-12. [http://dx.doi.org/10.1161/01.CIR.92.7.1808] [PMID: 7671365]

[81] Iwai N, Ohmichi N, Nakamura Y, Kinoshita M. DD genotype of the angiotensin-converting enzyme gene is a risk factor for left ventricular hypertrophy. Circulation 1994; 90(6): 2622-8. [http://dx.doi.org/10.1161/01.CIR.90.6.2622] [PMID: 7994801]

[82] Schunkert H, Hense HW, Holmer SR, *et al.* Association between a deletion polymorphism of the angiotensin-converting-enzyme gene and left ventricular hypertrophy. N Engl J Med 1994; 330(23): 1634-8. [http://dx.doi.org/10.1056/NEJM199406093302302] [PMID: 8177269]

[83] Myerson SG, Montgomery HE, Whittingham M, *et al.* Left ventricular hypertrophy with exercise and ACE gene insertion/deletion polymorphism: a randomized controlled trial with losartan. Circulation 2001; 103(2): 226-30. [http://dx.doi.org/10.1161/01.CIR.103.2.226] [PMID: 11208681]

[84] Clarkson PB, Prasad N, MacLeod C, Burchell B, MacDonald TM. Influence of the angiotensin converting enzyme I/D gene polymorphisms on left ventricular diastolic filling in patients with essential hypertension. J Hypertens 1997; 15(9): 995-1000. [http://dx.doi.org/10.1097/00004872-199715090-00010] [PMID: 9321747]

[85] Osono E, Kurihara S, Hayama N, *et al.* Insertion/deletion polymorphism in intron 16 of the ACE gene and left ventricular hypertrophy in patients with end-stage renal disease. Am J Kidney Dis 1998; 32(5): 725-30. [http://dx.doi.org/10.1016/S0272-6386(98)70126-X] [PMID: 9820440]

[86] Jalil JE, Piddo AM, Cordova S, *et al.* Prevalence of the angiotensin I converting enzyme insertion/deletion polymorphism, plasma angiotensin converting enzyme activity, and left ventricular mass in a normotensive Chilean population. Am J Hypertens 1999; 12(7): 697-704. [http://dx.doi.org/10.1016/S0895-7061(99)00040-0] [PMID: 10411367]

[87] Li X, Li Y, Jia N, Guo S, Chu S, Niu W. Angiotensin-converting enzyme gene deletion allele increases the risk of left ventricular hypertrophy: evidence from a meta-analysis. Mol Biol Rep 2012; 39(12): 10063-75. [http://dx.doi.org/10.1007/s11033-012-1875-6] [PMID: 22773337]

[88] Bai Y, Wang L, Hu S, Wei Y. Association of angiotensin-converting enzyme I/D polymorphism with heart failure: a meta-analysis. Mol Cell Biochem 2012; 361(1-2): 297-304. [http://dx.doi.org/10.1007/s11010-011-1115-8] [PMID: 22015653]

[89] McNamara DM. Emerging role of pharmacogenomics in heart failure. Curr Opin Cardiol 2008; 23(3): 261-8. [http://dx.doi.org/10.1097/HCO.0b013e3282fcd662] [PMID: 18382216]

[90] Carson P, Ziesche S, Johnson G, Cohn JN. Racial differences in response to therapy for heart failure: analysis of the vasodilator-heart failure trials. J Card Fail 1999; 5(3): 178-87. [http://dx.doi.org/10.1016/S1071-9164(99)90001-5] [PMID: 10496190]

[91] Raimundo S, Fischer J, Eichelbaum M, Griese EU, Schwab M, Zanger UM. Elucidation of the genetic basis of the common 'intermediate metabolizer' phenotype for drug oxidation by CYP2D6. Pharmacogenetics 2000; 10(7): 577-81. [http://dx.doi.org/10.1097/00008571-200010000-00001] [PMID: 11037799]

[92] Zanger UM, Fischer J, Raimundo S, *et al.* Comprehensive analysis of the genetic factors determining expression and function of hepatic CYP2D6. Pharmacogenetics 2001; 11(7): 573-85. [http://dx.doi.org/10.1097/00008571-200110000-00004] [PMID: 11668217]

[93] Rau T, Wuttke H, Michels LM, *et al.* Impact of the CYP2D6 genotype on the clinical effects of metoprolol: a prospective longitudinal study. Clin Pharmacol Ther 2009; 85(3): 269-72. [http://dx.doi.org/10.1038/clpt.2008.218] [PMID: 19037197]

[94] Bijl MJ, Visser LE, van Schaik RH, *et al.* Genetic variation in the CYP2D6 gene is associated with a lower heart rate and blood pressure in beta-blocker users. Clin Pharmacol Ther 2009; 85(1): 45-50. [http://dx.doi.org/10.1038/clpt.2008.172] [PMID: 18784654]

[95] Goryachkina K, Burbello A, Boldueva S, Babak S, Bergman U, Bertilsson L. CYP2D6 is a major determinant of metoprolol disposition and effects in hospitalized Russian patients treated for acute myocardial infarction. Eur J Clin Pharmacol 2008; 64(12): 1163-73. [http://dx.doi.org/10.1007/s00228-008-0525-3] [PMID: 18648788]

[96] Cappola TP, Li M, He J, *et al.* Common variants in HSPB7 and FRMD4B associated with advanced heart failure. Circ Cardiovasc Genet 2010; 3(2): 147-54. [http://dx.doi.org/10.1161/CIRCGENETICS.109.898395] [PMID: 20124441]

[97] Stark K, Esslinger UB, Reinhard W, *et al.* Genetic association study identifies HSPB7 as a risk gene for idiopathic dilated cardiomyopathy. PLoS Genet 2010; 6(10): e1001167. [http://dx.doi.org/10.1371/journal.pgen.1001167] [PMID: 20975947]

[98] Cappola TP, Matkovich SJ, Wang W, *et al.* Loss-of-function DNA sequence variant in the CLCNKA chloride channel implicates the cardio-renal axis in interindividual heart failure risk variation. Proc Natl Acad Sci USA 2011; 108(6): 2456-61. [http://dx.doi.org/10.1073/pnas.1017494108] [PMID: 21248228]

[99] Levy D, Larson MG, Vasan RS, Kannel WB, Ho KK. The progression from hypertension to congestive heart failure. JAMA 1996; 275(20): 1557-62. [http://dx.doi.org/10.1001/jama.1996.03530440037034] [PMID: 8622246]

[100] Wilhelmsen L, Rosengren A, Eriksson H, Lappas G. Heart failure in the general population of men--morbidity, risk factors and prognosis. J Intern Med 2001; 249(3): 253-61. [http://dx.doi.org/10.1046/j.1365-2796.2001.00801.x] [PMID: 11285045]

[101] Ehret GB, Munroe PB, Rice KM, *et al.* Genetic variants in novel pathways influence blood pressure and cardiovascular disease risk. Nature 2011; 478(7367): 103-9. [http://dx.doi.org/10.1038/nature10405] [PMID: 21909115]

[102] Teslovich TM, Musunuru K, Smith AV, *et al.* Biological, clinical and population relevance of 95 loci for blood lipids. Nature 2010; 466(7307): 707-13. [http://dx.doi.org/10.1038/nature09270] [PMID: 20686565]

[103] Ehret GB, Munroe PB, Rice KM, *et al.* Genetic variants in novel pathways influence blood pressure and cardiovascular disease risk. Nature 2011; 478(7367): 103-9. [http://dx.doi.org/10.1038/nature10405] [PMID: 21909115]

[104] Marenberg ME, Risch N, Berkman LF, Floderus B, de Faire U. Genetic susceptibility to death from coronary heart disease in a study of twins. N Engl J Med 1994; 330(15): 1041-6. [http://dx.doi.org/10.1056/NEJM199404143301503] [PMID: 8127331]

[105] Schunkert H, König IR, Kathiresan S, *et al.* Large-scale association analysis identifies 13 new susceptibility loci for coronary artery disease. Nat Genet 2011; 43(4): 333-8. [http://dx.doi.org/10.1038/ng.784] [PMID: 21378990]

[106] A genome-wide association study in Europeans and South Asians identifies five new loci for coronary artery disease. Nat Genet 2011; 43(4): 339-44. [http://dx.doi.org/10.1038/ng.782] [PMID: 21378988]

[107] Samani NJ, Erdmann J, Hall AS, *et al.* Genomewide association analysis of coronary artery disease. N Engl J Med 2007; 357(5): 443-53. [http://dx.doi.org/10.1056/NEJMoa072366] [PMID: 17634449]

[108] McPherson R, Pertsemlidis A, Kavaslar N, *et al.* A common allele on chromosome 9 associated with coronary heart disease. Science 2007; 316(5830): 1488-91. [http://dx.doi.org/10.1126/science.1142447] [PMID: 17478681]

[109] Helgadottir A, Thorleifsson G, Manolescu A, *et al.* A common variant on chromosome 9p21 affects the risk of myocardial infarction. Science 2007; 316(5830): 1491-3. [http://dx.doi.org/10.1126/science.1142842] [PMID: 17478679]

[110] Wild PS, Zeller T, Schillert A, *et al.* A genome-wide association study identifies LIPA as a susceptibility gene for coronary artery disease. Circ Cardiovasc Genet 2011; 4(4): 403-12. [http://dx.doi.org/10.1161/CIRCGENETICS.110.958728] [PMID: 21606135]

[111] Kleber ME, Renner W, Grammer TB, *et al.* Association of the single nucleotide polymorphism rs599839 in the vicinity of the sortilin 1 gene with LDL and triglyceride metabolism, coronary heart disease and myocardial infarction. The Ludwigshafen Risk and Cardiovascular Health Study. Atherosclerosis 2010; 209(2): 492-7.
[http://dx.doi.org/10.1016/j.atherosclerosis.2009.09.068] [PMID: 19837406]

[112] He J, Ogden LG, Bazzano LA, Vupputuri S, Loria C, Whelton PK. Risk factors for congestive heart failure in US men and women: NHANES I epidemiologic follow-up study. Arch Intern Med 2001; 161(7): 996-1002.
[http://dx.doi.org/10.1001/archinte.161.7.996] [PMID: 11295963]

[113] Voight BF, Scott LJ, Steinthorsdottir V, *et al.* Twelve type 2 diabetes susceptibility loci identified through large-scale association analysis. Nat Genet 2010; 42(7): 579-89.
[http://dx.doi.org/10.1038/ng.609] [PMID: 20581827]

[114] Dupuis J, Langenberg C, Prokopenko I, *et al.* New genetic loci implicated in fasting glucose homeostasis and their impact on type 2 diabetes risk. Nat Genet 2010; 42(2): 105-16.
[http://dx.doi.org/10.1038/ng.520] [PMID: 20081858]

[115] Morris AP. Fine mapping of type 2 diabetes susceptibility loci. Curr Diab Rep 2014; 14(11): 549.
[http://dx.doi.org/10.1007/s11892-014-0549-2] [PMID: 25239271]

[116] Towbin JA, Lowe AM, Colan SD, *et al.* Incidence, causes, and outcomes of dilated cardiomyopathy in children. JAMA 2006; 296(15): 1867-76.
[http://dx.doi.org/10.1001/jama.296.15.1867] [PMID: 17047217]

[117] Monserrat L, Hermida M, Bouzas B, *et al.* Familial dilated cardiomyopathy in patients transplanted for idiopathic dilated cardiomyopathy. Rev Esp Cardiol 2002; 55(7): 725-32.
[http://dx.doi.org/10.1016/S0300-8932(02)76691-8] [PMID: 12113700]

[118] Baig MK, Goldman JH, Caforio AL, Coonar AS, Keeling PJ, McKenna WJ. Familial dilated cardiomyopathy: cardiac abnormalities are common in asymptomatic relatives and may represent early disease. J Am Coll Cardiol 1998; 31(1): 195-201.
[http://dx.doi.org/10.1016/S0735-1097(97)00433-6] [PMID: 9426040]

[119] Garcia-Pavia P, Cobo-Marcos M, Guzzo-Merello G, *et al.* Genetics in dilated cardiomyopathy. Biomarkers Med 2013; 7(4): 517-33.
[http://dx.doi.org/10.2217/bmm.13.77] [PMID: 23905888]

[120] Marcus FI, Edson S, Towbin JA. Genetics of arrhythmogenic right ventricular cardiomyopathy: a practical guide for physicians. J Am Coll Cardiol 2013; 61(19): 1945-8.
[http://dx.doi.org/10.1016/j.jacc.2013.01.073] [PMID: 23500315]

[121] Maron BJ, Haas TS, Goodman JS. Hypertrophic cardiomyopathy: one gene — but many phenotypes. Am J Cardiol 2014; 113(10): 1772-3.
[http://dx.doi.org/10.1016/j.amjcard.2014.02.032] [PMID: 24792744]

[122] Charron P, Arad M, Arbustini E, *et al.* Genetic counselling and testing in cardiomyopathies: a position statement of the European Society of Cardiology Working Group on Myocardial and Pericardial Diseases. Eur Heart J 2010; 31(22): 2715-26.
[http://dx.doi.org/10.1093/eurheartj/ehq271] [PMID: 20823110]

[123] Ackerman MJ, Priori SG, Willems S, *et al.* HRS/EHRA expert consensus statement on the state of genetic testing for the channelopathies and cardiomyopathies this document was developed as a partnership between the Heart Rhythm Society (HRS) and the European Heart Rhythm Association (EHRA). Heart Rhythm 2011; 8(8): 1308-39. [http://dx.doi.org/10.1016/j.hrthm.2011.05.020] [PMID: 21787999]

[124] Geisterfer-Lowrance AA, Kass S, Tanigawa G, *et al.* A molecular basis for familial hypertrophic cardiomyopathy: a beta cardiac myosin heavy chain gene missense mutation. Cell 1990; 62(5): 999-1006. [http://dx.doi.org/10.1016/0092-8674(90)90274-I] [PMID: 1975517]

[125] Watkins H, Rosenzweig A, Hwang DS, *et al.* Characteristics and prognostic implications of myosin missense mutations in familial hypertrophic cardiomyopathy. N Engl J Med 1992; 326(17): 1108-14. [http://dx.doi.org/10.1056/NEJM199204233261703] [PMID: 1552912]

[126] Niimura H, Bachinski LL, Sangwatanaroj S, *et al.* Mutations in the gene for cardiac myosin-binding protein C and late-onset familial hypertrophic cardiomyopathy. N Engl J Med 1998; 338(18): 1248-57. [http://dx.doi.org/10.1056/NEJM199804303381802] [PMID: 9562578]

[127] Charron P, Dubourg O, Desnos M, *et al.* Clinical features and prognostic implications of familial hypertrophic cardiomyopathy related to the cardiac myosin-binding protein C gene. Circulation 1998; 97(22): 2230-6. [http://dx.doi.org/10.1161/01.CIR.97.22.2230] [PMID: 9631872]

[128] Gersh BJ, Maron BJ, Bonow RO, *et al.* 2011 ACCF/AHA guideline for the diagnosis and treatment of hypertrophic cardiomyopathy: executive summary: a report of the American College of Cardiology Foundation/American Heart Association Task Force on Practice Guidelines. Circulation 2011; 124(24): 2761-96. [http://dx.doi.org/10.1161/CIR.0b013e318223e230] [PMID: 22068435]

[129] Biagini E, Olivotto I, Iascone M, *et al.* Significance of sarcomere gene mutations analysis in the end-stage phase of hypertrophic cardiomyopathy. Am J Cardiol 2014; 114(5): 769-76. [http://dx.doi.org/10.1016/j.amjcard.2014.05.065] [PMID: 25037680]

[130] Morita H, Rehm HL, Menesses A, *et al.* Shared genetic causes of cardiac hypertrophy in children and adults. N Engl J Med 2008; 358(18): 1899-908. [http://dx.doi.org/10.1056/NEJMoa075463] [PMID: 18403758]

[131] Ingles J, Sarina T, Yeates L, *et al.* Clinical predictors of genetic testing outcomes in hypertrophic cardiomyopathy. Genet Med 2013; 15(12): 972-7. [http://dx.doi.org/10.1038/gim.2013.44] [PMID: 23598715]

[132] Girolami F, Ho CY, Semsarian C, *et al.* Clinical features and outcome of hypertrophic cardiomyopathy associated with triple sarcomere protein gene mutations. J Am Coll Cardiol 2010; 55(14): 1444-53. [http://dx.doi.org/10.1016/j.jacc.2009.11.062] [PMID: 20359594]

[133] Richard P, Villard E, Charron P, *et al.* The genetic bases of cardiomyopathies. J Am Coll Cardiol 2006; 48: A79-89. [http://dx.doi.org/10.1016/j.jacc.2006.09.014]

[134] Keren A, Syrris P, McKenna WJ. Hypertrophic cardiomyopathy: the genetic determinants of clinical

disease expression. Nat Clin Pract Cardiovasc Med 2008; 5(3): 158-68. [http://dx.doi.org/10.1038/ncpcardio1110] [PMID: 18227814]

[135] Olivotto I, Girolami F, Sciagrà R, *et al.* Microvascular function is selectively impaired in patients with hypertrophic cardiomyopathy and sarcomere myofilament gene mutations. J Am Coll Cardiol 2011; 58(8): 839-48. [http://dx.doi.org/10.1016/j.jacc.2011.05.018] [PMID: 21835320]

[136] Olivotto I, Girolami F, Ackerman MJ, *et al.* Myofilament protein gene mutation screening and outcome of patients with hypertrophic cardiomyopathy. Mayo Clin Proc 2008; 83(6): 630-8. [http://dx.doi.org/10.1016/S0025-6196(11)60890-2] [PMID: 18533079]

[137] Seydelmann N, Wanner C, Störk S, Ertl G, Weidemann F. Fabry disease and the heart. Best Pract Res Clin Endocrinol Metab 2015; 29(2): 195-204. [http://dx.doi.org/10.1016/j.beem.2014.10.003] [PMID: 25987173]

[138] Fukuda T, Roberts A, Plotz PH, Raben N. Acid alpha-glucosidase deficiency (Pompe disease). Curr Neurol Neurosci Rep 2007; 7(1): 71-7. [http://dx.doi.org/10.1007/s11910-007-0024-4] [PMID: 17217857]

[139] Tartaglia M, Gelb BD, Zenker M. Noonan syndrome and clinically related disorders. Best Pract Res Clin Endocrinol Metab 2011; 25(1): 161-79. [http://dx.doi.org/10.1016/j.beem.2010.09.002] [PMID: 21396583]

[140] Crombie DE, Pera MF, Delatycki MB, Pébay A. Using human pluripotent stem cells to study Friedreich ataxia cardiomyopathy. Int J Cardiol 2016; 212: 37-43. [http://dx.doi.org/10.1016/j.ijcard.2016.03.040] [PMID: 27019046]

[141] Manolio TA, Baughman KL, Rodeheffer R, *et al.* Prevalence and etiology of idiopathic dilated cardiomyopathy (summary of a National Heart, Lung, and Blood Institute workshop. Am J Cardiol 1992; 69(17): 1458-66. [http://dx.doi.org/10.1016/0002-9149(92)90901-A] [PMID: 1590237]

[142] Hershberger RE, Norton N, Morales A, Li D, Siegfried JD, Gonzalez-Quintana J. Coding sequence rare variants identified in MYBPC3, MYH6, TPM1, TNNC1, and TNNI3 from 312 patients with familial or idiopathic dilated cardiomyopathy. Circ Cardiovasc Genet 2010; 3(2): 155-61. b [http://dx.doi.org/10.1161/CIRCGENETICS.109.912345] [PMID: 20215591]

[143] Hershberger RE, Siegfried JD. Update 2011: clinical and genetic issues in familial dilated cardiomyopathy. J Am Coll Cardiol 2011; 57(16): 1641-9. [http://dx.doi.org/10.1016/j.jacc.2011.01.015] [PMID: 21492761]

[144] Petretta M, Pirozzi F, Sasso L, Paglia A, Bonaduce D. Review and metaanalysis of the frequency of familial dilated cardiomyopathy. Am J Cardiol 2011; 108(8): 1171-6. [http://dx.doi.org/10.1016/j.amjcard.2011.06.022] [PMID: 21798502]

[145] Herman DS, Lam L, Taylor MR, *et al.* Truncations of titin causing dilated cardiomyopathy. N Engl J Med 2012; 366(7): 619-28. [http://dx.doi.org/10.1056/NEJMoa1110186] [PMID: 22335739]

[146] Gupta P, Bilinska ZT, Sylvius N, *et al.* Genetic and ultrastructural studies in dilated cardiomyopathy patients: a large deletion in the lamin A/C gene is associated with cardiomyocyte nuclear envelope

disruption. Basic Res Cardiol 2010; 105(3): 365-77.
[http://dx.doi.org/10.1007/s00395-010-0085-4] [PMID: 20127487]

[147] Norton N, Li D, Rieder MJ, *et al.* Genome-wide studies of copy number variation and exome sequencing identify rare variants in BAG3 as a cause of dilated cardiomyopathy. Am J Hum Genet 2011; 88(3): 273-82. a
[http://dx.doi.org/10.1016/j.ajhg.2011.01.016] [PMID: 21353195]

[148] van Berlo JH, de Voogt WG, van der Kooi AJ, *et al.* Meta-analysis of clinical characteristics of 299 carriers of LMNA gene mutations: do lamin A/C mutations portend a high risk of sudden death? J Mol Med 2005; 83(1): 79-83.
[http://dx.doi.org/10.1007/s00109-004-0589-1] [PMID: 15551023]

[149] Meune C, Van Berlo JH, Anselme F, Bonne G, Pinto YM, Duboc D. Primary prevention of sudden death in patients with lamin A/C gene mutations. N Engl J Med 2006; 354(2): 209-10.
[http://dx.doi.org/10.1056/NEJMc052632] [PMID: 16407522]

[150] Fatkin D, MacRae C, Sasaki T, *et al.* Missense mutations in the rod domain of the lamin A/C gene as causes of dilated cardiomyopathy and conduction-system disease. N Engl J Med 1999; 341(23): 1715-24.
[http://dx.doi.org/10.1056/NEJM199912023412302] [PMID: 10580070]

[151] van Rijsingen IA, Arbustini E, Elliott PM, *et al.* Risk factors for malignant ventricular arrhythmias in lamin a/c mutation carriers a European cohort study. J Am Coll Cardiol 2012; 59(5): 493-500.
[http://dx.doi.org/10.1016/j.jacc.2011.08.078] [PMID: 22281253]

[152] McNair WP, Ku L, Taylor MR, *et al.* SCN5A mutation associated with dilated cardiomyopathy, conduction disorder, and arrhythmia. Circulation 2004; 110(15): 2163-7.
[http://dx.doi.org/10.1161/01.CIR.0000144458.58660.BB] [PMID: 15466643]

[153] Elliott P, O'Mahony C, Syrris P, *et al.* Prevalence of desmosomal protein gene mutations in patients with dilated cardiomyopathy. Circ Cardiovasc Genet 2010; 3(4): 314-22.
[http://dx.doi.org/10.1161/CIRCGENETICS.110.937805] [PMID: 20716751]

[154] Villard E, Perret C, Gary F, *et al.* A genome-wide association study identifies two loci associated with heart failure due to dilated cardiomyopathy. Eur Heart J 2011; 32(9): 1065-76.
[http://dx.doi.org/10.1093/eurheartj/ehr105] [PMID: 21459883]

[155] Schönberger J, Wang L, Shin JT, *et al.* Mutation in the transcriptional coactivator EYA4 causes dilated cardiomyopathy and sensorineural hearing loss. Nat Genet 2005; 37(4): 418-22.
[http://dx.doi.org/10.1038/ng1527] [PMID: 15735644]

[156] Theis JL, Sharpe KM, Matsumoto ME, *et al.* Homozygosity mapping and exome sequencing reveal GATAD1 mutation in autosomal recessive dilated cardiomyopathy. Circ Cardiovasc Genet 2011; 4(6): 585-94.
[http://dx.doi.org/10.1161/CIRCGENETICS.111.961052] [PMID: 21965549]

[157] Marcus FI, Fontaine GH, Guiraudon G, *et al.* Right ventricular dysplasia: a report of 24 adult cases. Circulation 1982; 65(2): 384-98.
[http://dx.doi.org/10.1161/01.CIR.65.2.384] [PMID: 7053899]

[158] Thiene G, Basso C. Arrhythmogenic right ventricular cardiomyopathy: An update. Cardiovasc Pathol

2001; 10(3): 109-17.
[http://dx.doi.org/10.1016/S1054-8807(01)00067-9] [PMID: 11485854]

[159] Hamid MS, Norman M, Quraishi A, *et al.* Prospective evaluation of relatives for familial arrhythmogenic right ventricular cardiomyopathy/dysplasia reveals a need to broaden diagnostic criteria. J Am Coll Cardiol 2002; 40(8): 1445-50.
[http://dx.doi.org/10.1016/S0735-1097(02)02307-0] [PMID: 12392835]

[160] Li D, Ahmad F, Gardner MJ, *et al.* The locus of a novel gene responsible for arrhythmogenic right-ventricular dysplasia characterized by early onset and high penetrance maps to chromosome 10p12-p14. Am J Hum Genet 2000; 66(1): 148-56.
[http://dx.doi.org/10.1086/302713] [PMID: 10631146]

[161] Matolweni LO, Bardien S, Rebello G, *et al.* Arrhythmogenic right ventricular cardiomyopathy type 6 (ARVC6): support for the locus assignment, narrowing of the critical region and mutation screening of three candidate genes. BMC Med Genet 2006; 7: 29.
[http://dx.doi.org/10.1186/1471-2350-7-29] [PMID: 16569242]

[162] Gallicano GI, Kouklis P, Bauer C, *et al.* Desmoplakin is required early in development for assembly of desmosomes and cytoskeletal linkage. J Cell Biol 1998; 143(7): 2009-22.
[http://dx.doi.org/10.1083/jcb.143.7.2009] [PMID: 9864371]

[163] Yang Z, Bowles NE, Scherer SE, *et al.* Desmosomal dysfunction due to mutations in desmoplakin causes arrhythmogenic right ventricular dysplasia/cardiomyopathy. Circ Res 2006; 99(6): 646-55.
[http://dx.doi.org/10.1161/01.RES.0000241482.19382.c6] [PMID: 16917092]

[164] Gerull B, Heuser A, Wichter T, *et al.* Mutations in the desmosomal protein plakophilin-2 are common in arrhythmogenic right ventricular cardiomyopathy. Nat Genet 2004; 36(11): 1162-4.
[http://dx.doi.org/10.1038/ng1461] [PMID: 15489853]

[165] Xu T, Yang Z, Vatta M, *et al.* Compound and digenic heterozygosity contributes to arrhythmogenic right ventricular cardiomyopathy. J Am Coll Cardiol 2010; 55(6): 587-97.
[http://dx.doi.org/10.1016/j.jacc.2009.11.020] [PMID: 20152563]

[166] Christensen AH, Benn M, Bundgaard H, Tybjaerg-Hansen A, Haunso S, Svendsen JH. Wide spectrum of desmosomal mutations in Danish patients with arrhythmogenic right ventricular cardiomyopathy. J Med Genet 2010; 47(11): 736-44. b
[http://dx.doi.org/10.1136/jmg.2010.077891] [PMID: 20864495]

[167] Bauce B, Nava A, Beffagna G, *et al.* Multiple mutations in desmosomal proteins encoding genes in arrhythmogenic right ventricular cardiomyopathy/dysplasia. Heart Rhythm 2010; 7(1): 22-9.
[http://dx.doi.org/10.1016/j.hrthm.2009.09.070] [PMID: 20129281]

[168] McKoy G, Protonotarios N, Crosby A, *et al.* Identification of a deletion in plakoglobin in arrhythmogenic right ventricular cardiomyopathy with palmoplantar keratoderma and woolly hair (Naxos disease). Lancet 2000; 355(9221): 2119-24.
[http://dx.doi.org/10.1016/S0140-6736(00)02379-5] [PMID: 10902626]

[169] Norgett EE, Hatsell SJ, Carvajal-Huerta L, *et al.* Recessive mutation in desmoplakin disrupts desmoplakin-intermediate filament interactions and causes dilated cardiomyopathy, woolly hair and keratoderma. Hum Mol Genet 2000; 9(18): 2761-6.
[http://dx.doi.org/10.1093/hmg/9.18.2761] [PMID: 11063735]

[170] Maron BJ, Towbin JA, Thiene G, *et al.* Contemporary definitions and classification of the cardiomyopathies: an American Heart Association Scientific Statement from the Council on Clinical Cardiology, Heart Failure and Transplantation Committee; Quality of Care and Outcomes Research and Functional Genomics and Translational Biology Interdisciplinary Working Groups; and Council on Epidemiology and Prevention. Circulation 2006; 113(14): 1807-16. [http://dx.doi.org/10.1161/CIRCULATIONAHA.106.174287] [PMID: 16567565]

[171] Monserrat L, Hermida-Prieto M, Fernandez X, *et al.* Mutation in the alpha-cardiac actin gene associated with apical hypertrophic cardiomyopathy, left ventricular non-compaction, and septal defects. Eur Heart J 2007; 28(16): 1953-61. [http://dx.doi.org/10.1093/eurheartj/ehm239] [PMID: 17611253]

[172] Hoedemaekers YM, Caliskan K, Michels M, *et al.* The importance of genetic counseling, DNA diagnostics, and cardiologic family screening in left ventricular noncompaction cardiomyopathy. Circ Cardiovasc Genet 2010; 3(3): 232-9. [http://dx.doi.org/10.1161/CIRCGENETICS.109.903898] [PMID: 20530761]

[173] Klaassen S, Probst S, Oechslin E, *et al.* Mutations in sarcomere protein genes in left ventricular noncompaction. Circulation 2008; 117(22): 2893-901. [http://dx.doi.org/10.1161/CIRCULATIONAHA.107.746164] [PMID: 18506004]

[174] Probst S, Oechslin E, Schuler P, *et al.* Sarcomere gene mutations in isolated left ventricular noncompaction cardiomyopathy do not predict clinical phenotype. Circ Cardiovasc Genet 2011; 4(4): 367-74. [http://dx.doi.org/10.1161/CIRCGENETICS.110.959270] [PMID: 21551322]

[175] Ichida F. Left ventricular noncompaction. Circ J 2009; 73(1): 19-26. [http://dx.doi.org/10.1253/circj.CJ-08-0995] [PMID: 19057090]

[176] Kaski JP, Syrris P, Burch M, *et al.* Idiopathic restrictive cardiomyopathy in children is caused by mutations in cardiac sarcomere protein genes. Heart 2008; 94(11): 1478-84. [http://dx.doi.org/10.1136/hrt.2007.134684] [PMID: 18467357]

[177] Mogensen J, Kubo T, Duque M, *et al.* Idiopathic restrictive cardiomyopathy is part of the clinical expression of cardiac troponin I mutations. J Clin Invest 2003; 111(2): 209-16. [http://dx.doi.org/10.1172/JCI200316336] [PMID: 12531876]

[178] van Spaendonck-Zwarts KY, van Hessem L, Jongbloed JD, *et al.* Desmin-related myopathy. Clin Genet 2011; 80(4): 354-66. [http://dx.doi.org/10.1111/j.1399-0004.2010.01512.x] [PMID: 20718792]

[179] Holmgren D, Wåhlander H, Eriksson BO, Oldfors A, Holme E, Tulinius M. Cardiomyopathy in children with mitochondrial disease; clinical course and cardiological findings. Eur Heart J 2003; 24(3): 280-8. [http://dx.doi.org/10.1016/S0195-668X(02)00387-1] [PMID: 12590906]

[180] Scaglia F, Towbin JA, Craigen WJ, *et al.* Clinical spectrum, morbidity, and mortality in 113 pediatric patients with mitochondrial disease. Pediatrics 2004; 114(4): 925-31. [http://dx.doi.org/10.1542/peds.2004-0718] [PMID: 15466086]

[181] Fayssoil A. Heart diseases in mitochondrial encephalomyopathy, lactic acidosis, and stroke syndrome.

Congest Heart Fail 2009; 15(6): 284-7.
[http://dx.doi.org/10.1111/j.1751-7133.2009.00108.x] [PMID: 19925507]

[182] Anan R, Nakagawa M, Miyata M, *et al.* Cardiac involvement in mitochondrial diseases. A study on 17 patients with documented mitochondrial DNA defects. Circulation 1995; 91(4): 955-61.
[http://dx.doi.org/10.1161/01.CIR.91.4.955] [PMID: 7850981]

[183] Wiles JR, Leslie N, Knilans TK, *et al.* Prolonged QTc interval in association with medium-chain acyl-coenzyme A dehydrogenase deficiency. Pediatrics 2014; 133(6): e1781-6.
[http://dx.doi.org/10.1542/peds.2013-1105]

[184] Abo Alrob O, Lopaschuk GD. Role of CoA and acetyl-CoA in regulating cardiac fatty acid and glucose oxidation. Biochem Soc Trans 2014; 42(4): 1043-51.
[http://dx.doi.org/10.1042/BST20140094] [PMID: 25110000]

[185] Adams DJ, Clark DA. Common genetic and epigenetic syndromes. Pediatr Clin North Am 2015; 62(2): 411-26.
[http://dx.doi.org/10.1016/j.pcl.2014.11.005] [PMID: 25836705]

[186] Hakim K, Boussaada R, Hamdi I, Msaad H. Cardiac events in Costello syndrome: One case and a review of the literature. J Saudi Heart Assoc 2014; 26(2): 105-9.
[http://dx.doi.org/10.1016/j.jsha.2013.11.002] [PMID: 24719541]

[187] Child AH, Aragon-Martin JA, Sage K. Genetic testing in Marfan syndrome. Br J Hosp Med (Lond) 2016; 77(1): 38-41.
[http://dx.doi.org/10.12968/hmed.2016.77.1.38] [PMID: 26903455]

[188] Papait R, Cattaneo P, Kunderfranco P, *et al.* Genome-wide analysis of histone marks identifying an epigenetic signature of promoters and enhancers underlying cardiac hypertrophy. Proc Natl Acad Sci USA 2013; 110(50): 20164-9.
[http://dx.doi.org/10.1073/pnas.1315155110] [PMID: 24284169]

[189] Pillai JB, Gupta M, Rajamohan SB, Lang R, Raman J, Gupta MP. Poly(ADP-ribose) polymerase---deficient mice are protected from angiotensin II-induced cardiac hypertrophy. Am J Physiol Heart Circ Physiol 2006; 291(4): H1545-53.
[http://dx.doi.org/10.1152/ajpheart.01124.2005] [PMID: 16632544]

[190] Xiao CY, Chen M, Zsengellér Z, *et al.* Poly(ADP-Ribose) polymerase promotes cardiac remodeling, contractile failure, and translocation of apoptosis-inducing factor in a murine experimental model of aortic banding and heart failure. J Pharmacol Exp Ther 2005; 312(3): 891-8.
[http://dx.doi.org/10.1124/jpet.104.077164] [PMID: 15523000]

[191] Han P, Hang CT, Yang J, Chang CP. Chromatin remodeling in cardiovascular development and physiology. Circ Res 2011; 108(3): 378-96.
[http://dx.doi.org/10.1161/CIRCRESAHA.110.224287] [PMID: 21293009]

[192] Hang CT, Yang J, Han P, *et al.* Chromatin regulation by Brg1 underlies heart muscle development and disease. Nature 2010; 466(7302): 62-7.
[http://dx.doi.org/10.1038/nature09130] [PMID: 20596014]

[193] Saxonov S, Berg P, Brutlag DL. A genome-wide analysis of CpG dinucleotides in the human genome distinguishes two distinct classes of promoters. Proc Natl Acad Sci USA 2006; 103(5): 1412-7.

[http://dx.doi.org/10.1073/pnas.0510310103] [PMID: 16432200]

[194] Deaton AM, Bird A. CpG islands and the regulation of transcription. Genes Dev 2011; 25(10): 1010-22.
[http://dx.doi.org/10.1101/gad.2037511] [PMID: 21576262]

[195] Movassagh M, Choy M-K, Knowles DA, *et al.* Distinct epigenomic features in end-stage failing human hearts. Circulation 2011; 124(22): 2411-22.
[http://dx.doi.org/10.1161/CIRCULATIONAHA.111.040071] [PMID: 22025602]

[196] Whayne TF. Epigenetics in the development, modification, and prevention of cardiovascular disease. Mol Biol Rep 2015; 42(4): 765-76.
[http://dx.doi.org/10.1007/s11033-014-3727-z] [PMID: 25205125]

[197] Watson CJ, Collier P, Tea I, *et al.* Hypoxia-induced epigenetic modifications are associated with cardiac tissue fibrosis and the development of a myofibroblast-like phenotype. Hum Mol Genet 2014; 23(8): 2176-88.
[http://dx.doi.org/10.1093/hmg/ddt614] [PMID: 24301681]

[198] Xiao D, Dasgupta C, Chen M, *et al.* Inhibition of DNA methylation reverses norepinephrine-induced cardiac hypertrophy in rats. Cardiovasc Res 2014; 101(3): 373-82.
[http://dx.doi.org/10.1093/cvr/cvt264] [PMID: 24272874]

[199] Ferguson BS, Harrison BC, Jeong MY, *et al.* Signal-dependent repression of DUSP5 by class I HDACs controls nuclear ERK activity and cardiomyocyte hypertrophy. Proc Natl Acad Sci USA 2013; 110(24): 9806-11.
[http://dx.doi.org/10.1073/pnas.1301509110] [PMID: 23720316]

[200] Kao YH, Liou JP, Chung CC, *et al.* Histone deacetylase inhibition improved cardiac functions with direct antifibrotic activity in heart failure. Int J Cardiol 2013; 168(4): 4178-83.
[http://dx.doi.org/10.1016/j.ijcard.2013.07.111] [PMID: 23931972]

[201] Nural-Guvener HF, Zakharova L, Nimlos J, Popovic S, Mastroeni D, Gaballa MA. HDAC class I inhibitor, Mocetinostat, reverses cardiac fibrosis in heart failure and diminishes CD90+ cardiac myofibroblast activation. Fibrogenesis Tissue Repair 2014; 7(1): 10.
[http://dx.doi.org/10.1186/1755-1536-7-10] [PMID: 25024745]

[202] Gupta MP, Samant SA, Smith SH, Shroff SG. HDAC4 and PCAF bind to cardiac sarcomeres and play a role in regulating myofilament contractile activity. J Biol Chem 2008; 283(15): 10135-46.
[http://dx.doi.org/10.1074/jbc.M710277200] [PMID: 18250163]

[203] Pedram A, Razandi M, Narayanan R, Dalton JT, McKinsey TA, Levin ER. Estrogen regulates histone deacetylases to prevent cardiac hypertrophy. Mol Biol Cell 2013; 24(24): 3805-18.
[http://dx.doi.org/10.1091/mbc.E13-08-0444] [PMID: 24152730]

[204] Haberland M, Montgomery RL, Olson EN. The many roles of histone deacetylases in development and physiology: implications for disease and therapy. Nat Rev Genet 2009; 10(1): 32-42.
[http://dx.doi.org/10.1038/nrg2485] [PMID: 19065135]

[205] Zhang CL, McKinsey TA, Chang S, Antos CL, Hill JA, Olson EN. Class II histone deacetylases act as signal-responsive repressors of cardiac hypertrophy. Cell 2002; 110(4): 479-88.
[http://dx.doi.org/10.1016/S0092-8674(02)00861-9] [PMID: 12202037]

[206] Antos CL, McKinsey TA, Dreitz M, *et al.* Dose-dependent blockade to cardiomyocyte hypertrophy by histone deacetylase inhibitors. J Biol Chem 2003; 278(31): 28930-7. [http://dx.doi.org/10.1074/jbc.M303113200] [PMID: 12761226]

[207] Chang S, McKinsey TA, Zhang CL, Richardson JA, Hill JA, Olson EN. Histone deacetylases 5 and 9 govern responsiveness of the heart to a subset of stress signals and play redundant roles in heart development. Mol Cell Biol 2004; 24(19): 8467-76. [http://dx.doi.org/10.1128/MCB.24.19.8467-8476.2004] [PMID: 15367668]

[208] Backs J, Song K, Bezprozvannaya S, Chang S, Olson EN. CaM kinase II selectively signals to histone deacetylase 4 during cardiomyocyte hypertrophy. J Clin Invest 2006; 116(7): 1853-64. [http://dx.doi.org/10.1172/JCI27438] [PMID: 16767219]

[209] Gusterson RJ, Jazrawi E, Adcock IM, Latchman DS. The transcriptional co-activators CREB-binding protein (CBP) and p300 play a critical role in cardiac hypertrophy that is dependent on their histone acetyltransferase activity. J Biol Chem 2003; 278(9): 6838-47. [http://dx.doi.org/10.1074/jbc.M211762200] [PMID: 12477714]

[210] Yanazume T, Hasegawa K, Morimoto T, *et al.* Cardiac p300 is involved in myocyte growth with decompensated heart failure. Mol Cell Biol 2003; 23(10): 3593-606. [http://dx.doi.org/10.1128/MCB.23.10.3593-3606.2003] [PMID: 12724418]

[211] Cao DJ, Wang ZV, Battiprolu PK, *et al.* Histone deacetylase (HDAC) inhibitors attenuate cardiac hypertrophy by suppressing autophagy. Proc Natl Acad Sci USA 2011; 108(10): 4123-8. [http://dx.doi.org/10.1073/pnas.1015081108] [PMID: 21367693]

[212] Teperino R, Schoonjans K, Auwerx J. Histone methyl transferases and demethylases; can they link metabolism and transcription? Cell Metab 2010; 12(4): 321-7. [http://dx.doi.org/10.1016/j.cmet.2010.09.004] [PMID: 20889125]

[213] Kaneda R, Takada S, Yamashita Y, *et al.* Genome-wide histone methylation profile for heart failure. Genes Cells 2009; 14(1): 69-77. [http://dx.doi.org/10.1111/j.1365-2443.2008.01252.x] [PMID: 19077033]

[214] Fabian MR, Sonenberg N, Filipowicz W. Regulation of mRNA translation and stability by microRNAs. Annu Rev Biochem 2010; 79: 351-79. [http://dx.doi.org/10.1146/annurev-biochem-060308-103103] [PMID: 20533884]

[215] Krol J, Loedige I, Filipowicz W. The widespread regulation of microRNA biogenesis, function and decay. Nat Rev Genet 2010; 11(9): 597-610. [PMID: 20661255]

[216] Thum T, Galuppo P, Wolf C, *et al.* MicroRNAs in the human heart: a clue to fetal gene reprogramming in heart failure. Circulation 2007; 116(3): 258-67. [http://dx.doi.org/10.1161/CIRCULATIONAHA.107.687947] [PMID: 17606841]

[217] Ikeda S, Kong SW, Lu J, *et al.* Altered microRNA expression in human heart disease. Physiol Genomics 2007; 31(3): 367-73. [http://dx.doi.org/10.1152/physiolgenomics.00144.2007] [PMID: 17712037]

[218] Sucharov C, Bristow MR, Port JD. miRNA expression in the failing human heart: functional correlates. J Mol Cell Cardiol 2008; 45(2): 185-92.

[http://dx.doi.org/10.1016/j.yjmcc.2008.04.014] [PMID: 18582896]

[219] Jessup M, Greenberg B, Mancini D, *et al.* Calcium Upregulation by Percutaneous Administration of Gene Therapy in Cardiac Disease (CUPID): a phase 2 trial of intracoronary gene therapy of sarcoplasmic reticulum Ca2+-ATPase in patients with advanced heart failure. Circulation 2011; 124(3): 304-13.
[http://dx.doi.org/10.1161/CIRCULATIONAHA.111.022889] [PMID: 21709064]

[220] Ikeda S, He A, Kong SW, *et al.* MicroRNA-1 negatively regulates expression of the hypertrophy-associated calmodulin and Mef2a genes. Mol Cell Biol 2009; 29(8): 2193-204.
[http://dx.doi.org/10.1128/MCB.01222-08] [PMID: 19188439]

[221] Fiore R, Schratt G. MicroRNAs in synapse development: tiny molecules to remember. Expert Opin Biol Ther 2007; 7(12): 1823-31.
[http://dx.doi.org/10.1517/14712598.7.12.1823] [PMID: 18034648]

[222] van Rooij E, Sutherland LB, Liu N, *et al.* A signature pattern of stress-responsive microRNAs that can evoke cardiac hypertrophy and heart failure. Proc Natl Acad Sci USA 2006; 103(48): 18255-60.
[http://dx.doi.org/10.1073/pnas.0608791103] [PMID: 17108080]

[223] Hosoda T, Zheng H, Cabral-da-Silva M, *et al.* Human cardiac stem cell differentiation is regulated by a merocrine mechanism. Circulation 2011; 123(12): 1287-96.
[http://dx.doi.org/10.1161/CIRCULATIONAHA.110.982918] [PMID: 21403094]

[224] Matkovich SJ, Hu Y, Eschenbacher WH, Dorn LE, Dorn GW II. Direct and indirect involvement of microRNA-499 in clinical and experimental cardiomyopathy. Circ Res 2012; 111(5): 521-31.
[http://dx.doi.org/10.1161/CIRCRESAHA.112.265736] [PMID: 22752967]

[225] Wahlquist C, Jeong D, Rojas-Muñoz A, *et al.* Inhibition of miR-25 improves cardiac contractility in the failing heart. Nature 2014; 508(7497): 531-5.
[http://dx.doi.org/10.1038/nature13073] [PMID: 24670661]

[226] Bostjancic E, Zidar N, Stajer D, Glavac D. MicroRNAs miR-1, miR-133a, miR-133b and miR-208 are dysregulated in human myocardial infarction. Cardiology 2010; 115(3): 163-9.
[http://dx.doi.org/10.1159/000268088] [PMID: 20029200]

[227] Carè A, Catalucci D, Felicetti F, *et al.* MicroRNA-133 controls cardiac hypertrophy. Nat Med 2007; 13(5): 613-8.
[http://dx.doi.org/10.1038/nm1582] [PMID: 17468766]

[228] Castaldi A, Zaglia T, Di Mauro V, *et al.* MicroRNA-133 modulates the β1-adrenergic receptor transduction cascade. Circ Res 2014; 115(2): 273-83.
[http://dx.doi.org/10.1161/CIRCRESAHA.115.303252] [PMID: 24807785]

[229] da Costa Martins PA, Salic K, Gladka MM, *et al.* MicroRNA-199b targets the nuclear kinase Dyrk1a in an auto-amplification loop promoting calcineurin/NFAT signalling. Nat Cell Biol 2010; 12(12): 1220-7.
[http://dx.doi.org/10.1038/ncb2126] [PMID: 21102440]

[230] Oliveira-Carvalho V, Carvalho VO, Silva MM, Guimarães GV, Bocchi EA. MicroRNAs: a new paradigm in the treatment and diagnosis of heart failure? Arq Bras Cardiol 2012; 98(4): 362-9.
[http://dx.doi.org/10.1590/S0066-782X2012000400011] [PMID: 22735911]

[231] Carninci P, Kasukawa T, Katayama S, *et al.* The transcriptional landscape of the mammalian genome. Science 2005; 309(5740): 1559-63.
[http://dx.doi.org/10.1126/science.1112014] [PMID: 16141072]

[232] Kumarswamy R, Bauters C, Volkmann I, *et al.* Circulating long noncoding RNA, LIPCAR, predicts survival in patients with heart failure. Circ Res 2014; 114(10): 1569-75.
[http://dx.doi.org/10.1161/CIRCRESAHA.114.303915] [PMID: 24663402]

[233] Schaefer AS, Bochenek G, Jochens A, *et al.* Genetic evidence for Plasminogen as a shared genetic risk factor of coronary artery disease and periodontitis. Circ Cardiovasc Genet 2015; 8(1): 159-67.
[http://dx.doi.org/10.1161/CIRCGENETICS.114.000554] [PMID: 25466412]

Frontiers in Heart Failure, 2016, *Vol. 1*, 122-172

CHAPTER 5

Clinical Manifestations, Co-existing Diseases, Patients' Investigation and Prognostication

John Skoularigis*, **Andreas Xanthopoulos**, **Gregory Giamouzis** and **Filippos Triposkiadis**

Department of Cardiology, University Hospital of Larissa, University of Thessaly, Larissa, Greece

Abstract: Heart failure is an important cause of morbidity and mortality worldwide and despite recent advances in therapeutic management, hospitalization rates remain high. The complex interactions of various physiologic, psychological, social, and health care delivery issues make heart failure a challenging chronic disease to manage. A better understanding of the underlying pathophysiological mechanisms, as well as novel diagnostic and therapeutic approaches, may result in cost-effective strategies achieving more drastic control of the epidemic. Prompt diagnosis and optimal treatment of heart failure can affect long-term outcome. A tool with diagnostic, prognostic, and treatment-guiding properties in this respect would be valuable. Recent evidence in the field of molecular biology and heart failure pathophysiology has led to the identification of novel biomarkers that may have significant advantages. Furthermore, heart failure is associated with several cardiac and non-cardiac comorbidities that play an integral role in its development, progression, and response to treatment. The comorbidity burden is highly associated with hospitalization rate in patients with heart failure and preserved left ventricular ejection fraction, as well as in those with heart failure and reduced ejection fraction. In the current review we address these issues and try to analyze this patient population focusing on the need for re-hospitalization and the poor prognosis.

Keywords: Bendopnea, Comorbidities, Dyspnea, Ejection fraction, Epidemiology, Fatigue, Heart failure, Peripheral edema, Prognosis, Re-hospitalization, Symptoms.

* **Corresponding author John Skoularigis:** Department of Cardiology, University Hospital of Larissa, Larissa, Greece; Tel: +30 2413 50 2977; Fax: +30 2413 50 1812; E-mail: iskoular@med.uth.gr, iskoular@gmail.com.

Panagiotis Georgoulias (Ed.)

INTRODUCTION

A widely used definition of heart failure (HF) states that "HF is a pathophysiological state in which an abnormality of cardiac function is responsible for the failure of the heart to pump blood at a rate commensurate with the requirements of the metabolizing tissues" [1]. Moreover, the ESC guidelines define HF clinically, as a syndrome in which patients have typical symptoms (*e.g.* breathlessness) and signs (*e.g.* increased jugular venous pressure) resulting from cardiac structural or functional abnormalities [2]. The prevalence of HF is estimated at 5.7 million people in the USA and it is expected to increase by 46% from 2012 to 2030, resulting in more than 8 million people with HF aged 18 or above [3, 4]. With respect to incidence, 870.000 new HF cases are emerging annually and the lifetime risk of developing HF, for both men and women at the age of 40, is 1 in 5 [3]. The reasons for this pandemic are multiple and include the aging of the population, the rising incidence of arterial hypertension (HT), diabetes mellitus (DM) and obesity, the expanding performance of primary percutaneous coronary intervention which improves survival after ST elevation myocardial infarction and the primary and secondary prophylaxis of sudden cardiac death with the use of implantable cardioverter defibrillators (ICDs). New therapies in HF are effective and improve outcomes based on a patient's thorough clinical assessment. Therefore, the physician should take a complete medical history and proceed to a focused physical examination in patients complaining for symptoms compatible with HF. This information guides the further investigation (invasive or non-invasive) and assists to risk stratification of the HF patients.

DIAGNOSTIC INVESTIGATION

Medical History

The diagnosis of HF [either with reduced ejection fraction (rEF) or with preserved EF (pEF)] is often challenging (Tables **1**, **2**). HF patients present with a variety of symptoms (Table **3**), although none of them is specific for this syndrome. For example, a patient complaining of acute dyspnea may have (apart from congestive HF) pneumonia, chronic obstructive pulmonary disease (COPD) exacerbation, pneumothorax or even pulmonary embolism. Thus, the initial diagnostic investigation, that involves the medical history, is of great importance. It is essential the physician to detect the patient's stage in the natural history of HF syndrome [5].

Table 1. Diagnosis of heart failure (European Society of Cardiology Guidelines).

Heart failure with reduced ejection fraction	Satisfaction of three conditions is required: • Symptoms typical of heart failure • Signs typical of heart failure • Reduced left ventricular ejection fraction
Heart failure with preserved ejection fraction	Satisfaction of four conditions is required: • Symptoms typical of heart failure • Signs typical of heart failure • Normal or only midely reduced left ventricular ejection fraction and left ventricle not dilated • Relevant structural heart disease (left ventricular hypertrophy / right atrial enlargement) and/or diastolic dysfunction

Table 2. Diagnosis of heart failure (Framingham Criteria).

Major criteria	• Paroxysmal nocturnal dyspnea • Weight loss of 4.5 kg in 5 days in response to treatment • Neck vein distention • Rales • Acute pulmonary edema • Hepatojugular reflux • S_3 gallop • Central venous pressure >16 cmH_2O • Circulation time of 25 seconds • Radiographic cardiomegaly • Pulmonary edema, visceral congestion, or cardiomegaly at autopsy
Minor criteria	• Nocturnal cough • Dyspnea on ordinary exertion • A decrease in vital capacity by one third of the maximal value recorded • Pleural effusion • Tachycardia (rate of 120 bpm) • Bilateral ankle edema **Note:** The Framingham criteria for the diagnosis of heart failure require the concurrent presence of either 2 major criteria or 1 major and 2 minor criteria.

The timely identification and management of HF risk factors, such as HT, coronary artery disease (CAD), exposure to cardiotoxins, and positive family history for DM or cardiomyopathy in asymptomatic patients, may prevent HF development. Therefore, a number of risk scores for the prediction of this syndrome have emerged over the last years, such as the Health ABC HF risk score and the ARIC HF risk score [6, 7]. Stage A includes all asymptomatic cases at high risk for HF. Furthermore, asymptomatic patients with structural and functional abnormalities of the heart are classified in stage B, whereas those with HF symptoms adequately controlled under medical therapy in stage C. Finally, HF patients who have symptoms refractory to conventional treatment are classified in stage D [8].

Table 3. Symptoms of heart failure due to left ventricular and/or right ventricular failure.

Symptoms of left and right ventricular failure	• Chest pain / pressure and palpitations • Fatigue and weakness • Nocturia and oliguria • Loss of appetite • Anorexia, weight loss / gain, nausea • Central or peripheral cyanosis, pallor • Somnolence or diminished mental acuity
Symptoms of left ventricular failure	• Cough • Exertional dyspnea • Bendopnea • Paroxysmal nocturnal dyspnea • Orthopnea • Acute pulmonary edema
Symptoms of right ventricular failure	• Edema (extremities, scrotum, or other parts of the body) • Increasing abdominal girth or bloating • Abdominal pain

One of the most important information that physicians can gain from the medical history is patient's functional capacity during the last days or even weeks. A subjective, but widely used, tool is the New York Heart Association (NYHA) classification system (Table **4**) which categorizes HF patients based on a scale I – IV. NYHA system guides HF management and defines prognosis in HF patients [9].

Searching for factors (Table **5**) that may precipitate worsening of HF should be an integral part of the medical history. In a prospective study that assessed which factors were related to short-term worsening of HF in a population of 215 patients, poor compliance (21%) and infection (12%) were the most frequent, while in 40%

of the patients no precipitating factors were identified [10].

Table 4. The New York Heart Association classification system.

Class I (mild)	1. No limitation of physical activity. 2. Ordinary physical activity does not cause undue fatigue, palpitation, or dyspnea (shortness of breath).
Class II (mild)	1. Slight limitation of physical activity. 2. Comfortable at rest, but ordinary physical activity results in fatigue, palpitation, or dyspnea.
Class III (moderate)	1. Marked limitation of physical activity. 2. Comfortable at rest, but less than ordinary activity causes fatigue, palpitation, or dyspnea.
Class IV (severe)	1. Unable to carry out any physical activity without discomfort. 2. Symptoms of cardiac insufficiency at rest. 3. If any physical activity is undertaken, discomfort is increased.

Table 5. Precipitating factors for heart failure exacerbation.

• Myocardial ischemia or infarction	
• Dietary sodium excess or excess fluid intake	
• Iatrogenic volume overload	
• Arrhythmias	tachyarrhythmias, bradyarrhythmias
• Uncontrolled hypertension	
• Worsening valvular dysfunction	
• Comorbidities	fever, infections / sepsis, thyroid dysfunction, anemia, renal insufficiency, nutritional deficiencies, pulmonary diseases (including chronic obstructive pulmonary disease, pulmonary embolism)
• Inappropriate reduction of heart failure medications	
• Medication non-compliance	
• Adverse drug effects	negative inotropic agents (such as b-blockers), antiarrhythmics, non-steroidal anti-inflammatory drugs, corticosteroids, alcohol, cocaine

Main Symptoms in Heart Failure (HF)

Dyspnea

The cardinal symptom of congestive HF is dyspnea. It is defined as the abnormal sensation of an uncomfortable awareness of breathing. When it occurs at rest or at a level of physical activity in which it is not expected, breathing discomfort is abnormal. Dyspnea, breathlessness and shortness of breath are interchangeable terms used by health care professionals to describe breathing discomfort. The pathophysiological mechanism of dyspnea remains debatable on whether it is the result of pulmonary venous congestion or stems from decreased forward cardiac output [11].

Other manifestations of congestion include cough, exertional dyspnea, orthopnea, paroxysmal nocturnal dyspnea, dyspnea at rest and acute pulmonary edema. A dry, hacking cough, is often the initial symptom of acute HF (*de novo* or chronic HF decompensation), especially when the patient is lying down. Exertional dyspnea is abnormal if it occurs during activity that is normally expected to be well tolerated by the patient. Orthopnea is the sensation of breathing difficulty while patient is supine and it is relieved in the upright posture. Paroxysmal nocturnal dyspnea is the symptom of breathlessness that awakens the HF patient, usually 3 hours after going to bed. Lastly, acute pulmonary edema is a life threatening clinical manifestation of left HF. Patients present with sudden onset of extreme breathlessness, anxiety, and feelings of drowning. As dyspnea is a completely subjective sensation and there is no objective method to quantify its severity, a visual analog scale (VAS) score and the relative dyspnea score are used in HF patients.

Fatigue

Similar to dyspnea, the pathophysiological mechanism of fatigue remains controversial. While some physicians believed that fatigue in HF patients stemmed exclusively from low cardiac output, there is a growing perception over the last 2 decades that abnormalities of skeletal muscles, compensatory vascular and autonomic responses, and other non-cardiac comorbidities such as anemia may contribute importantly to fatigue [12, 13]. In a recent study, investigators examined the relationship between fatigue and clinical outcomes, using dyspnea as a comparative parameter, in patients with LVEF ≤35% enrolled in the CORONA (Controlled Rosuvastatin Multinational Trial in Heart Failure) study [14]. They concluded that patients with systolic HF and greater fatigue (and/or an increase in fatigue) had worse clinical outcomes. Patients with congestive HF and fatigue (either general or during exercise) experience poor HF self-care, which cannot be attributed to sleep problems or mood symptoms and is independent of clinical severity indicators. Treatment of fatigue may improve HF self-care skills and quality of life, and also cardiovascular prognosis.

Peripheral Edema

Peripheral edema is a common manifestation of right HF either *de novo* or as a result of left HF. The underlying mechanism includes increased hydrostatic venous pressure [15]. The main localization of peripheral edema is the ankle and the feet. Patients often complain about swollen feet that get worse after a long day in the upright position and substantially improve when they wake up in the morning. Various methods quantitatively measuring peripheral edema have been proposed (*e.g.* volumetry and ankle circumference) but their use in the daily clinical practice is generally limited. The most common technique is a subjective clinical assessment in which the health care provider applies constantly pressure with his index finger to a single location on the patient's ankle. This technique provides an estimation of pit depth and the time needed for the skin to return to its original appearance, as a single edema score ranging from 0 to 4 [16]. Weighing the HF patient every 2 to 3 days is an indirect way to estimate fluid accumulation in the body, usually before the manifestation of peripheral edema.

Bendopnea: A Novel Symptom in Advanced Heart Failure (HF)

Bendopnea is defined as shortness of breath which occurs when a HF patient bends forward (*e.g.* when he/she puts on his/her shoes). It was first described by Thibodeau *et al.* who conducted a prospective study in 102 patients with systolic HF. Investigators showed that bendopnea was reproduced *via* a further increase in filling pressures during bending when filling pressures were already high, especially if cardiac index was reduced [17]. A similar observation was made by Brandon *et al.* who used ultrasound for the estimation of pulmonary capillary wedge pressures [18].

Other Symptoms

Patients with HF can sometimes complain of palpitations, lightheadedness, pre-syncope or syncope. The cause in most cases is attributed to underlying arrhythmia or outflow tract obstruction, and less commonly to low output states [5]. Anorexia, weight loss or weight gain, somnolence or diminished mental acuity and nocturnal angina are also part of the full picture.

Physical Examination

Following medical history, the physical examination is the next step in the diagnostic evaluation of a patient with suspected HF. Patient's general appearance is often, for the examiner, a source of valuable information. For example, a labored breathing during rest or when the patient is lying down (orthopnea) may guide further diagnostic assessment. In addition, typical respiration patterns, such as the Cheyne-Stokes pattern, or cyanosis may be observed. With respect to cyanosis, the peripheral localization is the most common form and indicates reduced perfusion or low cardiac output while the central cyanosis is less frequent and may result from an intracardiac or intrapulmonary shunting.

Other findings during inspection are peripheral edema and ascites, characteristic features of volume overload. The latter can also be manifested as a variety of signs during physical examination, such as jugular venous distention, "V waves", rales, pleural effusion, S3 (gallop rhythm), hyperdynamic and displaced leftward or inferiorly LV apex. One of the most reliable clinical findings for detecting increased filling pressure is jugular venous distention [19]. The abdomino-jugular reflux is a useful sign for the diagnosis of right HF. In patients with advanced HF, the Kussmaul sign is frequent and denotes paradoxical increase in jugular venous pressure during inspiration [20]. Giant "V waves" of tricuspid insufficiency may also be seen and occur simultaneously with the carotid pulse. The auscultation of the lung fields and the heart may reveal rales or reduced alveolar ventilation (pleural effusion) and S3 (or gallop rhythm), respectively, whereas their absence cannot exclude the diagnosis of congestive HF. A systolic murmur is often audible at the apex indicating mitral valve regurgitation. When it is heard in the left parasternal border, it indicates tricuspid valve regurgitation. Palpation often reveals hyperdynamic or sustained precordial pulsation due to left/right ventricular volume or pressure overload and parasternal lift. In addition to congestion, which is the most common reason for HF hospitalization and readmission, low cardiac output as the presenting feature of acute decompensated HF is another, although uncommon, cause of hospitalization [21, 22]. Patients with HF and low cardiac output often present with tachycardia, borderline or low blood pressure, narrow pulse pressure, cool skin, pallor or cyanosis.

Examination of the arterial pulse is a fundamental part of the evaluation of a HF patient. Pulsus alternans (alternating strong and weak beats) is virtually diagnostic of severe HF. Pulsus paradoxus is an exacerbation of a physiologic phenomenon and is defined as a substantial diminishment in the amplitude of the arterial pulse of more than 10 mmHg, during inspiration. It is found in disorders such as pericardial tamponade, pulmonary embolism, asthma, pregnancy, obesity, sleep apnea, superior vena cava syndrome and advanced HF. A carotid pulse, which is weak (parvus) with a delayed upstroke (tardus), is evident among patients with aortic stenosis and denotes impaired flow. Conversely, patients with severe, chronic aortic regurgitation manifest accentuated pulses and a series of findings related to a large stroke volume (Corrigan pulse). Lastly, coarctation of aorta is typically accompanied with diminished or absent pulses of the lower limbs [23].

Sensitivity and Specificity of Heart Failure (HF) Symptoms and Signs

There is no symptom or sign that is both sensitive and specific for the diagnosis of congestive HF, and a purely clinical diagnosis is problematic (Table **6**). Therefore, the patient's initial approach (medical history and physical examination) is often complemented with the laboratory investigation.

Table 6. Sensitivity, specificity and predictive accuracy (diagnostic value) of symptoms and signs for the diagnosis (investigation) of heart failure [24].

Symptoms of heart failure			
	Sensitivity	**Specificity**	**Predictive Accuracy**
Exertional dyspnea	66%	52%	23
Orthopnea	21%	81%	02
Paroxysmal nocturnal dyspnea	33%	76%	26
History of edema	23%	80%	22

(Table 6) contd.....

Signs of heart failure			
	Sensitivity	**Specificity**	**Predictive Accuracy**
Resting heart rate	07%	99%	06%
Rales	13%	91%	21%
Third heart sound	31%	95%	61%
Jugular venous distention	10%	97%	02%
Edema (on examination)	10%	93%	03%

Laboratory Tests

The routine laboratory assessment of the patient consists of the full blood count and the standard biochemical tests, such as urea, creatinine, e-glomerular filtration rate (e-GFR), liver enzymes and the electrolytes. In addition, thyroid function should be evaluated as thyroid dysfunction is a common cause of HF exacerbation or sometimes mimics the latter [2]. Blood glucose and glycosylated hemoglobin percentage (HbA1c), should also be part of the routine laboratory assessment because undiagnosed DM is common among HF patients [2].

Biomarkers constitute an integral part of the patient's laboratory investigation as they provide incremental diagnostic and prognostic information. Braunwald classified biomarkers of HF in the following categories [25]:

a. myocyte injury
b. myocyte stretch
c. renal dysfunction
d. inflammation
e. oxidative stress
f. extracellular matrix remodeling
g. neurohumoral activation

Probably, the most used biomarkers in HF are the natriuretic peptides [*i.e.* B-type natriuretic peptide (BNP), N-terminal prohormone of BNP (NT-proBNP), midregional pro-atrial natriuretic peptide (MR-proANP)]. BNP and its prodromal aminoterminal fragment (NT-proBNP) are hormones, which are secreted by the wall of heart chambers (ventricles) as a response to pressure or volume overload. Factors that influence circulating levels of BNP and NT-proBNP are shown in

Table 7. Although the sensitivity of BNP and NT-proBNP is relatively high, their specificity is relatively low [26, 27]. Therefore, they are currently used in the diagnostic work-up for the exclusion of HF. In the acute setting, BNP values < 100 pg/ml and NT-proBNP <300 pg/ml are unlikely in HF. Respectively, BNP values <125 pg/ml and NT-proBNP <35 pg/ml are unlikely in the non-acute setting [2].

Table 7. Factors that influence BNP/NT-proBNP levels.

Factors that can account for lower than expected BNP/NT-proBNP when HF is present	• Obesity • Flash pulmonary edema • Stable NYHA class I patients • Pericardial constriction • Acute mitral regurgitation • Atrial myxoma • Mitral stenosis • Cardiac tamponade
Factors associated with higher BNP/NT-proBNP	• Advanced age • Myocardial infarction • Renal failure • Lung disease with right sided failure • High output states • Cardiotoxic drugs (*i.e.* anthracyclines) • Arrhythmias (*i.e.* atrial fibrillation) • LV dysfunction (*i.e.* Takotsubo, valvular heart disease, amyloidosis, myocarditis)

BNP: B-type natriuretic peptide; NT-proBNP: N-terminal prohormone of BNP; LV: left ventricle; NYHA: New York Heart Association.

Galectin-3 (GAL-3) and soluble ST2 (sST2) are two relative novel biomarkers in HF. GAL-3 is a b-galactoside-binding protein with the ability to interact with surface receptors of the macrophages, and also with collagen receptors [28]. The sST2 is a member of the Toll-like/IL-1-receptor superfamily and is expressed by mast and T-helper 2 cells, and also the hematopoietic organs [29]. GAL-3 and sST2 have additive prognostic and diagnostic value when they are combined with BNP or NT-proBNP. They have also lower intra-individual variability compared to natriuretic peptides. The latter are affected by renal dysfunction and body mass index, contrary to sST2 levels. However, both GAL-3 and sST2 have inferior diagnostic sensitivity than natriuretic peptides [30].

Electrocardiogram (ECG)

In patients with suspected HF, ECG is a valuable diagnostic tool. In those presenting acutely, a normal ECG almost excludes the possibility of HF (likelihood of HF <2%), whereas in the non-acute setting a normal ECG has a lower predictive value (likelihood of HF <10-14%) [2]. The ECG often manifests a structural abnormality of the heart, such as LV hypertrophy due to HT, hypertrophic obstructive cardiomyopathy, or even valvular heart disease. Other ECG findings suggesting structural heart disease are biphasic P wave in lead V_1 (a sensitive indicator of left atrial enlargement) and increased P wave duration and amplitude in lead II (indicating left and right atrial enlargement, respectively). Sinus tachycardia may result from HF decompensation, fever, or anemia. In contrast, sinus bradycardia stems from hypothyroidism, sick sinus syndrome and the use of drugs with negative chronotropic effect. Low QRS voltage is encountered in patients with pericardial effusion, amyloidosis, COPD, or obese people.

ECG sometimes determines the cause of HF, for example CAD (Q waves, ST elevation), even in the presence of left bundle branch block (LBBB) [31]. Patients with LV systolic dysfunction may complain for palpitations or syncope due to supraventricular or ventricular arrhythmias, which can be imprinted on a simple ECG tracing or even longer tracings such as those depicted by the Holter monitor or implantable loop recorders. ECG may guide the management of HF patients with broad QRS complex (> 120 msec) and LBBB morphology to cardiac resynchronization therapy (CRT-D or CRT-P). A recent study in patients with LBBB evaluated for resynchronization therapy showed that ECG predicts a poor response to resynchronization therapy based on 3 ECG findings that can be helpful in diagnosing RV disease: a) low voltage in the extremity leads, b) R/S ratio below 1 in lead V5 and c) a positive terminal R in lead aVR [32].

Chest X-ray

The importance of chest X-ray in the diagnostic assessment of patients with suspected HF is relatively low. Nonetheless, it is helpful for the exclusion of alternative causes of dyspnea such as COPD, pneumonia or pneumothorax [2].

The pathophysiological progression of congestive HF, as depicted in the chest X-ray, consists of 3 stages (Table **8**).

Table 8. Chest X-ray findings in different stages of congestive heart failure.

Stage I	• Cardiomegaly. • Pulmonary vasculature redistribution (cephalization). • Increased mediastinal width. • Pulmonary artery to bronchus ratio > 1.
Stage II	• Kerley B lines. • Thickened interlobar fissure. • Peribronchial cuffing. • Less distinct vessels (surrounding edema).
Stage III	• Butterfly appearance. • Air bronchograms. • Pleural effusion.

Physical or radiographic signs have poor predictive value for identifying patients with congestion (pulmonary capillary wedge pressure, PCWP ≥30 mm Hg) [33]. In addition, there is no correlation between very high BNP levels (>400 pg/mL) and a finding of congestive HF on chest X-ray [34]. Therefore, after medical history, physical examination, blood tests and chest x-ray, patients should often undergo further diagnostic evaluation.

Echocardiography

Echocardiography (transthoracic (TTE) and/or transesophageal (TEE)) plays a pivotal role in the diagnostic algorithm of patients with probable HF. It is a source of valuable information with regard to cardiac anatomy and function. In daily clinical practice, the categorization of patients into two distinct groups [HF with reduced EF (HFrEF) *vs.* HF with preserved EF (HFpEF)] is based on the echocardiographic evaluation. The estimation of LVEF using the M-mode echocardiography (fractional shortening) is more of historical value because its accuracy is limited. It is based on the assumption that there is a uniform wall thickness and normal concentric wall motion. This is not the case in the majority of patients with HFrEF, who have CAD and thus wall motion abnormalities [2]. In contrast, 2D echocardiography is the most frequently used and important diagnostic imaging modality in HFrEF or HFpEF. The Simpson's Biplane method uses tracing of the endocardial border at end diastole and end systole to estimate LVEF. An alternative method is a visual estimation of LVEF; although the accuracy is operator dependent. The stroke volume is calculated subtracting LV systolic volume from LV diastolic volume. The assessment of RV systolic function is also an integral part of the echocardiographic examination. The most commonly used methods are tricuspid annular plane systolic excursion (TAPSE) and tissue Doppler imaging TDI of the RV. Estimation of the LV diastolic function in a patient with normal systolic function is a diagnostic challenge and defines the group of patients with HFpEF [35].

Measurement of ventricular (or atrial) volumes, diameters and mass by using the 2-D echocardiography has poor reproducibility according to a recent meta-analysis [36]. In contrast, a number of echocardiographic studies showed that adequate reproducibility, with respect to LV volume and mass, could be obtained following interventional procedures [37, 38]. Finally, the use of Doppler technique helps the examiner to assess valvular area, valvular abnormalities, such as stenosis or regurgitation, shunts, cardiac output and the diastolic function (E/A ratio).

New Echocardiographic Techniques

The implementation of 3D echocardiography complements 2D in the daily clinical practice. The estimation of LV mass, volume and EF with the real time 3D echocardiography correlates well with the cardiac magnetic resonance (CMR) findings, not only in sinus rhythm but also in patients with atrial fibrillation [39, 40]. Another promising indication of 3D echocardiography is the evaluation of valvular and congenital anomalies, in which 3D echocardiography has been proved to be very useful in guiding percutaneous procedures and intraoperative surgical interventions [41].

A relative new echocardiographic technique is the speckle tracking, which measures myocardial strain (longitudinal, circumferential, radial), strain rate, torsion and twist. In general, speckle-tracking's echocardiography main application is the evaluation of myocardial systolic and diastolic function in normal or pathological conditions. Speckle tracking echocardiography is used in

HT, DM, CAD, valvular heart disease, mechanical dyssynchrony, cardiomyopathies and HF [42]. Longitudinal strain allows the detection of early systolic dysfunction in patients with a pEF. In patients with HF and arterial HT longitudinal strain progressively deteriorates from NYHA class I to IV [43]. The same is true for patients with HFpEF [44]. In transplant patients without CAD who exhibit normal EF, deformation parameters are reduced suggesting that strain analysis is more sensitive than assessment of systolic function using EF [45].

Consideration of stress-strain relationships (LV size, arterial HT and LV wall thickness) is mandatory when interpreting strain [46]. 3D strain is an emerging echocardiographic technique that seems to be more reproducible, less time consuming and more accurate than 2D speckle tracking for the estimation of LV function [47].

Table 9. Estimation of myocardial viability in stress echocardiography [52].

Resting segmental function (at rest)	Low dobutamine dose	High dobutamine dose (maximal stress)	Type of response to dobutamine	Clinical interpretation	Likelihood for recovery of function
Abnormal	Improved	Worse than low dose	Biphasic	Viable -ischemic myocardium	Very high
Abnormal	Worse than rest or no change	Worse than rest or low dose	Worsening in function	Viable - ischemic myocardium	Medium
Abnormal	Improved	Further or continued improvement	Sustained (maintained) improvement in function	Viable - non-ischemic myocardium	Low
Abnormal	No change	No change	No change in function	Non-viable myocardium	Low

Stress Echocardiography

Stress echocardiography was first presented in 1979 and its main indication was the identification of patients with CAD. The basic principle of this technique is that stress (either physical or pharmacologic) induces ischemia, which in turn is depicted as a regional wall motion abnormality distal to an obstructive coronary artery. The sensitivity of exercise echocardiography ranges from 80 to 85% whereas the specificity from 80 to 88% [48]. Similar sensitivity and specificity exhibit the dobutamine stress echocardiography. Besides CAD investigation, stress echocardiography can be used for the assessment of post-acute myocardial infarction prognosis, preoperative risk, myocardial viability (Table **9**), severity of valvular heart disease and occult pulmonary hypertension, conditions that are often encountered in HF patients. Stress echocardiography has been recently used for the selection between left ventricular assist devices (LVAD) and biventricular assist devices (BiVAD) in patients with moderate RV dysfunction, the identification of factors that predict response to cardiac resynchronization therapy [49] and the estimation of prognosis in mild HF [49 - 51].

Magnetic Resonance Imaging (MRI)

Cardiac MR (CMR) has an emerging role in the non-invasive diagnostic assessment of HF. It is considered as the gold standard for the quantification of LV and RV volumes and EF. Therefore, it is often used in patients with inadequate acoustic window (*i.e.* COPD, obese) during the echocardiographic examination. Other indication of CMR is the assessment of LV diastolic function. Almost half of the patients with HF have pEF and diastolic dysfunction. The E/E′ ratio mentioned earlier correlates well with elevated filling pressures. Another application of CMR in HF patients is the determination of the cause of HF, whether it is CAD or cardiomyopathies and the differential diagnosis of the hypertensive, hypertrophic cardiomyopathy and amyloidosis [53, 54]. Lastly, the CMR can be used for the evaluation of myocardial viability, which is an important predictor of prognosis in patients with HF and CAD. In patients presenting with symptoms and signs of acute HF and normal coronary arteries, CMR is suggested as a part of the regular diagnostic algorithm in order to elucidate the underlying mechanism of HF. A recent study showed that assessment of LV dyssynchrony in advanced HF with MRI and myocardial strain can predict major cardiovascular events [55].

Cardiopulmonary Exercise Testing (CPX)

The role of CPX for the diagnostic and prognostic stratification of patients with preserved and reduced EF, is crucial. Functional capacity is measured in metabolic equivalents (METs), where 1 MET represents 3.5 mL O_2 / kg*/min. Exercise test is indicated in HF patients who are candidates for heart transplantation and those who need to undergo quantitative assessment of functional capacity. Among the variables used in CPX in patients with HFrEF, the most extensively studied are peak VO_2 and the VE/VO_2 slope [56]. A VE/VCO_2 slope ≥ 45 and a peak VO_2 < 10.0 mL $O_2 \cdot kg^{-1} \cdot min^{-1}$ are predictors of poor survival over the 4 year period following CPX test [57]. Other variables of poor prognosis are the presence of exercise oscillatory ventilation, a low rest/exercise partial pressure of end-tidal carbon dioxide ($P_{ET}CO_2$), a drop in systolic blood pressure during exercise test, ST changes, a low heart rate recovery at one minute post-exercise test and symptoms such as dyspnea [58 - 60]. In patients with HFpEF, the CPX is used for the grading of diastolic function and the assessment of prognosis. Patients with HF irrespective of the EF share common CPX variables.

Nuclear Imaging Techniques

The information needed for the diagnosis, staging, guidance of therapy and prognosis of HF patients is often depicted by nuclear non-invasive imaging techniques, such as single photon emission computed tomography (SPECT) and positron emission tomography (PET). Myocardial perfusion imaging (MPI) remains the cornerstone of diagnostic evaluation in HF and CAD. The etiology of HF (ischemic or non-ischemic) is often challenging. The traditional SPECT with thallium-201 (^{201}Tl) has a sensitivity that ranges from 73 to 92% and a specificity of 63-87% for the detection of CAD, whereas the vasodilator stress PET has sensitivity and specificity of 81–97% and 74-91%, respectively [61]. The evaluation of myocardial wall motion is another application of SPECT and PET. ^{99m}Tc-sestamibi SPECT under exercise stress can determine more accurately the etiology of HF (ischemic or not) [62]. The latter can be assessed with the combination of ^{13}N-NH_3 PET for perfusion and ^{18}F-FDG PET for glucose metabolism, with 100% sensitivity and 80% specificity [63]. Another very important indication of SPECT and PET is the detection of viable myocardium. ^{201}Tl imaging is often used for the detection of myocardial viability. A meta-analysis showed that the mean sensitivity and specificity of ^{201}Tl SPECT for the prediction of regional LV function improvement after revascularization were 86% and 59%, respectively [64]. 18F-FDG PET viability imaging is regarded as the gold standard for myocardial viability assessment [65]. The FDG PET imaging is also indicated for the identification of right HF and pulmonary HT [66]. The PET radiotracer ^{11}C-hydroxyephedrine is applicable in the investigation of the myocardial sympathetic innervations and not only provides valuable information on patient outcome but also guides the decision to implant an ICD in patients with a considerable risk for sudden cardiac death.

Computed Tomography (CT)

CT has potentially multiple indications in HF patients (Table **10**), its use is generally limited. There are various reasons for the limited use of CT in HF. Firstly, the lack of adequate image acquisition due to extra beats (ventricular or supraventricular), which are common in HF patients. In addition, the presence of atrial fibrillation, a frequent arrhythmia in HF, is another cause of poor quality CT images. The administration of b-blockers, in order to keep the heart rate as low as possible, is often problematic in HF patients with low blood pressure. Breathhold can also be an issue in patients with shortness of breath and contrast dye may cause harm in those with renal dysfunction. Finally, the radiation exposure is probably the main limitation for the routine use of CT in HF patients that need to undergo multiple times the same non-invasive test for the estimation of LVEF, LV volume or mass [67].

Table 10. Indications of computed tomography (CT) in heart failure.

• LV/RV volume estimation. • Estimation of LV or RV ejection fraction. • Viability assessment. • Cardiac dyssynchrony assessment.	• Coronary artery imaging. • Detection of specific cardiomyopathies. • Evaluation of myocardial cell therapy.

LV: left ventricle; RV: right ventricle.

Cardiac Catheterization

Despite the tremendous development of non-invasive techniques, such as the echocardiography or the MRI, the cardiac catheterization (right or left) remains the gold standard for the accurate estimation of hemodynamics in heart disease

[68]. The three main reasons to proceed to invasive evaluation in HF patients are: a) to clarify the diagnosis in patients with atypical symptoms, b) to assess pulmonary HT and c) to investigate if a candidate is suitable for advanced chronic HF therapies. The parameters that are commonly estimated during the invasive catheterization is the right atrial and ventricular pressure, the pulmonary capillary wedge pressure which reflects the left atrial pressure, the LV pressure, the cardiac output using either the Fick or the thermodilution method and the central venous pressure. The investigators of the ESCAPE randomized trial examined the safety and effectiveness of pulmonary artery catheterization (PAC) in patients hospitalized with severe symptomatic and recurrent HF [69]. They concluded that, although safe, there was no indication for routine performance of PACs to guide therapy during hospitalization for decompensation of chronic HF [69]. In the subgroup of patients, in whom signs and symptoms of congestion do not resolve with initial therapy, the implementation of PAC monitoring, at experienced centers, appears reasonable as the information derived from PAC may guide further therapeutic management [68].

In a recent study that compared the results derived from CPX test and right heart catheterization in ambulatory HF patients, the investigators demonstrated discordant findings with these two tests in 47% of the cohort [70]. Low cardiac index was independently related to poor outcomes. Other factors linked to poor outcomes were %VO2, LV size, and exercise time. In HF patients, the elevated pressures of the left heart are passively transmitted back into the pulmonary circulation, leading to elevated pulmonary arterial pressures (secondary pulmonary HT). This pathophysiological mechanism is common in HF and is a marker of disease severity and increased mortality [71]. All patients who are candidates for mechanical circulatory support should have invasive hemodynamics obtained to confirm the severity of HF, to measure pulmonary pressures and vascular resistance, and to assess RV function. Severe irreversible RV failure is a contraindication for LVAD implantation [2]. Although in patients who receive LVADs the survival is very good, not all patients progress smoothly, due to early right HF and failure to thrive, despite hemodynamic improvements [72]. Post-implantation RV failure either early or late has multiple causes, such as improved left-sided forward flow with mechanical unloading which often exacerbates the RV preload, in conjunction with perioperative transfusions of blood products that lead to leftward bowing of the septum, worsening of tricuspid regurgitation and ventriculo-arterial uncoupling [73]. The Interagency Registry for Mechanically Assisted Circulatory Support (INTERMACS) showed that although the majority of the hemodynamic factors are predictive factors of RV failure post-implantation, the multivariate analyses failed to demonstrate this notion. Continuous flow ventricular assist devices (VADs), such as the HeartMate II device, are now the predominant devices used for durable long-term mechanical circulatory support. LVAD documentation should be assessed at regular intervals [74].

Telemonitoring is a relative new diagnostic modality that seems to be beneficial in HF patients [75]. It includes the recording of variables such as body weight, heart rate, arterial blood pressure, and ECG, by portable devices that transmit remotely these data (*i.e. via* a telephone line) to a server where they can be stored, reviewed and analyzed by the investigator team. Implantable monitors include RV leads that measure intrathoracic impedance and pressure, wireless pulmonary artery pressure monitors, and left atrial pressure sensors [76].

Endomyocardial Biopsy

A recent study suggests that the diagnostic capability of CMR in patients with HF is similar or even better to endomyocardial biopsy [77]. Although the role of myocardial biopsy has diminished over the last years in HF patients, it remains important in a subgroup of patients with specific types of cardiomyopathy. Bennett MK *et al.* investigated the value of endomyocardial biopsy in 851 patients with unexplained HF from 2000 - 2009 and concluded that myocardial biopsy is useful in acute onset unexplained HF and rare clinical scenarios, such as suspected hypersensitivity myocarditis, anthracycline cardiomyopathy, cardiac tumors, and arrhythmogenic right ventricular dysplasia. However, it is rarely used in the usual care [78]. Furthermore, Cooper LT *et al.* reported 14 clinical scenarios in which endomyocardial biopsy should be highly considered [79]. If acute inflammatory myocarditis is the probable cause of HF, endomyocardial biopsy should be a part of the diagnostic algorithm, especially with the current availability of newer molecular markers. The management and prognosis is different with respect to various types of myocarditis. For example, patients with giant cell myocarditis experience rapid clinical deterioration and have poor prognosis. The management includes immunosuppressive therapy and often heart transplantation. On the contrary; patients with fulminant myocarditis may fully recover under hemodynamic support. Thus, the endomyocardial biopsy should be performed under strict indications in order to guide the diagnostic and therapeutic assessment of HF patient.

Genetic Evaluation

The reasons for implementation of genetic evaluation in the diagnostic algorithm of HF patients are multiple. Firstly, the conventional phenotype classification has limitations due to overlapping manifestations and genetic diversity of each cardiomyopathy. Despite genetic heterogeneity, homogeneity of cellular mechanisms may be used as a base to common therapy. In addition, genetic cascade screening is a cost-effective way of identifying the family members who need clinical assessment [80]. Cardiomyopathies with known genetic cause include hypertrophic, dilated, restrictive, arrhythmogenic right ventricular dysplasia/cardiomyopathy and left ventricular non-compaction [81]. The main indication of genetic testing remains the identification of high-risk individuals for these inherited cardiomyopathies who require careful evaluation and close monitoring. There is increasing evidence that the risk of HF depends on genetic predisposition; however, the genetic contribution to HF is heterogeneous and complex. The evaluation of pathogenicity remains problematic and it is likely to become worse as multiple rare variants emerge in cardiomyopathy genes from next-generation sequencing. With the progress of genetics, our understanding in pathophysiological and cellular mechanisms of HF becomes deeper. Pharmacogenomic-guided therapy is still under clinical investigation and genetic polymorphisms in the adrenergic receptors may be one of the earliest targets of personalized medicine [82].

COEXISTING CARDIOVASCULAR DISEASES

Comorbidities are defined as chronic conditions coexisting with HF that significantly affect its development, progression and response to treatment [83].

Comorbidities are divided into two main categories: a) cardiovascular and b) non-cardiovascular. The first group includes HT, CAD, peripheral artery disease, cerebrovascular disease, arrhythmias and valvular heart disease. Non-cardiovascular comorbidities include respiratory, endocrine, metabolic, nutritional, renal, hematopoietic, neurological, as well as musculoskeletal conditions [84]. The majority of patients with chronic HF (74%) had at least one comorbidity mainly renal disease, anemia, and DM according to data from the European Society of Cardiology Heart Failure Pilot Survey [85].

Although patients with HFpEF have an increased burden of comorbidities, such as anemia, DM, obesity and COPD, compared to patients with HFrEF, the increased risk of morbidity and mortality is general the same in these two populations [86]. However, unlike the numerous clinical studies for HFrEF, there is a lack of robust evidence for HFpEF and new clinical studies are needed to guide the treatment of comorbidities in these patients [87]. Apart from chronic HF, comorbidities are also evident in patients with acute HF who represent a heterogeneous cohort, affecting substantially the morbidity and mortality of this population. Attention to the diagnosis and management of comorbidities represents a critical step in the integrated care of patients with acute HF [88]. In summary, comorbidities whether cardiovascular or non-cardiovascular should prompt a proper investigation and treatment in patients with HFrEF or HFpEF, in order to reduce morbidity and improve prognosis and outcome.

Cardiovascular Comorbidities

Hypertension

Arterial HT is one of the most common risk factors for the development of HF. The presence of arterial HT is associated with a 2 – 3-fold higher risk of HF in the general population with a synergic effect with other causes of HF, such as valvular heart disease and CAD [89]. The prevalence of HT in trials ranges from 42% in the SOLVD trial to 64% in the more recent I-PRESERVE trial [90, 91]. Hypertension is often the substrate for the development of HF as it leads to LV hypertrophy and to LV diastolic dysfunction. Thus, HFpEF patients are often hypertensive. Nevertheless, HT and LV hypertrophy may also cause LV systolic dysfunction and HF when linked to other conditions, such as CAD and acute myocardial infarction. In patients with preserved LV systolic function, HT is a risk factor for symptomatic HF and, frequently, for acute HF. In contrast, in patients with LV systolic dysfunction, hypotension, rather than HT, is a risk factor of higher mortality and morbidity [92].

Coronary Artery Disease/Peripheral Artery Disease

CAD is the main cause of HF, especially when HT coexists [93]. It may be the initiating cause in almost 70% of cases of HF. Thus, in patients with HF symptoms of unknown etiology, the diagnostic algorithm should encompass the exclusion of ischemia with invasive (coronary angiography) or non-invasive (*i.e.* SPECT, stress echo, stress MRI) tests [2]. Peripheral artery disease is associated with a 2-fold increase in the prevalence of HF. Its prevalence in patients with HF is generally estimated 15 – 20% [94].

Cerebrovascular Disease

The most common cerebrovascular disease in patients with HF is ischemic stroke, which is often the result of atrial fibrillation, atrial flutter or even endocavitary thrombus. A meta-analysis by Witt BJ *et al.* showed that the stroke rate during the first year of HF, was 18.4 per 1,000 and tended to increase to a maximum of 47.4 strokes per 1,000 cases of HF after 4 to 5 years of follow-up [95]. Apart from patients with atrial fibrillation (both HFrEF and HFpEF), there is no evidence that an oral anticoagulant leads to lower mortality and morbidity compared to placebo or aspirin [96].

Arrhythmias

Arrhythmias (supraventricular or ventricular) are common in patients with HF. Multiple parameters trigger pathophysiologic mechanisms leading HF patients to arrhythmia, such as electrolyte abnormalities, ventricular remodeling, myocardial fibrosis and drugs with pro-arrhythmic effects. The most common supraventricular arrhythmia in patients with HF is atrial fibrillation, which increases the risk of thrombo-embolic complications and may lead to HF decompensation. Whether atrial fibrillation is an independent predictor of mortality and if it can cause systolic HF ('tachycardiomyopathy'), are less certain. Ventricular arrhythmias in patients with HF are life-threatening conditions. Therefore, in patients with symptomatic HF and EF ≤35%, an ICD is recommended for primary prevention according to more recent ESC guidelines.

Valvular Heart Disease

Valvular heart disease may cause or aggravate HF. The main issue in patients with HFrEF is the entity of 'low-flow, low-gradient' aortic stenosis (valve area <1 cm^2, EF <40%, mean gradient <40 mmHg). Some patients may have severe aortic stenosis and others 'pseudo-aortic stenosis'. Dobutamine stress echocardiography is the examination of choice and often discriminates these two conditions.

LV dilatation and remodeling lead to reduced leaflet coaptation and to secondary (or functional) mitral valve regurgitation. There is a bidirectional interaction between the secondary mitral valve regurgitation and the LV enlargement. Thus, the worsening of HF leads to the augmentation of the regurgitant blood volume and vice versa. The estimation of the mitral valve regurgitation in patients with low EF is often challenging. Independently of myocardial function, mitral and tricuspid regurgitation are known risk factors of mortality [97]. Medical therapy and cardiac resynchronization therapy may decrease mitral and tricuspid regurgitation based on LV reverse remodelling [98]. The role of surgery on outcomes is less clear. New techniques (mitra-Clip) of percutaneous treatment of mitral regurgitation may offer another therapeutic option.

Non-cardiovascular Comorbidities

Anemia

Anemia, which is defined according to WHO as a hemoglobin (Hb) concentration <13 g/dL in men and <12 g/dL in women, is common in HF, particularly in hospitalized patients. Data from the Framingham study showed that lower hematocrit correlates with increased risk of developing HF [99]. Anemia is more frequent in women, the elderly, and in patients with impaired renal function and it is linked to more symptoms, worse functional status, greater risk of HF hospitalization, and poorer survival [2]. In HF, multiple pathophysiological mechanisms, including the renin-angiotensin system, hematinic abnormalities (mainly iron deficiency), chronic inflammation, hemodilution and co-existent chronic kidney disease, may lead to anemia. The diagnostic evaluation is the same in HF patients with or without anemia and the correctable causes should be treated accordingly. Sometimes, the cause remains unclear.

The best evidence on whether treatment with erythropoietin-stimulating agents in patients with HF and anemia is beneficial comes from the Reduction of Events with Darbepoetin Alfa in Heart Failure (RED-HF) trial, the largest multicenter, randomized, controlled trial to date [100]. In this study, 2,278 patients with systolic HF (LVEF ≤40%, NYHA functional class ≥2) and anemia (Hb 9–12 g/dL) were randomized into two groups (darbepoetin alfa administration or placebo group). After a median follow up period of 28 months, Hb in the darbepoetin alfa group rose, but remained stable in the placebo group. However, there was no significant difference between the darbepoetin alfa and placebo groups for the primary composite outcome of death from any cause or first HF hospitalization [101]. On the contrary, the FAIR-HF study showed that treatment with intravenous ferric carboxymaltose in patients with chronic HF and iron deficiency, with or without anemia, improves symptoms, functional capacity and quality of life; with acceptable side effects [102].

Chronic Obstructive Pulmonary Disease (COPD)

The incidence of COPD in patients with HF ranges from 9 to 52% and its adverse effects are similar both in HFrEF and HFpEF [103]. Common risk factors such as smoking and systemic inflammation may explain the interaction between HF and COPD [104]. It is often difficult to differentiate whether the cause of dyspnea is the HFpEF or the COPD [105]. The symptoms are similar and the ECG, chest X-ray, echocardiography and spirometry are sometimes not diagnostic. The natriuretic peptides (BNP, NT-proBNP and MR-proANP) may be helpful. HF and COPD patients are related to worse functional status and a less favorable prognosis. In addition, COPD is an independent predictor of worse outcomes in HF [2]. Beta-blockers are contraindicated in asthma but not in COPD. In the latter, a selective beta-1 adrenoreceptor antagonist (*i.e.* bisoprolol, metoprolol succinate, or nebivolol) is generally indicated [106]. Oral corticosteroids should be avoided in patients with HF and COPD, as they can lead sodium and water retention.

Cachexia

The definition of cachexia is not universally accepted. Probably, the most widely accepted one is proposed by Akashi YJ *et al.* and defines cachexia as involuntary non-edematous weight loss ≥ 6% of total body weight within the previous 6 – 12 months [107]. It is a generalized process; wasting affects all body compartments, especially lean tissue, fat tissue and bone tissue and occurs in 10–15% of patients with HF. The pathophysiology of cachexia includes poor nutrition, malabsorption, impaired calorie and protein balance, hormone resistance, immune activation, neurohormonal disorders, and reduced anabolic drive. The terms malnutrition and cachexia are frequently used interchangeably, and most researchers do not discriminate between the 2 conditions in their clinical studies, as they are phenotypically similar and often coexist [108]. The nutrition risk that is not combined with an inflammatory condition is defined as starvation-related malnutrition (such as anorexia nervosa), whereas the presence of either chronic or acute inflammation results in malnutrition, traditionally known as cachexia [109]. Cachexia treatments, although not evidence based, include appetite stimulants, exercise training, and anabolic agents (insulin, anabolic steroids) in combination with nutritional supplements.

Obesity

Obesity is a very common comorbidity in the HF population. Some studies have shown that up to 32 - 49% of patients with HF are obese and 31% to 40% are overweight (body mass index, BMI=25.0-29.9 kg/m^2) [110, 111]. A small number of patients with HF are classified as underweight. Patients who are overweight and obese present with symptomatology of HF 10 years earlier than their leaner counterparts [112]. Interestingly, obesity is significantly more prevalent in patients with HFpEF compared with those with HFrEF [113].

"The cardiomyopathy of obesity" was first described back in 1992 by Kasper *et al.*, based on hemodynamic and endomyocardial biopsy abnormalities associated with marked obesity when compared with lean controls [114]. The mechanisms linking obesity to HF include HT, DM and dyslipidemia, all of which augment the risk of myocardial infarction, altered LV remodeling, cardiac steatosis, lipoapoptosis and obstructive sleep apnea (OSA). Notably, HT and DM independently increase the risk of HF [115]. The diagnosis of HF in obese patients is often challenging. Obese patients, even in the absence of HF, often present with dyspnea, effort intolerance, and ankle swelling. On top of that, obese HF patients have reduced natriuretic peptide levels and poor-quality echocardiographic images. The increased survival observed in obese patients with HF is called the "obesity paradox". A common explanation for this phenomenon is that the additional adipose tissue offers greater reserves against the catabolic changes related to the disease process that can lead to cardiac cachexia.

Cancer

Cancer is an expanding pandemic disease. It is estimated that more than 1.6 million new cases of cancer in the USA will be diagnosed in 2015, according to the American Cancer Society. Among women, breast cancer is the most common cancer (29%). Current cancer treatment consists of a combination of chemotherapy, radiotherapy, and surgery to prolong life and provide cure. However, some of these treatments are linked to cardiovascular complications, such as HF. Main risk factors for LV dysfunction and cardiomyopathy are the cumulative dose, the administration schedule, and the concomitant use of other cardiotoxic therapies [116]. The best recognized cardiotoxic chemotherapeutic agents are the anthracyclines (*e.g.* doxorubicin), and trastuzumab, which are used for the treatment of breast cancer [117]. Cardiotoxicity associated with anthracycline administration has been categorized into acute, early-onset chronic progressive, and late-onset chronic progressive. Free radical formation is generally considered as the main mechanism of anthracycline-induced cardiotoxicity. Cardiotoxicity caused by trastuzumab is probably secondary to inhibition of ErbB2 signaling, thereby affecting normal growth and survival of cardiomyocytes [118].

Timely evaluation of EF is crucial in patients receiving cardiotoxic chemotherapy. Preventative measures include minimization of the patient's lifetime cumulative dose, changing the anthracycline administration (*e.g.*, continuous infusion *vs.*

bolus administration), use of liposomal anthracyclines or anthracycline analogues (*e.g.*, idarubicin), and also the addition of cardioprotectants (*e.g.*, dexrazoxane) to anthracycline treatment [119]. In patients who develop LV systolic dysfunction, chemotherapy should be discontinued and guidelines recommended treatment for HFrEF should be initiated.

Depression

Depression affects negatively patients with cardiovascular diseases [120]. It is an independent risk factor for the future development of HF [121]. Furthermore, the presence of depression is independently associated with severe functional impairment, increased risk of mortality and hospital readmission and thus poor prognosis for patients with already existing HF [122, 123]. Plasma B-type natriuretic peptide and interleukin-10 levels predict adverse clinical outcome in depressed HF patients [124]. In the elderly, a high index of suspicion is required to make the diagnosis. Validated questionnaires are used to identify patients with mood disorders or depression. The treatment consists of psychosocial intervention and pharmacological agents. The latter are mostly represented by selective serotonin reuptake inhibitors, which are considered to be safe in HF patients [2]. Tricyclic antidepressants should be avoided, because they may cause hypotension, worsening of HF, and arrhythmias [125].

Diabetes Mellitus (DM)

DM is an established risk factor for HF. The prevalence of DM in the general population is 6 – 8%, but it is higher in people with symptomatic HF (12 – 30%). Among hospitalized HF patients, DM prevalence is increasing towards 40% [126]. In the CHARM study, DM proved to be an independent negative prognostic factor in HF patients [127]. Diabetic patients have an almost two-fold increased risk (adjusted for all the other known risk factors) of HF [128]. There is a correlation between plasma glucose levels, the HbA1c percentage, and the risk of developing HF [129]. Thus, each 1% increase in HbA1c is associated with an 8% increased risk of HF [130]. The DM leads to HF through multiple mechanisms, such as the CAD, obesity and HT. In addition, hyperglycemia is, by itself, a cause of myocardial damage (diabetic cardiomyopathy). Endothelial dysfunction, increased circulating free fatty acids and pro-inflammatory state may all contribute to the development of myocardial dysfunction and HF. The OPTIMIZE-HF study revealed a high prevalence of DM in hospitalized patients with HF [131]. Although HF patients with DM experienced similar short-term mortality compared to patients without DM, the presence of DM was related to a higher risk of rehospitalization [131]. The diagnosis of diabetic cardiomyopathy is based on the echocardiographic findings of diastolic dysfunction [129]. Diastolic dysfunction may progress in a time-dependent fashion, leading to systolic dysfunction. Angiotensin converting enzyme inhibitor (ACE-I) is indicated in DM and HF, because it improves symptoms and reduces mortality, while a beta-blocker should be administered to all patients with an LVEF $\leq$40%. If the symptoms persist, despite ACE-I and beta-blocker administration, a mineralocorticoid receptor antagonist should be added [132]. The target HbA_1C should be approximately 7% while metformin is the recommended first-hand glucose lowering treatment [132].

Hyperlipidemia

An elevated level of low-density lipoprotein (LDL) is an unusual finding in patients with HFrEF [2]. In addition, patients with advanced HFrEF and cachexia, often have low concentrations of LDL, which is a marker of poor prognosis [133]. The same is true for the elderly people with advanced HF [134]. Low total cholesterol is not an independent prognostic factor in dilated cardiomyopathy [135]. Dyslipidemia may play a role in the etiology and pathogenesis of unknown cause HF. Rosuvastatin failed to show benefit with respect to morbidity and mortality in HF patients in two recent randomized trials [136, 137]. Based on the findings of the GISSI-HF and CORONA trials, statins were not confirmed to be beneficial in patients with non-ischemic HF. In patients with ischemic HF, CORONA reported a morbidity benefit with lower hospitalizations for cardiovascular causes. Therefore, it may be advisable to prescribe statins in patients with ischemic HF, especially if their LDL cholesterol levels are significantly increased and/or their congestive HF is mild [138].

Gout

Hyperuricaemia and gout are common comorbidities in HF and may be caused or worsened by diuretic treatment or renal dysfunction or even the combination of these two factors. Patients with HFrEF and hyperuricaemia have worse prognosis than those with HFrEF without hyperuricaemia [139]. Gout is also related to higher risk for clinical HF, subclinical findings of systolic dysfunction and mortality. Non-steroidal anti-inflammatory drugs (NSAIDs) should be avoided in patients with HF and gout attacks because these drugs may decompensate the HF patient. Xanthine oxidase inhibitors (*i.e.* allopurinol) may assist in the prevention of gout attacks. The "Efficacy and Safety Study of Oxypurinol Added to Standard Therapy in Patients with NYHA Class III-IV Congestive Heart Failure" (OPT-CHF) has reported a favorable functional clinical effect of the medication oxypurinol in HF patients with initially high serum levels of uric acid [140]. Some other studies have shown an improvement in both LV hypertrophy and endothelial function and also in clinical outcomes of HF among patients with hyperuricaemia who receive allopurinol treatment [141 - 143]. Another medication used for the prevention of gout attacks is colchicine, which should not be used in patients with renal dysfunction due to the risk of diarrhea. Lastly, systemic corticosteroids are contraindicated because they cause water and sodium retention, with the exception of the intra-articular corticosteroids which can be used as second line therapy in mono-articular gout [2].

Erectile Dysfunction

Almost 30% of the HF population is totally absent of sexual activity due to the concern about the potential corresponding risks [144]. Erectile dysfunction and HF share common risk factors such as age, HT, dyslipidemia, DM, smoking, obesity, depression and alcohol consumption. Causes of erectile dysfunction in patients with HF include endothelial dysfunction, atherosclerosis, cardiac drugs, exercise tolerance reduction, psychogenic factors and HF related hypogonadism [145]. The management of these patients consists of the risk factors modification, the guideline directed pharmacological therapy for HF (drugs with no or low effect on patient's erectile function) and the use of phosphodiesterase V inhibitors which are not contraindicated in patients not receiving nitrates. In patients with stable HF, sexual activity is not contraindicated, as it is a form of moderate physical exertion [145].

Thyroid Dysfunction

Thyroid hormones affect every cell, tissue, and organ in the body and their normal secretion, absorption and metabolism are essential for the optimal functioning of the heart. Thyroid dysfunction is present in 5% to 10% of the population, mostly in women and patients over 60 years of age [146]. Hyperthyroidism is associated with supraventricular arrhythmias and especially atrial fibrillation [147]. The cardiac and hemodynamic consequences of hyperthyroidism include the reduction of the systemic vascular resistance, decrease in renal perfusion, decrease in afterload, peripheral vasodilatation, concentric cardiac hypertrophy, reduced functional cardiac reserve and physical load tolerance, pulmonary HT and increase in sympathetic tone [148]. On the contrary, hypothyroidism often features negative chronotropic and inotropic state, ventricular tachyarrhythmias because of bradycardia and hypothermia, peripheral vasoconstriction, pericarditis, increase in arterial stiffness, reduction in myocardial contractility and bradycardia [148]. The effects of hypothyroidism on HF risk and mortality rates are discrepant [149 - 151]. Patients with ischemic or non-ischemic HF who participated in SCD-HeFT (Sudden Cardiac Death in Heart Failure Trial) were randomized to placebo or amiodarone or ICD therapy [152]. Thyroid-stimulating hormone was measured at baseline and at 6-month intervals throughout the 5-year study. This trial showed that impaired thyroid function in patients with symptomatic HF and EF ≤35% was associated with significantly elevated risk for death, even after adjustment for known mortality predictors [152].

Sleep Disturbance and Sleep-disordered Breathing

Patients with HF often complain for sleep disturbances. The main causes are pulmonary congestion, which leads to orthopnea and paroxysmal nocturnal dyspnea, diuretic therapy that provokes or augments nocturnal diuresis, anxiety and other psychological problems [2]. Approximately, one-third of patients with HF have sleep-disordered breathing [153]. Sleep apnea (SA) is an independent risk factor for both HFrEF and HFpEF [154]. SA is characterized by repetitive apneas and hypopneas leading to adverse cardiovascular events. The two main phenotypes of SA, obstructive (OSA) and central sleep apnea (CSA), are related to similar pathophysiologic consequences in HF and increase both morbidity and mortality [155, 156]. SA leads to intermittent hypoxemia, hypercapnia and sympathetic excitation. In particular, OSA causes recurrent episodes of negative intrathoracic pressure and LV afterload increases. Patients are obese and snore or exhibit daytime somnolence. However, not all patients with OSA are obese. The prevalence of CSA in HF (Cheyne–Stokes respiration) is uncertain and may have declined since the widespread use of modern HF therapies such as b-blockers and CRT. The test for diagnosing sleep disorders is called polysomnography (PSG). PSG includes the continuous recording of brain waves, nasal and oral airflow, thoracoabdominal excursions, pulse oximetry, ECG and anterior tibialis muscle electromyogram. By interpreting these tracings, the physician can obtain valuable information such as the total sleep time, sleep onset, rapid-eye-movement (REM) sleep, non-REM and sleep-related breathing patterns. Apnea is defined as a breathing cessation for at least 10 sec [157]. OSA treatment is mainly continuous positive airway pressure (C-PAP), whereas treatment of CSA includes optimization of HF treatment, night oxygen therapy and non-invasive positive pressure ventilation [158]. Adaptive servo-ventilation improves exercise capacity, quality of life, and cardiac function in HF patients with CSA [159].

Renal Dysfunction

Renal dysfunction (RD) is a frequent coexisting disease and a major prognostic parameter in the HF population [160, 161]. The majority of HF patients have mild or moderate RD [162]. In a meta-analysis enrolling 80,098 hospitalized and non-hospitalized HF patients, 63% had some degree of RD [163]. In the Candesartan in Heart Failure Assessment of Reduction in Mortality and Morbidity (CHARM) study, RD was reported in 36% of HF patients [164]. In addition, the Acute Decompensated Heart Failure National Registry (ADHERE) showed renal impairment in the majority of patients hospitalized with acute decompensated HF [165]. Sodium and water depletion and hypotension are well-recognized causes of renal dysfunction. Notably, volume overload, right HF, and renal venous congestion may also cause RD. Other causes of RD are prostatic obstruction and nephrotoxic drugs such as NSAIDs and certain antibiotics (*e.g.* trimethoprim) [2].

There is a strong interplay between the heart and the kidneys. The term "cardiorenal syndrome" refers to a clinical condition that includes a broad spectrum of acute and chronic impairments, in which the primary failing organ could be either the heart or the kidneys. Any primary impairment in one of the two organs promotes and causes a combination of feedback mechanisms that further worsen the function of both the heart and the kidney. The pathophysiological mechanisms of cardiorenal syndrome include hemodynamic imbalance, neurohormonal signaling and inflammatory activation [166]. However, they are not fully understood. Transient increases of creatinine in patients with acute HF are not prognostically important, whereas persistent deterioration is associated with a higher mortality in this patient population. Congestion plays a pivotal role in the course of renal function deterioration and the combination of congestion and renal dysfunction is the most important clinical prognostic factor in acute and chronic HF patients [167].

Thiazide diuretics seem to be less effective in patients with a very low e-GFR and certain renally excreted drugs (*e.g.* digoxin, insulin, and low molecular weight heparins) may accumulate in patients with RD and should be avoided. A rise in urea and creatinine is expected after the implementation of ACE-I. If creatinine increases by >100% or to >3.5 mg/dL (or e-GFR <20 mL/min/1.73 m^2), ACE-I (or angiotensin-receptor blocker) administration should be discontinued and specialist advice sought [2]. With regard to mineralocorticoid receptor antagonists, if creatinine rises to 2.5 mg/dL or e-GFR <30 mL/min/1.73 m^2, the physician should halve the dose and monitor blood chemistry closely. If creatinine increases to >3.5 mg/dL or e-GFR <20 mL/min/1.73 m^2 the mineralocorticoid receptor antagonist should be stopped immediately and specialist advice is needed [2].

PROGNOSTICATION OF HEART FAILURE (HF) PATIENTS

The prognostic evaluation of patients with HF is an integral part of the clinical assessment, as it often guides the management of these patients. For example, the decision for transplantation or implantation of VADs highly depends on the expected outcome of patients with end stage HF. On the contrary, those with poor prognosis should receive palliative care.

A number of variables provide prognostic information in HF [2]. Among them, age, sex, ethnicity, NYHA functional class, body mass index, signs of congestion, presence of S_3, low systolic blood pressure, DM, depression, COPD and CAD are the most common parameters regarding demographics, patient's history and physical examination. In addition, routine laboratory tests such as liver enzymes, urea, creatinine, e-GFR, red cell distribution width and high sensitive troponin (either T or I) are of prognostic significance. Furthermore, a thorough laboratory evaluation should encompass the neurohormones. In clinical practice the most commonly measured neurohormones are the cytokines, renin activity, angiotensin II, aldosterone, catecholamines, natriuretic peptides and copeptin. Serum prolactin is related to neurohormonal activation and depressive symptoms and is an independent prognostic factor in advanced HF [168]. Recently, a growing interest in two biomarkers, namely sST-2 and galectin-3 has emerged, with respect to their prognostic value both in acute and chronic HF [169 - 171]. Apart from medical history, physical examination and laboratory tests, the physician can receive valuable prognostic information from the ECG. Augmented QRS width, LV hypertrophy, atrial fibrillation, complex ventricular arrhythmias and low heart rate variability are markers of poor prognosis. On top of the ECG findings, imaging parameters such as LVEF, left atrial size, restrictive filling pattern, right ventricular function and wall motion index may assist in the prediction of patient's outcome. Equally important are the exercise test parameters or hemodynamic variables such as the $VO_{2,}$ VE/VCO2 slope, 6-min walk distance, pulmonary artery wedge pressure and cardiac index.

Several "risk scores" models have been developed over the past decades for both acute and chronic HF. The "Seattle Heart Failure Model" is a calculator of projected survival at baseline and after interventions for patients with HF. Therefore, it provides an accurate estimation of mean, 1-, 2-, and 3-year survival based on easily obtained clinical, pharmacological, device, and laboratory characteristics [172]. It was developed from a database of 1,125 patients in the PRAISE-1 clinical trial, confined to patients with severe HF (NYHA class III B or IV and EF ≤30%). Recently, a new risk score, the "MAGGIC Risk Score", has been developed for the prognostic assessment in HF, based on the MAGGIC meta-analysis [173]. The latter includes individual data on 39,372 patients with

HF with reduced and preserved EF. The model includes 13 independent predictors of mortality in the following order of predictive strength: age, lower EF, NYHA class, serum creatinine, DM, not prescribed beta-blocker, lower systolic blood pressure, lower body mass, time since diagnosis, current smoker, COPD, male gender, and not prescribed ACE-I or angiotensin-receptor blockers. The simplified integer risk score can be easily used in the daily practice. The "Mortality Risk Score for Heart Failure" is a statistical model developed from chart-abstracted data from the National Heart Care Project and it is intended for use in patients aged 65 and older [174]. Another risk score, which is valid in acute decompensated HF and predicts patients' in-hospital mortality, is the "ADHERE CART Risk Score" [175]. The risk stratification is based on the estimation of 3 parameters: a) blood urea nitrogen (BUN), b) serum creatinine level and c) systolic blood pressure at admission, which proved to be independent predictors of high risk for in-hospital mortality in the current CART analysis. Thus, acute decompensated HF patients can be readily stratified into groups of low, intermediate, and high risk for in-hospital mortality, with mortality risks ranging from 2.1% to 21.9%. Lastly, the "Readmission score" estimates the risk of 30-day readmission rates after discharge for HF [176]. This score can be a measure of health system's performance and facilitates tracking of improvement over time. However, the use of these prognostic variables and risk scores in routine clinical practice remains challenging. Yet, there is no universally accepted algorithm to triage HF therapeutic approaches based on prognostic evaluation.

CONCLUDING REMARKS

Despite major treatment improvements in virtually all cardiac disorders, HF is an exception. Its prevalence is increasing, and only short prolongations in survival are occurring. Given this trend, attention is being directed to identifying high risk individuals for developing HF. The diagnosis of HF is predominantly based on history and physical examination, although echocardiography and cardiac catheterization can be beneficial. Furthermore, HF is characterized by the presence of complex bidirectional associations with multiple cardiac and non-cardiac comorbidities. Nevertheless, these complex associations are not necessarily due to direct organ to organ interactions and may be linked to several confounding factors that affect their development. Determination of the etiology of a HF exacerbation is crucial to guide patients' treatment in order to improve the current HF symptoms, as well as to prevent recurrence.

CONFLICT OF INTEREST

The authors confirm that they have no conflict of interest to declare for this publication.

ACKNOWLEDGEMENTS

Declared none.

REFERENCES

[1] Braunwald E. Clinical manifestations of heart failure. In: Braunwald E, Ed. Braunwald's Heart Disease: A Textbook of Cardiovascular Medicine. Philadelphia: Saunders 1988; pp. 471-84.

[2] McMurray JJ, Adamopoulos S, Anker SD, *et al.* ESC Guidelines for the diagnosis and treatment of acute and chronic heart failure 2012: The Task Force for the Diagnosis and Treatment of Acute and Chronic Heart Failure 2012 of the European Society of Cardiology. Developed in collaboration with the Heart Failure Association (HFA) of the ESC. Eur Heart J 2012; 33(14): 1787-847. [http://dx.doi.org/10.1093/eurheartj/ehs104] [PMID: 22611136]

[3] Mozaffarian D, Benjamin EJ, Go AS, *et al.* Heart disease and stroke statistics--2015 update: a report from the American Heart Association. Circulation 2015; 131(4): e29-e322. [http://dx.doi.org/10.1161/CIR.0000000000000152] [PMID: 25520374]

[4] Heidenreich PA, Albert NM, Allen LA, *et al.* Forecasting the impact of heart failure in the United States: a policy statement from the American Heart Association. Circ Heart Fail 2013; 6(3): 606-19. [http://dx.doi.org/10.1161/HHF.0b013e318291329a] [PMID: 23616602]

[5] Tang WH, Francis GS. Clinical Evaluation of Heart Failure. In: Mann DL, Felker GM, Eds. Heart Failure: A Companion to Braunwald's Heart Disease. Philadelphia: Elsevier 2015; p. 421.

[6] Butler J, Kalogeropoulos A, Georgiopoulou V, *et al.* Incident heart failure prediction in the elderly: the health ABC heart failure score. Circ Heart Fail 2008; 1(2): 125-33. [http://dx.doi.org/10.1161/CIRCHEARTFAILURE.108.768457] [PMID: 19777072]

[7] Agarwal SK, Chambless LE, Ballantyne CM, *et al.* Prediction of incident heart failure in general practice: the Atherosclerosis Risk in Communities (ARIC) Study. Circ Heart Fail 2012; 5(4): 422-9. [http://dx.doi.org/10.1161/CIRCHEARTFAILURE.111.964841] [PMID: 22589298]

[8] Ammar KA, Jacobsen SJ, Mahoney DW, *et al.* Prevalence and prognostic significance of heart failure stages: application of the American College of Cardiology/American Heart Association heart failure staging criteria in the community. Circulation 2007; 115(12): 1563-70. [http://dx.doi.org/10.1161/CIRCULATIONAHA.106.666818] [PMID: 17353436]

[9] The Criteria Committee of the New York Heart Association. Nomenclature and Criteria for Diagnosis of Diseases of the Heart and Great Vessels. 9th ed. Boston, Mass: Little, Brown & Co; 1994: 253-256.

[10] Opasich C, Rapezzi C, Lucci D, *et al.* Precipitating factors and decision-making processes of short-term worsening heart failure despite "optimal" treatment (from the IN-CHF Registry). Am J Cardiol 2001; 88(4): 382-7.
[http://dx.doi.org/10.1016/S0002-9149(01)01683-6] [PMID: 11545758]

[11] Chatterjee NA, Fifer MA. Clinical Manifestations. In: Lilly LS, Ed. Pathophysiology of Heart Disease. 5th ed. Philadelphia: Lippincott Williams & Wilkins 2014; pp. 232-3.

[12] Wilson JR, Mancini DM. The mechanism of exertional fatigue in heart failure. Cardioscience 1990; 1(1): 13-7.
[PMID: 2102792]

[13] Lunde PK, Verburg E, Vøllestad NK, Sejersted OM. Skeletal muscle fatigue in normal subjects and heart failure patients. Is there a common mechanism? Acta Physiol Scand 1998; 162(3): 215-28.
[http://dx.doi.org/10.1046/j.1365-201X.1998.0343f.x] [PMID: 9578367]

[14] Perez-Moreno AC, Jhund PS, Macdonald MR, *et al.* Fatigue as a predictor of outcome in patients with heart failure: analysis of CORONA (Controlled Rosuvastatin Multinational Trial in Heart Failure). JACC Heart Fail 2014; 2(2): 187-97.
[http://dx.doi.org/10.1016/j.jchf.2014.01.001] [PMID: 24720928]

[15] Navas JP, Martinez-Maldonado M. Pathophysiology of edema in congestive heart failure. Heart Dis Stroke 1993; 2(4): 325-9.
[PMID: 8156185]

[16] Malacco E, Varì N, Capuano V, Spagnuolo V, Borgnino C, Palatini P. A randomized, double-blind, active-controlled, parallel-group comparison of valsartan and amlodipine in the treatment of isolated systolic hypertension in elderly patients: the Val-Syst study. Clin Ther 2003; 25(11): 2765-80.
[http://dx.doi.org/10.1016/S0149-2918(03)80332-6] [PMID: 14693303]

[17] Thibodeau JT, Turer AT, Gualano SK, *et al.* Characterization of a novel symptom of advanced heart failure: bendopnea. JACC Heart Fail 2014; 2(1): 24-31.
[http://dx.doi.org/10.1016/j.jchf.2013.07.009] [PMID: 24622115]

[18] Brandon N, Mehra MR. "Flexo-dyspnea": A novel clinical observation in the heart failure syndrome. J Heart Lung Transplant 2013; 32(8): 844-5.
[http://dx.doi.org/10.1016/j.healun.2013.06.006] [PMID: 23856222]

[19] Badgett RG, Lucey CR, Mulrow CD. Can the clinical examination diagnose left-sided heart failure in adults? JAMA 1997; 277(21): 1712-9.
[http://dx.doi.org/10.1001/jama.1997.03540450068038] [PMID: 9169900]

[20] Nadir AM, Beadle R, Lim HS. Kussmaul physiology in patients with heart failure. Circ Heart Fail 2014; 7(3): 440-7.
[http://dx.doi.org/10.1161/CIRCHEARTFAILURE.113.000830] [PMID: 24619369]

[21] Gheorghiade M, Filippatos G, De Luca L, Burnett J. Congestion in acute heart failure syndromes: an essential target of evaluation and treatment. Am J Med 2006; 119(12) (Suppl. 1): S3-S10.
[http://dx.doi.org/10.1016/j.amjmed.2006.09.011] [PMID: 17113398]

[22] Gheorghiade M, Abraham WT, Albert NM, *et al.* Relationship between admission serum sodium concentration and clinical outcomes in patients hospitalized for heart failure: an analysis from the

OPTIMIZE-HF registry. Eur Heart J 2007; 28(8): 980-8.
[http://dx.doi.org/10.1093/eurheartj/ehl542] [PMID: 17309900]

[23] Ohlow MA, Lauer B. Coarctation of aorta with complete aortic occlusion. J Geriatr Cardiol 2013; 10(4): 383-5.
[PMID: 24454333]

[24] Harlan WR, Oberman A, Grimm R, Rosati RA. Chronic congestive heart failure in coronary artery disease: clinical criteria. Ann Intern Med 1977; 86(2): 133-8.
[http://dx.doi.org/10.7326/0003-4819-86-2-133] [PMID: 835934]

[25] Braunwald E. Heart failure. JACC Heart Fail 2013; 1(1): 1-20.
[http://dx.doi.org/10.1016/j.jchf.2012.10.002] [PMID: 24621794]

[26] Maisel AS, Krishnaswamy P, Nowak RM, *et al.* Rapid measurement of B-type natriuretic peptide in the emergency diagnosis of heart failure. N Engl J Med 2002; 347(3): 161-7.
[http://dx.doi.org/10.1056/NEJMoa020233] [PMID: 12124404]

[27] Januzzi JL Jr, Camargo CA, Anwaruddin S, *et al.* The N-terminal Pro-BNP investigation of dyspnea in the emergency department (PRIDE) study. Am J Cardiol 2005; 95(8): 948-54.
[http://dx.doi.org/10.1016/j.amjcard.2004.12.032] [PMID: 15820160]

[28] de Boer RA, Yu L, van Veldhuisen DJ. Galectin-3 in cardiac remodeling and heart failure. Curr Heart Fail Rep 2010; 7(1): 1-8.
[http://dx.doi.org/10.1007/s11897-010-0004-x] [PMID: 20425490]

[29] Kakkar R, Lee RT. The IL-33/ST2 pathway: therapeutic target and novel biomarker. Nat Rev Drug Discov 2008; 7(10): 827-40.
[http://dx.doi.org/10.1038/nrd2660] [PMID: 18827826]

[30] Karayannis G, Triposkiadis F, Skoularigis J, Georgoulias P, Butler J, Giamouzis G. The emerging role of Galectin-3 and ST2 in heart failure: practical considerations and pitfalls using novel biomarkers. Curr Heart Fail Rep 2013; 10(4): 441-9.
[http://dx.doi.org/10.1007/s11897-013-0169-1] [PMID: 24142671]

[31] Josephson ME, Wellens HJ. The ECG in left bundle branch block and heart failure. Heart Rhythm 2015; 12(1): 250-1.
[http://dx.doi.org/10.1016/j.hrthm.2014.08.024] [PMID: 25542713]

[32] Van Bommel R, Marsan N, Delgado V, *et al.* ECG in detecting right ventricular dilatation in the presence of left bundle branch block. Am J Cardiol 2011; 107: 736.
[http://dx.doi.org/10.1016/j.amjcard.2010.10.051] [PMID: 21185006]

[33] Chakko S, Woska D, Martinez H, *et al.* Clinical, radiographic, and hemodynamic correlations in chronic congestive heart failure: conflicting results may lead to inappropriate care. Am J Med 1991; 90(3): 353-9.
[http://dx.doi.org/10.1016/0002-9343(91)80016-F] [PMID: 1825901]

[34] Aleman C, Chan SB, Kordick MF. Correlation between chest x-ray and B-type natriuretic peptide in congestive heart failure. Am J Emerg Med 2005; 23(4): 501-3.
[http://dx.doi.org/10.1016/j.ajem.2004.12.009] [PMID: 16032620]

[35] Little WC, Oh JK. Echocardiographic evaluation of diastolic function can be used to guide clinical

care. Circulation 2009; 120(9): 802-9.
[http://dx.doi.org/10.1161/CIRCULATIONAHA.109.869602] [PMID: 19720946]

[36] Thavendiranathan P, Grant AD, Negishi T, Plana JC, Popović ZB, Marwick TH. Reproducibility of echocardiographic techniques for sequential assessment of left ventricular ejection fraction and volumes: application to patients undergoing cancer chemotherapy. J Am Coll Cardiol 2013; 61(1): 77-84.
[http://dx.doi.org/10.1016/j.jacc.2012.09.035] [PMID: 23199515]

[37] Tang AS, Wells GA, Talajic M, *et al.* Cardiac-resynchronization therapy for mild-to-moderate heart failure. N Engl J Med 2010; 363(25): 2385-95.
[http://dx.doi.org/10.1056/NEJMoa1009540] [PMID: 21073365]

[38] Curtis AB, Worley SJ, Adamson PB, *et al.* Biventricular pacing for atrioventricular block and systolic dysfunction. N Engl J Med 2013; 368(17): 1585-93.
[http://dx.doi.org/10.1056/NEJMoa1210356] [PMID: 23614585]

[39] Lang RM, Badano LP, Tsang W, *et al.* EAE/ASE recommendations for image acquisition and display using three-dimensional echocardiography. Eur Heart J Cardiovasc Imaging 2012; 13(1): 1-46.
[http://dx.doi.org/10.1093/ehjci/jer316] [PMID: 22275509]

[40] Thavendiranathan P, Liu S, Verhaert D, *et al.* Feasibility, accuracy, and reproducibility of real-time full-volume 3D transthoracic echocardiography to measure LV volumes and systolic function: a fully automated endocardial contouring algorithm in sinus rhythm and atrial fibrillation. JACC Cardiovasc Imaging 2012; 5(3): 239-51.
[http://dx.doi.org/10.1016/j.jcmg.2011.12.012] [PMID: 22421168]

[41] Vujisić-Tešić B, Trifunović D. Real time three-dimensional echocardiography: The importance of the third dimension in everyday clinical practice. Heart and Blood Vessels. Journal of the Cardiology Society of Serbia 2013; 31(4): 258.

[42] Blessberger H, Binder T. Two dimensional speckle tracking echocardiography: clinical applications. Heart 2010; 96(24): 2032-40.
[http://dx.doi.org/10.1136/hrt.2010.199885] [PMID: 21088126]

[43] Kosmala W, Plaksej R, Strotmann JM, *et al.* Progression of left ventricular functional abnormalities in hypertensive patients with heart failure: an ultrasonic two-dimensional speckle tracking study. J Am Soc Echocardiogr 2008; 21(12): 1309-17.
[http://dx.doi.org/10.1016/j.echo.2008.10.006] [PMID: 19041574]

[44] Liu YW, Tsai WC, Su CT, Lin CC, Chen JH. Evidence of left ventricular systolic dysfunction detected by automated function imaging in patients with heart failure and preserved left ventricular ejection fraction. J Card Fail 2009; 15(9): 782-9.
[http://dx.doi.org/10.1016/j.cardfail.2009.05.006] [PMID: 19879465]

[45] Syeda B, Höfer P, Pichler P, *et al.* Two-dimensional speckle-tracking strain echocardiography in long-term heart transplant patients: a study comparing deformation parameters and ejection fraction derived from echocardiography and multislice computed tomography. Eur J Echocardiogr 2011; 12(7): 490-6.
[http://dx.doi.org/10.1093/ejechocard/jer064] [PMID: 21636605]

[46] Uematsu M. Speckle Tracking Echocardiography - Quo Vadis? Circ J 2015; 79(4): 735-41.
[PMID: 25766514]

[47] Xu TY, Sun JP, Lee AP, *et al.* Three-dimensional speckle strain echocardiography is more accurate and efficient than 2D strain in the evaluation of left ventricular function. Int J Cardiol 2014; 176(2): 360-6.
[http://dx.doi.org/10.1016/j.ijcard.2014.07.015] [PMID: 25088155]

[48] Heijenbrok-Kal MH, Fleischmann KE, Hunink MG. Stress echocardiography, stress single-photo--emission computed tomography and electron beam computed tomography for the assessment of coronary artery disease: a meta-analysis of diagnostic performance. Am Heart J 2007; 154(3): 415-23.
[http://dx.doi.org/10.1016/j.ahj.2007.04.061] [PMID: 17719283]

[49] Ammirati E, Cipriani M, De Chiara B, *et al.* Left ventricular or Biventricular assist device? How dobutamine stress echocardiography can untie the dilemma of right ventricular dysfunction. Int J Cardiol 2014; 177(1): 6-8.
[http://dx.doi.org/10.1016/j.ijcard.2014.07.194] [PMID: 25499322]

[50] Murín P, Mitro P, Valocik G, Spurný P. Global myocardial contractile reserve assessed by high-dose dobutamine stress echocardiography predicts response to the cardiac resynchronization therapy. Echocardiography 2015; 32(3): 490-5.
[http://dx.doi.org/10.1111/echo.12694] [PMID: 25059770]

[51] Yamada H, Kusunose K, Nishio S, *et al.* Pre-load stress echocardiography for predicting the prognosis in mild heart failure. JACC Cardiovasc Imaging 2014; 7(7): 641-9.
[http://dx.doi.org/10.1016/j.jcmg.2014.04.009] [PMID: 24954460]

[52] Armstrong WF, Zoghbi WA. Stress echocardiography: current methodology and clinical applications. J Am Coll Cardiol 2005; 45(11): 1739-47.
[http://dx.doi.org/10.1016/j.jacc.2004.12.078] [PMID: 15936598]

[53] Muzzarelli S, Ordovas K, Higgins CB. Cardiovascular MRI for the assessment of heart failure: focus on clinical management and prognosis. J Magn Reson Imaging 2011; 33(2): 275-86.
[http://dx.doi.org/10.1002/jmri.22433] [PMID: 21274968]

[54] Takeda M, Amano Y, Tachi M, Tani H, Mizuno K, Kumita S. MRI differentiation of cardiomyopathy showing left ventricular hypertrophy and heart failure: differentiation between cardiac amyloidosis, hypertrophic cardiomyopathy, and hypertensive heart disease. Jpn J Radiol 2013; 31(10): 693-700.
[http://dx.doi.org/10.1007/s11604-013-0238-0] [PMID: 23996116]

[55] Nagao M, Yamasaki Y, Yonezawa M, *et al.* Geometrical characteristics of left ventricular dyssynchrony in advanced heart failure. Myocardial strain analysis by tagged MRI. Int Heart J 2014; 55(6): 512-8.
[http://dx.doi.org/10.1536/ihj.14-137] [PMID: 25310930]

[56] Guazzi M, Adams V, Conraads V, *et al.* EACPR/AHA Scientific Statement. Clinical recommendations for cardiopulmonary exercise testing data assessment in specific patient populations. Circulation 2012; 126(18): 2261-74.
[http://dx.doi.org/10.1161/CIR.0b013e31826fb946] [PMID: 22952317]

[57] Arena R, Myers J, Abella J, *et al.* Defining the optimal prognostic window for cardiopulmonary exercise testing in patients with heart failure. Circ Heart Fail 2010; 3(3): 405-11.
[http://dx.doi.org/10.1161/CIRCHEARTFAILURE.109.906446] [PMID: 20200329]

[58] Chase P, Arena R, Myers J, *et al.* Prognostic usefulness of dyspnea *versus* fatigue as reason for exercise test termination in patients with heart failure. Am J Cardiol 2008; 102(7): 879-82. [http://dx.doi.org/10.1016/j.amjcard.2008.05.031] [PMID: 18805115]

[59] Arena R, Myers J, Abella J, *et al.* The prognostic value of the heart rate response during exercise and recovery in patients with heart failure: influence of beta-blockade. Int J Cardiol 2010; 138(2): 166-73. [http://dx.doi.org/10.1016/j.ijcard.2008.08.010] [PMID: 18804882]

[60] Bilsel T, Terzi S, Akbulut T, Sayar N, Hobikoglu G, Yesilcimen K. Abnormal heart rate recovery immediately after cardiopulmonary exercise testing in heart failure patients. Int Heart J 2006; 47(3): 431-40. [http://dx.doi.org/10.1536/ihj.47.431] [PMID: 16823249]

[61] Montalescot G, Sechtem U, Achenbach S, *et al.* 2013 ESC guidelines on the management of stable coronary artery disease: the Task Force on the management of stable coronary artery disease of the European Society of Cardiology. Eur Heart J 2013; 34(38): 2949-3003. [http://dx.doi.org/10.1093/eurheartj/eht296] [PMID: 23996286]

[62] Danias PG, Ahlberg AW, Clark BA III, *et al.* Combined assessment of myocardial perfusion and left ventricular function with exercise technetium-99m sestamibi gated single-photon emission computed tomography can differentiate between ischemic and nonischemic dilated cardiomyopathy. Am J Cardiol 1998; 82(10): 1253-8. [http://dx.doi.org/10.1016/S0002-9149(98)00609-2] [PMID: 9832104]

[63] Mody FV, Brunken RC, Stevenson LW, Nienaber CA, Phelps ME, Schelbert HR. Differentiating cardiomyopathy of coronary artery disease from nonischemic dilated cardiomyopathy utilizing positron emission tomography. J Am Coll Cardiol 1991; 17(2): 373-83. [http://dx.doi.org/10.1016/S0735-1097(10)80102-0] [PMID: 1991893]

[64] Schinkel AF, Poldermans D, Elhendy A, Bax JJ. Assessment of myocardial viability in patients with heart failure. J Nucl Med 2007; 48(7): 1135-46. [http://dx.doi.org/10.2967/jnumed.106.038851] [PMID: 17574986]

[65] Rischpler C, Nekolla S, Schwaiger M. PET and SPECT in heart failure. Curr Cardiol Rep 2013; 15(3): 337. [http://dx.doi.org/10.1007/s11886-012-0337-z] [PMID: 23338719]

[66] Ahmadi A, Ohira H, Mielniczuk LM. FDG PET imaging for identifying pulmonary hypertension and right heart failure. Curr Cardiol Rep 2015; 17(1): 555. [http://dx.doi.org/10.1007/s11886-014-0555-7] [PMID: 25504422]

[67] Mangalat D, Kalogeropoulos A, Georgiopoulou V, Stillman A, Butler J. Value of Cardiac CT in Patients With Heart Failure. Curr Cardiovasc Imaging Rep 2009; 2(6): 410-7. [http://dx.doi.org/10.1007/s12410-009-0052-3] [PMID: 20369033]

[68] Yancy CW, Jessup M, Bozkurt B, *et al.* 2013 ACCF/AHA guideline for the management of heart failure: a report of the American College of Cardiology Foundation/American Heart Association task force on practice guidelines. J Am Coll Cardiol 2013; 62(16): e147-239. [http://dx.doi.org/10.1016/j.jacc.2013.05.019] [PMID: 23747642]

[69] Binanay C, Califf RM, Hasselblad V, *et al.* Evaluation study of congestive heart failure and pulmonary

artery catheterization effectiveness: the ESCAPE trial. JAMA 2005; 294(13): 1625-33. [http://dx.doi.org/10.1001/jama.294.13.1625] [PMID: 16204662]

[70] Patel CB, DeVore AD, Felker GM, *et al.* Characteristics and outcomes of patients with heart failure and discordant findings by right-sided heart catheterization and cardiopulmonary exercise testing. Am J Cardiol 2014; 114(7): 1059-64.
[http://dx.doi.org/10.1016/j.amjcard.2014.07.022] [PMID: 25212547]

[71] Fang JC, DeMarco T, Givertz MM, *et al.* World Health Organization Pulmonary Hypertension group 2: pulmonary hypertension due to left heart disease in the adult--a summary statement from the Pulmonary Hypertension Council of the International Society for Heart and Lung Transplantation. J Heart Lung Transplant 2012; 31(9): 913-33.
[http://dx.doi.org/10.1016/j.healun.2012.06.002] [PMID: 22884380]

[72] Spiliopoulos K, Giamouzis G, Karayannis G, *et al.* Current status of mechanical circulatory support: a systematic review. Cardiol Res Pract 2012.
[http://dx.doi.org/10.1155/2012/574198]

[73] Fida N, Loebe M, Estep JD, Guha A. Predictors and management of right heart failure after left ventricular assist device implantation. Methodist DeBakey Cardiovasc J 2015; 11(1): 18-23. r
[http://dx.doi.org/10.14797/mdcj-11-1-18] [PMID: 25793025]

[74] Estep JD, Trachtenberg BH, Loza LP, Bruckner BA. Continuous flow left ventricular assist devices: shared care goals of monitoring and treating patients. Methodist DeBakey Cardiovasc J 2015; 11(1): 33-44.
[http://dx.doi.org/10.14797/mdcj-11-1-33] [PMID: 25793028]

[75] Abraham WT. Disease management: remote monitoring in heart failure patients with implantable defibrillators, resynchronization devices, and haemodynamic monitors. Europace 2013; 15 (Suppl. 1): i40-6.
[http://dx.doi.org/10.1093/europace/eut105] [PMID: 23737229]

[76] Giamouzis G, Mastrogiannis D, Koutrakis K, *et al.* Telemonitoring in chronic heart failure: a systematic review. Cardiol Res Pract 2012.
[http://dx.doi.org/10.1155/2012/410820]

[77] Yoshida A, Ishibashi-Ueda H, Yamada N, *et al.* Direct comparison of the diagnostic capability of cardiac magnetic resonance and endomyocardial biopsy in patients with heart failure. Eur J Heart Fail 2013; 15(2): 166-75.
[http://dx.doi.org/10.1093/eurjhf/hfs206] [PMID: 23329703]

[78] Bennett MK, Gilotra NA, Harrington C, *et al.* Evaluation of the role of endomyocardial biopsy in 851 patients with unexplained heart failure from 2000-2009. Circ Heart Fail 2013; 6(4): 676-84. l
[http://dx.doi.org/10.1161/CIRCHEARTFAILURE.112.000087] [PMID: 23733916]

[79] Cooper LT, Baughman KL, Feldman AM, *et al.* The role of endomyocardial biopsy in the management of cardiovascular disease: a scientific statement from the American Heart Association, the American College of Cardiology, and the European Society of Cardiology. J Am Coll Cardiol 2007; 50(19): 1914-31.
[http://dx.doi.org/10.1016/j.jacc.2007.09.008] [PMID: 17980265]

[80] Cahill TJ, Ashrafian H, Watkins H. Genetic cardiomyopathies causing heart failure. Circ Res 2013;

113(6): 660-75.
[http://dx.doi.org/10.1161/CIRCRESAHA.113.300282] [PMID: 23989711]

[81] Hershberger RE, Lindenfeld J, Mestroni L, Seidman CE, Taylor MR, Towbin JA. Genetic evaluation of cardiomyopathy--a Heart Failure Society of America practice guideline. J Card Fail 2009; 15(2): 83-97.
[http://dx.doi.org/10.1016/j.cardfail.2009.01.006] [PMID: 19254666]

[82] Triposkiadis F, Karayannis G, Giamouzis G, Skoularigis J, Louridas G, Butler J. The sympathetic nervous system in heart failure physiology, pathophysiology, and clinical implications. J Am Coll Cardiol 2009; 54(19): 1747-62.
[http://dx.doi.org/10.1016/j.jacc.2009.05.015] [PMID: 19874988]

[83] Lang CC, Mancini DM. Non-cardiac comorbidities in chronic heart failure. Heart 2007; 93(6): 665-71.
[http://dx.doi.org/10.1136/hrt.2005.068296] [PMID: 16488925]

[84] Metra M, Zacà V, Parati G, *et al.* Heart Failure Study Group of the Italian Society of Cardiology. Cardiovascular and non-cardiovascular comorbidities in patients with chronic heart failure. J Cardiovasc Med (Hagerstown) 2011; 12(2): 76-84.
[http://dx.doi.org/10.2459/JCM.0b013e32834058d1] [PMID: 20962666]

[85] van Deursen VM, Urso R, Laroche C, *et al.* Co-morbidities in patients with heart failure: an analysis of the European Heart Failure Pilot Survey. Eur J Heart Fail 2014; 16(1): 103-11.
[http://dx.doi.org/10.1002/ejhf.30] [PMID: 24453099]

[86] Mentz RJ, Kelly JP, von Lueder TG, *et al.* Noncardiac comorbidities in heart failure with reduced *versus* preserved ejection fraction. J Am Coll Cardiol 2014; 64(21): 2281-93.
[http://dx.doi.org/10.1016/j.jacc.2014.08.036] [PMID: 25456761]

[87] Liu M, Fang F, Yu CM. Non-cardiac Comorbidities in Heart Failure With Preserved Ejection Fraction. Circ J 2015. advance publication
[http://dx.doi.org/10.1253/circj.CJ-15-0056]

[88] Mentz RJ, Felker GM. Noncardiac comorbidities and acute heart failure patients. Heart Fail Clin 2013; 9(3): 359-367, vii.
[http://dx.doi.org/10.1016/j.hfc.2013.04.003] [PMID: 23809421]

[89] Levy D, Larson MG, Vasan RS, Kannel WB, Ho KK. The progression from hypertension to congestive heart failure. JAMA 1996; 275(20): 1557-62.
[http://dx.doi.org/10.1001/jama.1996.03530440037034] [PMID: 8622246]

[90] The SOLVD Investigators. Effect of enalapril on survival in patients with reduced left ventricular ejection fractions and congestive heart failure. N Engl J Med 1991; 325(5): 293-302.
[http://dx.doi.org/10.1056/NEJM199108013250501] [PMID: 2057034]

[91] Massie BM, Carson PE, McMurray JJ, *et al.* Irbesartan in patients with heart failure and preserved ejection fraction. N Engl J Med 2008; 359(23): 2456-67.
[http://dx.doi.org/10.1056/NEJMoa0805450] [PMID: 19001508]

[92] Kalantar-Zadeh K, Block G, Horwich T, Fonarow GC. Reverse epidemiology of conventional cardiovascular risk factors in patients with chronic heart failure. J Am Coll Cardiol 2004; 43(8): 1439-44.

[http://dx.doi.org/10.1016/j.jacc.2003.11.039] [PMID: 15093881]

[93] Allman KC, Shaw LJ, Hachamovitch R, Udelson JE. Myocardial viability testing and impact of revascularization on prognosis in patients with coronary artery disease and left ventricular dysfunction: a meta-analysis. J Am Coll Cardiol 2002; 39(7): 1151-8. [http://dx.doi.org/10.1016/S0735-1097(02)01726-6] [PMID: 11923039]

[94] Henkel DM, Redfield MM, Weston SA, Gerber Y, Roger VL. Death in heart failure: a community perspective. Circ Heart Fail 2008; 1(2): 91-7. [http://dx.doi.org/10.1161/CIRCHEARTFAILURE.107.743146] [PMID: 19300532]

[95] Witt BJ, Gami AS, Ballman KV, *et al.* The incidence of ischemic stroke in chronic heart failure: a meta-analysis. J Card Fail 2007; 13(6): 489-96. [http://dx.doi.org/10.1016/j.cardfail.2007.01.009] [PMID: 17675064]

[96] Homma S, Thompson JL, Pullicino PM, *et al.* Warfarin and aspirin in patients with heart failure and sinus rhythm. N Engl J Med 2012; 366(20): 1859-69. [http://dx.doi.org/10.1056/NEJMoa1202299] [PMID: 22551105]

[97] Bursi F, Barbieri A, Grigioni F, *et al.* Prognostic implications of functional mitral regurgitation according to the severity of the underlying chronic heart failure: a long-term outcome study. Eur J Heart Fail 2010; 12(4): 382-8. [http://dx.doi.org/10.1093/eurjhf/hfq014] [PMID: 20197266]

[98] St John Sutton M, Ghio S, Plappert T, *et al.* Cardiac resynchronization induces major structural and functional reverse remodeling in patients with New York Heart Association class I/II heart failure. Circulation 2009; 120(19): 1858-65. [http://dx.doi.org/10.1161/CIRCULATIONAHA.108.818724] [PMID: 19858419]

[99] Kannel WB. Epidemiology and prevention of cardiac failure: Framingham Study insights. Eur Heart J 1987; 8 (Suppl. F): 23-6. [http://dx.doi.org/10.1093/eurheartj/8.suppl_F.23] [PMID: 3665963]

[100] Gaggin HK, Dec GW. The Role of Treatment for Anemia as a Therapeutic Target in the Management of Chronic Heart Failure: Insights After RED-HF. Curr Treat Options Cardiovasc Med 2014; 16(1): 279. [http://dx.doi.org/10.1007/s11936-013-0279-9] [PMID: 24346853]

[101] Swedberg K, Young JB, Anand IS, *et al.* Treatment of anemia with darbepoetin alfa in systolic heart failure. N Engl J Med 2013; 368(13): 1210-9. [http://dx.doi.org/10.1056/NEJMoa1214865] [PMID: 23473338]

[102] Anker SD, Comin Colet J, Filippatos G, *et al.* Ferric carboxymaltose in patients with heart failure and iron deficiency. N Engl J Med 2009; 361(25): 2436-48. [http://dx.doi.org/10.1056/NEJMoa0908355] [PMID: 19920054]

[103] Kwon BJ, Kim DB, Jang SW, *et al.* Prognosis of heart failure patients with reduced and preserved ejection fraction and coexistent chronic obstructive pulmonary disease. Eur J Heart Fail 2010; 12(12): 1339-44. [http://dx.doi.org/10.1093/eurjhf/hfq157] [PMID: 20861127]

[104] Triposkiadis FK, Skoularigis J. Prevalence and importance of comorbidities in patients with heart

failure. Curr Heart Fail Rep 2012; 9(4): 354-62.
[http://dx.doi.org/10.1007/s11897-012-0110-z] [PMID: 22918666]

[105] Rutten FH, Moons KG, Cramer MJ, *et al.* Recognising heart failure in elderly patients with stable chronic obstructive pulmonary disease in primary care: cross sectional diagnostic study. BMJ 2005; 331(7529): 1379.
[http://dx.doi.org/10.1136/bmj.38664.661181.55] [PMID: 16321994]

[106] Düngen HD, Apostolovic S, Inkrot S, *et al.* Titration to target dose of bisoprolol *vs.* carvedilol in elderly patients with heart failure: the CIBIS-ELD trial. Eur J Heart Fail 2011; 13(6): 670-80.
[http://dx.doi.org/10.1093/eurjhf/hfr020] [PMID: 21429992]

[107] Akashi YJ, Springer J, Anker SD. Cachexia in chronic heart failure: prognostic implications and novel therapeutic approaches. Curr Heart Fail Rep 2005; 2(4): 198-203.
[http://dx.doi.org/10.1007/BF02696650] [PMID: 16332313]

[108] Rahman A, Jafry S, Jeejeebhoy K, Nagpal AD, Pisani B, Agarwala R. Malnutrition and Cachexia in Heart Failure. J Parenter Enteral Nutr 2015.

[109] White JV, Guenter P, Jensen G, Malone A, Schofield M. Consensus statement: Academy of Nutrition and Dietetics and American Society for Parenteral and Enteral Nutrition: characteristics recommended for the identification and documentation of adult malnutrition (undernutrition). JPEN J Parenter Enteral Nutr 2012; 36(3): 275-83.
[http://dx.doi.org/10.1177/0148607112440285] [PMID: 22535923]

[110] Kenchaiah S, Pocock SJ, Wang D, *et al.* Body mass index and prognosis in patients with chronic heart failure: insights from the Candesartan in Heart failure: Assessment of Reduction in Mortality and morbidity (CHARM) program. Circulation 2007; 116(6): 627-36.
[http://dx.doi.org/10.1161/CIRCULATIONAHA.106.679779] [PMID: 17638930]

[111] Horwich TB, Broderick S, Chen L, *et al.* Relation among body mass index, exercise training, and outcomes in chronic systolic heart failure. Am J Cardiol 2011; 108(12): 1754-9.
[http://dx.doi.org/10.1016/j.amjcard.2011.07.051] [PMID: 21907317]

[112] Gupta PP, Fonarow GC, Horwich TB. Obesity and the obesity paradox in heart failure. Can J Cardiol 2015; 31(2): 195-202.
[http://dx.doi.org/10.1016/j.cjca.2014.08.004] [PMID: 25661554]

[113] Kapoor JR, Heidenreich PA. Obesity and survival in patients with heart failure and preserved systolic function: a U-shaped relationship. Am Heart J 2010; 159(1): 75-80.
[http://dx.doi.org/10.1016/j.ahj.2009.10.026] [PMID: 20102870]

[114] Kasper EK, Hruban RH, Baughman KL. Cardiomyopathy of obesity: a clinicopathologic evaluation of 43 obese patients with heart failure. Am J Cardiol 1992; 70(9): 921-4.
[http://dx.doi.org/10.1016/0002-9149(92)90739-L] [PMID: 1529947]

[115] Alpert MA, Omran J, Mehra A, Ardhanari S. Impact of obesity and weight loss on cardiac performance and morphology in adults. Prog Cardiovasc Dis 2014; 56(4): 391-400.
[http://dx.doi.org/10.1016/j.pcad.2013.09.003] [PMID: 24438730]

[116] Yeh ET, Bickford CL. Cardiovascular complications of cancer therapy: incidence, pathogenesis, diagnosis, and management. J Am Coll Cardiol 2009; 53(24): 2231-47.

[http://dx.doi.org/10.1016/j.jacc.2009.02.050] [PMID: 19520246]

[117] Eschenhagen T, Force T, Ewer MS, *et al.* Cardiovascular side effects of cancer therapies: a position statement from the Heart Failure Association of the European Society of Cardiology. Eur J Heart Fail 2011; 13(1): 1-10.
[http://dx.doi.org/10.1093/eurjhf/hfq213] [PMID: 21169385]

[118] Ewer MS, O'Shaughnessy JA. Cardiac toxicity of trastuzumab-related regimens in HER2-overexpressing breast cancer. Clin Breast Cancer 2007; 7(8): 600-7.
[http://dx.doi.org/10.3816/CBC.2007.n.017] [PMID: 17592672]

[119] Wouters KA, Kremer LC, Miller TL, Herman EH, Lipshultz SE. Protecting against anthracycline-induced myocardial damage: a review of the most promising strategies. Br J Haematol 2005; 131(5): 561-78.
[http://dx.doi.org/10.1111/j.1365-2141.2005.05759.x] [PMID: 16351632]

[120] Mastrogiannis D, Giamouzis G, Dardiotis E. Depression in patients with cardiovascular disease. Cardiol Res Pract 2012.
[http://dx.doi.org/10.1155/2012/794762]

[121] Williams SA, Kasl SV, Heiat A, Abramson JL, Krumholz HM, Vaccarino V. Depression and risk of heart failure among the elderly: a prospective community-based study. Psychosom Med 2002; 64(1): 6-12.
[http://dx.doi.org/10.1097/00006842-200201000-00002] [PMID: 11818580]

[122] Clarke SP, Frasure-Smith N, Lespérance F, Bourassa MG. Psychosocial factors as predictors of functional status at 1 year in patients with left ventricular dysfunction. Res Nurs Health 2000; 23(4): 290-300.
[http://dx.doi.org/10.1002/1098-240X(200008)23:4<290::AID-NUR5>3.0.CO;2-0] [PMID: 10940954]

[123] Jiang W, Alexander J, Christopher E, *et al.* Relationship of depression to increased risk of mortality and rehospitalization in patients with congestive heart failure. Arch Intern Med 2001; 161(15): 1849-56.
[http://dx.doi.org/10.1001/archinte.161.15.1849] [PMID: 11493126]

[124] Parissis JT, Farmakis D, Nikolaou M, *et al.* Plasma B-type natriuretic peptide and anti-inflammatory cytokine interleukin-10 levels predict adverse clinical outcome in chronic heart failure patients with depressive symptoms: a 1-year follow-up study. Eur J Heart Fail 2009; 11(10): 967-72.
[http://dx.doi.org/10.1093/eurjhf/hfp125] [PMID: 19789400]

[125] O'Connor CM, Jiang W, Kuchibhatla M, *et al.* Safety and efficacy of sertraline for depression in patients with heart failure: results of the SADHART-CHF (Sertraline Against Depression and Heart Disease in Chronic Heart Failure) trial. J Am Coll Cardiol 2010; 56(9): 692-9.
[http://dx.doi.org/10.1016/j.jacc.2010.03.068] [PMID: 20723799]

[126] MacDonald MR, Petrie MC, Hawkins NM, *et al.* Diabetes, left ventricular systolic dysfunction, and chronic heart failure. Eur Heart J 2008; 29(10): 1224-40.
[http://dx.doi.org/10.1093/eurheartj/ehn156] [PMID: 18424786]

[127] MacDonald MR, Petrie MC, Varyani F, *et al.* Impact of diabetes on outcomes in patients with low and preserved ejection fraction heart failure: an analysis of the Candesartan in Heart failure: Assessment of

Reduction in Mortality and morbidity (CHARM) programme. Eur Heart J 2008; 29(11): 1377-85. [http://dx.doi.org/10.1093/eurheartj/ehn153] [PMID: 18413309]

[128] He J, Ogden LG, Bazzano LA, Vupputuri S, Loria C, Whelton PK. Risk factors for congestive heart failure in US men and women: NHANES I epidemiologic follow-up study. Arch Intern Med 2001; 161(7): 996-1002. [http://dx.doi.org/10.1001/archinte.161.7.996] [PMID: 11295963]

[129] Barzilay JI, Kronmal RA, Gottdiener JS, *et al.* The association of fasting glucose levels with congestive heart failure in diabetic adults > or =65 years: the Cardiovascular Health Study. J Am Coll Cardiol 2004; 43(12): 2236-41. [http://dx.doi.org/10.1016/j.jacc.2003.10.074] [PMID: 15193686]

[130] Iribarren C, Karter AJ, Go AS, *et al.* Glycemic control and heart failure among adult patients with diabetes. Circulation 2001; 103(22): 2668-73. [http://dx.doi.org/10.1161/01.CIR.103.22.2668] [PMID: 11390335]

[131] Greenberg BH, Abraham WT, Albert NM, *et al.* Influence of diabetes on characteristics and outcomes in patients hospitalized with heart failure: a report from the Organized Program to Initiate Lifesaving Treatment in Hospitalized Patients with Heart Failure (OPTIMIZE-HF). Am Heart J 2007; 154(2): 277.e1-8. [http://dx.doi.org/10.1016/j.ahj.2007.05.001] [PMID: 17643576]

[132] Rydén L, Grant PJ, Anker SD, *et al.* ESC Guidelines on diabetes, pre-diabetes, and cardiovascular diseases developed in collaboration with the EASD: the Task Force on diabetes, pre-diabetes, and cardiovascular diseases of the European Society of Cardiology (ESC) and developed in collaboration with the European Association for the Study of Diabetes (EASD). Eur Heart J 2013; 34(39): 3035-87. [http://dx.doi.org/10.1093/eurheartj/eht108] [PMID: 23996285]

[133] Rauchhaus M, Clark AL, Doehner W, *et al.* The relationship between cholesterol and survival in patients with chronic heart failure. J Am Coll Cardiol 2003; 42(11): 1933-40. [http://dx.doi.org/10.1016/j.jacc.2003.07.016] [PMID: 14662255]

[134] Charach G, Rabinovich A, Ori A, *et al.* Low levels of low-density lipoprotein cholesterol: a negative predictor of survival in elderly patients with advanced heart failure. Cardiology 2014; 127(1): 45-50. [http://dx.doi.org/10.1159/000355164] [PMID: 24217704]

[135] Skwarek M, Bilińska ZT, Mazurkiewicz Ł, *et al.* Significance of dyslipidaemia in patients with heart failure of unexplained aetiology. Kardiol Pol 2008; 66(5): 515-22. [PMID: 18537059]

[136] Kjekshus J, Apetrei E, Barrios V, *et al.* Rosuvastatin in older patients with systolic heart failure. N Engl J Med 2007; 357(22): 2248-61. [http://dx.doi.org/10.1056/NEJMoa0706201] [PMID: 17984166]

[137] Tavazzi L, Maggioni AP, Marchioli R, *et al.* Effect of rosuvastatin in patients with chronic heart failure (the GISSI-HF trial): a randomised, double-blind, placebo-controlled trial. Lancet 2008; 372(9645): 1231-9. [http://dx.doi.org/10.1016/S0140-6736(08)61240-4] [PMID: 18757089]

[138] Kosmas CE, Alkhawam H, El-Hunjul M, *et al.* Statin-mediated low-density lipoprotein lowering in chronic congestive heart failure. Am J Med Sci 2014; 347(1): 14-22.

[http://dx.doi.org/10.1097/MAJ.0b013e318273514c] [PMID: 23154655]

[139] Ketchum ES, Levy WC. Establishing prognosis in heart failure: a multimarker approach. Prog Cardiovasc Dis 2011; 54(2): 86-96.
[http://dx.doi.org/10.1016/j.pcad.2011.03.003] [PMID: 21875508]

[140] Hare JM, Mangal B, Brown J, *et al.* Impact of oxypurinol in patients with symptomatic heart failure. Results of the OPT-CHF study. J Am Coll Cardiol 2008; 51(24): 2301-9.
[http://dx.doi.org/10.1016/j.jacc.2008.01.068] [PMID: 18549913]

[141] George J, Carr E, Davies J, Belch JJ, Struthers A. High-dose allopurinol improves endothelial function by profoundly reducing vascular oxidative stress and not by lowering uric acid. Circulation 2006; 114(23): 2508-16.
[http://dx.doi.org/10.1161/CIRCULATIONAHA.106.651117] [PMID: 17130343]

[142] Xu X, Hu X, Lu Z, *et al.* Xanthine oxidase inhibition with febuxostat attenuates systolic overload-induced left ventricular hypertrophy and dysfunction in mice. J Card Fail 2008; 14(9): 746-53.
[http://dx.doi.org/10.1016/j.cardfail.2008.06.006] [PMID: 18995179]

[143] Wei L, Fahey T, Struthers AD, MacDonald TM. Association between allopurinol and mortality in heart failure patients: a long-term follow-up study. Int J Clin Pract 2009; 63(9): 1327-33.
[http://dx.doi.org/10.1111/j.1742-1241.2009.02118.x] [PMID: 19691616]

[144] Bocchi EA, Guimarães G, Mocelin A, Bacal F, Bellotti G, Ramires JF. Sildenafil effects on exercise, neurohormonal activation, and erectile dysfunction in congestive heart failure: a double-blind, placebo-controlled, randomized study followed by a prospective treatment for erectile dysfunction. Circulation 2002; 106(9): 1097-103.
[http://dx.doi.org/10.1161/01.CIR.0000027149.83473.B6] [PMID: 12196335]

[145] Alberti L, Torlasco C, Lauretta L, *et al.* Erectile dysfunction in heart failure patients: a critical reappraisal. Andrology 2013; 1(2): 177-91.
[http://dx.doi.org/10.1111/j.2047-2927.2012.00048.x] [PMID: 23339018]

[146] Helfand M. Screening for subclinical thyroid dysfunction in nonpregnant adults: a summary of the evidence for the U.S. Preventive Services Task Force. Ann Intern Med 2004; 140(2): 128-41.
[http://dx.doi.org/10.7326/0003-4819-140-2-200401200-00015] [PMID: 14734337]

[147] Heeringa J, Hoogendoorn EH, van der Deure WM, *et al.* High-normal thyroid function and risk of atrial fibrillation: the Rotterdam study. Arch Intern Med 2008; 168(20): 2219-24.
[http://dx.doi.org/10.1001/archinte.168.20.2219] [PMID: 19001198]

[148] Vargas-Uricoechea H, Bonelo-Perdomo A, Sierra-Torres CH. Effects of thyroid hormones on the heart. Clin Investig Arterioscler 2014; 26(6): 296-309.
[http://dx.doi.org/10.1016/j.arteri.2014.07.003] [PMID: 25438971]

[149] Rodondi N, Newman AB, Vittinghoff E, *et al.* Subclinical hypothyroidism and the risk of heart failure, other cardiovascular events, and death. Arch Intern Med 2005; 165(21): 2460-6.
[http://dx.doi.org/10.1001/archinte.165.21.2460] [PMID: 16314541]

[150] Rodondi N, Bauer DC, Cappola AR, *et al.* Subclinical thyroid dysfunction, cardiac function, and the risk of heart failure. The Cardiovascular Health study. J Am Coll Cardiol 2008; 52(14): 1152-9.
[http://dx.doi.org/10.1016/j.jacc.2008.07.009] [PMID: 18804743]

[151] Gencer B, Collet TH, Virgini V, *et al.* Subclinical thyroid dysfunction and the risk of heart failure events: an individual participant data analysis from 6 prospective cohorts. Circulation 2012; 126(9): 1040-9.
[http://dx.doi.org/10.1161/CIRCULATIONAHA.112.096024] [PMID: 22821943]

[152] Mitchell JE, Hellkamp AS, Mark DB, *et al.* Thyroid function in heart failure and impact on mortality. JACC Heart Fail 2013; 1(1): 48-55.
[http://dx.doi.org/10.1016/j.jchf.2012.10.004] [PMID: 24159562]

[153] Kasai T, Bradley TD. Obstructive sleep apnea and heart failure: pathophysiologic and therapeutic implications. J Am Coll Cardiol 2011; 57(2): 119-27.
[http://dx.doi.org/10.1016/j.jacc.2010.08.627] [PMID: 21211682]

[154] Herrscher TE, Akre H, Øverland B, Sandvik L, Westheim AS. High prevalence of sleep apnea in heart failure outpatients: even in patients with preserved systolic function. J Card Fail 2011; 17(5): 420-5.
[http://dx.doi.org/10.1016/j.cardfail.2011.01.013] [PMID: 21549300]

[155] Bradley TD, Floras JS. Sleep apnea and heart failure: Part I: obstructive sleep apnea. Circulation 2003; 107(12): 1671-8.
[http://dx.doi.org/10.1161/01.CIR.0000061757.12581.15] [PMID: 12668504]

[156] Garcia-Touchard A, Somers VK, Olson LJ, Caples SM. Central sleep apnea: implications for congestive heart failure. Chest 2008; 133(6): 1495-504.
[http://dx.doi.org/10.1378/chest.07-0871] [PMID: 18574295]

[157] Javaheri S, Javaheri S, Javaheri A. Sleep apnea, heart failure, and pulmonary hypertension. Curr Heart Fail Rep 2013; 10(4): 315-20.
[http://dx.doi.org/10.1007/s11897-013-0167-3] [PMID: 24097114]

[158] Momomura S. Treatment of Cheyne-Stokes respiration-central sleep apnea in patients with heart failure. J Cardiol 2012; 59(2): 110-6.
[http://dx.doi.org/10.1016/j.jjcc.2011.12.008] [PMID: 22370166]

[159] Sharma BK, Bakker JP, McSharry DG, Desai AS, Javaheri S, Malhotra A. Adaptive servoventilation for treatment of sleep-disordered breathing in heart failure: a systematic review and meta-analysis. Chest 2012; 142(5): 1211-21.
[http://dx.doi.org/10.1378/chest.12-0815] [PMID: 22722232]

[160] Cole RT, Masoumi A, Triposkiadis F, *et al.* Renal dysfunction in heart failure. Med Clin North Am 2012; 96(5): 955-74.
[http://dx.doi.org/10.1016/j.mcna.2012.07.005] [PMID: 22980058]

[161] Giamouzis G, Kalogeropoulos A, Georgiopoulou V, *et al.* Hospitalization epidemic in patients with heart failure: risk factors, risk prediction, knowledge gaps, and future directions. J Card Fail 2011; 17(1): 54-75.
[http://dx.doi.org/10.1016/j.cardfail.2010.08.010] [PMID: 21187265]

[162] Cleland JG, Carubelli V, Castiello T, Yassin A, Pellicori P, Antony R. Renal dysfunction in acute and chronic heart failure: prevalence, incidence and prognosis. Heart Fail Rev 2012; 17(2): 133-49.
[http://dx.doi.org/10.1007/s10741-012-9306-2] [PMID: 22426973]

[163] Smith GL, Lichtman JH, Bracken MB, *et al.* Renal impairment and outcomes in heart failure:

systematic review and meta-analysis. J Am Coll Cardiol 2006; 47(10): 1987-96. [http://dx.doi.org/10.1016/j.jacc.2005.11.084] [PMID: 16697315]

[164] Hillege HL, Nitsch D, Pfeffer MA, *et al.* Renal function as a predictor of outcome in a broad spectrum of patients with heart failure. Circulation 2006; 113(5): 671-8. [http://dx.doi.org/10.1161/CIRCULATIONAHA.105.580506] [PMID: 16461840]

[165] Heywood JT, Fonarow GC, Costanzo MR, Mathur VS, Wigneswaran JR, Wynne J. High prevalence of renal dysfunction and its impact on outcome in 118,465 patients hospitalized with acute decompensated heart failure: a report from the ADHERE database. J Card Fail 2007; 13(6): 422-30. [http://dx.doi.org/10.1016/j.cardfail.2007.03.011] [PMID: 17675055]

[166] Triposkiadis F, Starling RC, Boudoulas H, Giamouzis G, Butler J. The cardiorenal syndrome in heart failure: cardiac? renal? syndrome? Heart Fail Rev 2012; 17(3): 355-66. [http://dx.doi.org/10.1007/s10741-011-9291-x] [PMID: 22086438]

[167] Giamouzis G, Kalogeropoulos AP, Butler J, *et al.* Epidemiology and importance of renal dysfunction in heart failure patients. Curr Heart Fail Rep 2013; 10(4): 411-20. [http://dx.doi.org/10.1007/s11897-013-0164-6] [PMID: 24097112]

[168] Parissis JT, Farmakis D, Fountoulaki K, *et al.* Clinical and neurohormonal correlates and prognostic value of serum prolactin levels in patients with chronic heart failure. Eur J Heart Fail 2013; 15(10): 1122-30. [http://dx.doi.org/10.1093/eurjhf/hft070] [PMID: 23639781]

[169] Filipe MD, Meijers WC, Rogier van der Velde A, de Boer RA. Galectin-3 and heart failure: prognosis, prediction & clinical utility. Clin Chim Acta 2015; 443: 48-56. [http://dx.doi.org/10.1016/j.cca.2014.10.009] [PMID: 25446877]

[170] Bayes-Genis A, Zhang Y, Ky B. ST2 and patient prognosis in chronic heart failure. Am J Cardiol 2015; 115(7) (Suppl.): 64B-9B. [http://dx.doi.org/10.1016/j.amjcard.2015.01.043] [PMID: 25665758]

[171] Januzzi JL, Mebazaa A, Di Somma S. ST2 and prognosis in acutely decompensated heart failure: the International ST2 Consensus Panel. Am J Cardiol 2015; 115(7) (Suppl.): 26B-31B. [http://dx.doi.org/10.1016/j.amjcard.2015.01.037] [PMID: 25665762]

[172] Levy WC, Mozaffarian D, Linker DT, *et al.* The Seattle Heart Failure Model: prediction of survival in heart failure. Circulation 2006; 113(11): 1424-33. [http://dx.doi.org/10.1161/CIRCULATIONAHA.105.584102] [PMID: 16534009]

[173] Pocock SJ, Ariti CA, McMurray JJ, *et al.* Predicting survival in heart failure: a risk score based on 39 372 patients from 30 studies. Eur Heart J 2013; 34(19): 1404-13. [http://dx.doi.org/10.1093/eurheartj/ehs337] [PMID: 23095984]

[174] Krumholz HM, Wang Y, Mattera JA, *et al.* An administrative claims model suitable for profiling hospital performance based on 30-day mortality rates among patients with heart failure. Circulation 2006; 113(13): 1693-701. [http://dx.doi.org/10.1161/CIRCULATIONAHA.105.611194] [PMID: 16549636]

[175] Fonarow GC, Adams KF Jr, Abraham WT, Yancy CW, Boscardin WJ. Risk stratification for in-hospital mortality in acutely decompensated heart failure: classification and regression tree analysis.

JAMA 2005; 293(5): 572-80.
[http://dx.doi.org/10.1001/jama.293.5.572] [PMID: 15687312]

[176] Keenan PS, Normand SL, Lin Z, *et al.* An administrative claims measure suitable for profiling hospital performance on the basis of 30-day all-cause readmission rates among patients with heart failure. Circ Cardiovasc Qual Outcomes 2008; 1(1): 29-37.
[http://dx.doi.org/10.1161/CIRCOUTCOMES.108.802686] [PMID: 20031785]

CHAPTER 6

Laboratory Variables and Biochemical Markers

Christos A. Zivlas* and **Dennis V. Cokkinos**

Biomedical Research Foundation of the Academy of Athens, Athens, Greece

Abstract: Heart failure is a syndrome affecting not only the heart, but in fact all the organs and systems of the body. Therefore, common serum laboratory variables, such as creatinine, play an important role in diagnosis and follow-up of specific organ dysfunction in heart failure. Actually, treatment is tailored according to these variables. More recently, natriuretic peptides were suggested as a valuable tool for the diagnosis of acute and chronic heart failure, substituting echocardiography at the emergency department. Furthermore, these peptides are used for the prognosis of heart failure patients. Many newer biochemical markers related to a variety of pathophysiological processes, such as inflammation, oxidative stress, remodeling of the extracellular matrix and neurohormones, have been investigated in the past few years. Some of them have shown promising characteristics, not only as diagnostic tools, but also as potential treatment targets. Finally, manipulation of genes *via* micro-RNAs has emerged as a vast new era in the understanding and treatment of heart failure. In this chapter, the majority of laboratory variables and biochemical markers used in heart failure will be discussed. Moreover, information will be given for the clinical benefits of an integrated approach in the management of heart failure patients. Latest advances regarding novel biomarkers will be also presented.

Keywords: Biomarker, Cystatin-C, Galectin-3, Heart failure, Interleukin-1β, Micro-RNAs, Natriuretic peptide, NGAL, Osteopontin, Prolactin, ST2.

INTRODUCTION

Laboratory variables and biomarkers are widely used in heart failure (HF) patients, for diagnostic and treatment purposes. In this chapter biological substan-

* **Corresponding author Christos A. Zivlas:** Biomedical Research Foundation of the Academy of Athens, Athens, Greece; Tel: +44 777 419 9134; Fax: +30 210 659 7545; E-mail: christosazivlas@hotmail.com.

Panagiotis Georgoulias (Ed.)

ces, enzymes, hormones and other markers detected in the blood will be discussed, reflecting the pathophysiological alterations that occur in cardiac myocytes, cardiac interstitium and many other organs. All these changes result from increased tissue/organ water and decreased tissue/organ perfusion [1]. Six categories of biomarkers (plus one category of novel biomarkers) in HF have been generally proposed. Each category is related to a distinct pathophysiological process (Table **1**). Certainly, there are no boundaries in the living organism and different pathophysiological pathways have been recently elucidated to interact with each other, such as the ST2 – interleukin-33 (IL-33) system responsible for inflammation, as well as fibrosis.

Table 1. Categories of biomarkers in heart failure [1].

Biomarkers in alphabetical order	**Categories based on pathophysiological process***						
	INF	**OXS**	**EMR**	**NEH**	**MIA**	**MYS**	**NBM**
Adiponectin							x
Aldosterone				x			
Angiotensin II				x			
Antidiuretic hormone				x			
Biopyrins (urinary)		x					
Brain natriuretic peptide						x	
C-reactive protein	x						
Cardiac-specific troponin I					x		
Cardiac-specific troponin T					x		
Creatine kinase MB fraction					x		
Cystatin C			x				
Endothelin				x			
Fas (APO-1)	x						
Galectin 3			x				
Growth differentiation factor 15							x
Heart-type fatty-acid protein					x		
Interleukin 1	x						
Interleukin 6	x						
Interleukin 18	x						
Isoprostanes (plasma, urinary)		x					

(Table 1) contd.....

Biomarkers in alphabetical order	**Categories based on pathophysiological process***						
	INF	**OXS**	**EMR**	**NEH**	**MIA**	**MYS**	**NBM**
Malondialdehyde (plasma)		x					
Matrix metalloproteinases			x				
Micro-RNAs							x
Midregional fragment of proadrenomedullin						x	
Myeloperoxidase		x					
Myosin light-chain kinase I					x		
N-terminal pro-brain natriuretic peptide						x	
Norepinephrine				x			
Osteoprotegerin	x						
Osteopontin			x				
Oxidized low-density lipoproteins		x					
Procollagen type I			x				
Procollagen type III			x				
Prolactin				x			
Renin				x			
sFas					x		
Suppression of Tumorgenicity 2 (ST2)						x	
Tissue inhibitors of metalloproteinases			x				
Tumor necrosis factor a	x						

* INF: inflammation; OXS: oxidative stress; EMR: extracellular-matrix remodeling; NEH: neurohormones; MIA: myocyte injury/apoptosis; MYS: myocyte stress; NBM: new biomarkers.

Independently of the pathway, the main characteristics of useful biomarkers include reasonable cost with short turn-around times, provision of information not already available through a careful clinical assessment, and significant aid in decision making [2]. According to the National Institutes of Health making group, a biomarker is defined as "a characteristic that is objectively measured and evaluated as an indicator of normal biological processes, pathogenic processes, or pharmacologic responses to a therapeutic intervention" [3]. Multi-marker approaches for better risk stratification of HF patients are more commonly used recently, as the use of a single biomarker provides less information [4]. Finally, many biomarkers are potential therapeutic targets, thus their study may lead to new developments in HF therapy [2]. Below, classic laboratory variables used in HF will be presented, followed by novel biomarkers. Last but not least, it should always keep in mind that the value of clinical examination and the physician's judgment should never be underestimated or replaced by a single biomarker.

CLASSIC LABORATORY VARIABLES

Haematocrit and Haemoglobin

Haematocrit and haemoglobin are routinely assessed in HF patients, in order not only to detect anaemia, but also for prognostic purposes. Anaemia, defined as haemoglobin concentration <13g/dl in men and <12g/dl in women, is associated with more symptoms, worse functional status, greater risk of HF hospitalization, and reduced survival [5]. It is more common in elderly patients, in women and in patients with impaired renal function. Correctable causes should be extensively investigated and treated, although this is not always feasible. In a recent study of 2,278 patients, administration of darbepoetin alfa, an erythropoietin-stimulating agent, as a treatment for mild to moderate anaemia in systolic HF patients, did not improve the primary composite end point of death from any cause or the secondary endpoint of hospitalization because of the syndrome worsening [6]. On the other hand, the treatment of HF patients with reduced left ventricular ejection fraction (LVEF) and iron deficiency with intravenous (i.v.) iron administration, has been investigated in 2 multicenter studies, with very positive results [7, 8]. Iron treatment sustainably improved functional capacity and quality of life (QoL). Moreover, it was associated with lower risk of hospitalization for worsening HF, although no mortality reduction was observed. Interestingly, elevated red cell distribution width (RDW) is also considered as a strong, independent (and inexpensive) predictor of adverse outcome in chronic HF, probably indicating inflammatory stress and impaired iron mobilization [9].

Creatinine and Creatinine Clearance

Creatinine blood levels reflect renal function and constitute a valuable prognostic marker in HF patients. Its measurement is recommended in HF patients in order to evaluate patient suitability for diuretic, renin–angiotensin–aldosterone antagonist, and anticoagulant therapy and also for treatment monitoring [5]. The estimated glomerular filtration rate (eGFR) is a more accurate marker of renal function and should be calculated in all HF patients, since when serum creatinine levels are elevated above the normal limit, at least 50% of functioning nephrons have been already lost [10]. The close interactions (crosstalk) between the heart and the kidneys are well established and defined as "cardiorenal syndrome" or "renocardiac syndrome", depending on which organ dysfunctions first. These terms reflect the concomitant renal dysfunction, worsening of renal function and diuretic resistance during heart failure therapy. Additionally, they reflect the subsequent cardiac dysfunction (*e.g.*, HF, arrhythmia, ischemia) after kidney function worsening [11, 12]. The pathophysiology of this syndrome is complex and comprises reduced renal perfusion, kidney venous congestion, and neurohormonal pathways alterations (activation of renin-angiotensin-aldosterone system – RAAS, sympathetic activation, arginine vasopressin – AVP and natriuretic peptides release) [12]. Novel and more accurate biomarkers for the diagnosis of this syndrome, such as cystatin-C and neutrophil gelatinase-associated lipocalin (NGAL), will be discussed later in this chapter.

Electrolytes: Sodium and Potassium

Sodium and water retention are major factors leading to peripheral oedema and other signs in HF. Serum sodium level measurement is indicated in routine laboratory tests of HF patients [5]. In the ESC-HF Pilot survey, hyponatremia was an independent and simple prognostic marker for high mortality rate at 1 year [13]. Of premium importance is the differentiation between depletional *versus* dilutional hyponatremia, the former caused by diuretic therapy - induced sodium excretion, while the latter is due to water retention. Treatment is relevant to each type. In depletional hyponatremia, treatment should include isotonic saline, possibly accompanied with administration of potassium/magnesium. Dilutional hyponatremia is treated with loop diuretics or acetazolamide. Thiazide-type diuretic agents and mineralocorticoid receptor antagonists should be avoided [14]. Vasopressin receptor antagonists (VRAs), mainly tolvaptan (a V-2 receptor antagonist), could also be used for treating dilutional hyponatremia, with relative safety [5, 15].

Hyper- or hypo-kalaemia are common and possibly life-threatening conditions in

HF patients. Therefore, serial measurements of serum potassium are recommended [5]. Adjustments to treatment (dose reduction) should be made, whenever a patient receiving RAAS antagonists develops hyperkalaemia. On the other hand, in case of hypokalaemia, potassium supplements, increase of RAAS antagonists dose or adding a potassium sparing diuretic, can resolve this problem. In other words, maintenance of normal potassium homeostasis should be always considered in the HF therapy [16].

Liver Enzymes

In contrast to cardiorenal syndrome, "cardiohepatic" interactions are not clearly delineated. Liver dysfunction is not uncommon in acute and chronic HF, and is caused of a combination of inferior vena cava congestion (as a result of elevated right sided cardiac pressures) coupled with impaired perfusion (due to left sided cardiac failure) and drug toxicity [17]. Terms such as "ischemic hepatitis" or "shock liver" have been used in the past to describe this pathophysiology. However, the new term "acute cardiogenic liver injury (ACLI)" should be used, because it corresponds more accurately to these pathophysiological mechanisms [18]. Biochemical findings in patients with ACLI originate either from the hepatic cells necrosis (initially from zone 3) and the subsequent release of cellular substances and enzymes to circulation, or from diminished protein production by liver [19]. Similarly, in chronic HF the liver is affected, a pathological condition called "congestive hepatopathy" (previously called "nutmeg liver"), attributing the main principle of hepatopathy to venous congestion [17].

Aminotransferases and Lactate Dehydrogenase

Aminotranferases and lactate dehydrogenase (LDH) levels are both elevated in ACLI, 10 to 20 fold, usually within 1 to 3 days [17]. A very useful marker, the ratio of serum alanine aminotranferase (ALT) to LDH (values <1.5) early in the course of hepatic injury, is characteristic of ACLI, in contrast to other forms of hepatitis [20]. Nikolaou *et al.* have demonstrated recently that abnormal transaminases in acutely decompensated heart failure (ADHF) were associated with increased 31- and 180-day mortality [21]. Nevertheless, it seems that in chronic HF hepatic enzymes associated with cholestasis play a more important role in patients' prognosis [17].

Alkaline Phosphatase, Gamma-Glutamyl Transpeptidase and Total Bilirubin

Alkaline phosphatase (ALP) and gamma-glutamyl transpeptidase (γ-GT) have been independently correlated with adverse prognosis, not only in ADHF, but also in chronic HF [17, 21]. Moreover, high levels of ALP in HF patients indicate elevated right-sided filling pressures, peripheral oedema, ascites, and tricuspid regurgitation. These abnormalities are associated with high serum levels of creatinine and B-type natriuretic peptide (BNP) [21]. In CHARM (Candesartan in Heart Failure: Assessment of Reduction in Mortality and Morbidity program) trial, total bilirubin was also demonstrated to be independently associated with morbidity and mortality in chronic HF patients [22]. Moreover, total bilirubin is used as a marker for worse outcomes after left ventricular assist device (LVAD) implantation, and has been incorporated into risk models for LVAD implantation and heart transplantation [17]. Lastly, γ-GT levels are associated with HF severity and may provide prognostic information for subclinical or mild HF [23].

Albumin

Hypoalbuminemia is one of the most common abnormal liver function tests in chronic HF patients [22]. It mainly signifies systemic inflammation, rather than poor nutritional status. It is also an independent predictor of death in HF (acute and chronic). Furthermore, albumin predicts the outcome in patients after LVAD implantation, and therefore is incorporated into risk scores [17].

Prothrombin Time

Prolongation of prothrombin time may occur in more than 80% of ACLI patients, while it is unusual in viral hepatitis [18]. It is important to know that these alterations are not reversed by parenteral vitamin K administration. Thus, special caution is needed in HF patients who receive oral anticoagulation (*e.g.* patients with atrial fibrillation).

Uric Acid (UA)

Hyperuricemia (*i.e.*, serum uric acid ≥9.5mg/dL) is present in ≈25% of patients with HF and reduced LVEF. It predisposes to worse outcomes in patients with moderate to severe HF. Uric acid (UA) levels reflect the degree of circulating xanthine oxidase (XO) activity; it is postulated that it stimulates the formation of reactive oxygen species. In addition, UA is a general biomarker of cell death, *via* degradation of accumulated purines, a marker of hyperinsulinemia, inflammation and impaired vascular function [24]. Moreover, higher UA levels have been associated with hemodynamic parameters, such as lower cardiac index (CI) and LV stroke work index, and higher right atrial, pulmonary arterial and pulmonary capillary wedge (PCW) pressures, regardless of N-terminal proBNP (NT-proBNP) levels [25]. Hence, XO inhibition in HF patients with hyperuricemia has provided promising results, regarding improvement in cardiac function and overall survival [26]. The Xanthine Oxidase Inhibition for Hyperuricemic Heart Failure Patients (EXACT-HF) study will more consistently address these issues and its results are anticipated soon [27].

Troponins

The importance of cardiac troponins in HF, as markers of ongoing myocardial damage and disease severity, has been demonstrated since 1999 [28]. More recently, in the Valsartan Heart Failure Trial (Val-HeFT), which enrolled more than 4,000 patients with chronic stable HF, the prognostic value of plasma concentrations of the traditional troponin T (cTnT) and the highly sensitive assay (hs-cTnT) in mortality and morbidity was also reported [29]. Actually, higher levels of these markers correlated with more severe HF, lower LVEF, higher New York Heart Association (NYHA) Class, diabetes, higher incidence of atrial fibrillation (AF), renal and hepatic dysfunction, and higher levels of BNP, C-reactive protein (CRP), norepinephrine, renin and aldosterone. Interestingly, in patients with undetectable baseline cTnT, hs-cTnT was the main predictor of death. The combination of troponin and BNP levels improved further the prognostic discrimination of mortality and hospitalization in the same study. Lately, the prognostic value of over time changes in the levels of hs-cTnT in 5,284 patients with chronic and symptomatic HF was shown, based on data from 2 large randomized clinical trials, the Val-HeFT trial and the Gruppo Italiano per lo Studio della Sopravvivenza nell'Insufficienza Cardiaca-Heart Failure (GISSI-HF) trial. These data suggested that even small changes in troponin levels have prognostic significance and may help to identify patients at long-term risk for adverse events [30]. The pathophysiological mechanisms behind these fluctuations in troponin levels are not fully understood yet, and may involve, apart from death of cardiac myocytes, increased wall stress and transient loss of cell membrane integrity, neurohormonal activation, inflammation, oxidative stress, altered calcium handling and epicardial coronary artery disease progression [29, 30].

Natriuretic Peptides

Since the initial discovery of atrial natriuretic peptide (ANP), BNP and NT-proBNP, the field in HF has dramatically changed, not only regarding diagnosis, but also prognosis and treatment [31, 32]. NT-proBNP has been proved to be the single strongest predictor of 1-year death, in patients treated for breathlessness in the emergency department [33]. Subsequently, the prognostic value of over time changes in the natriuretic peptides levels was demonstrated [34]. Surprisingly, HF patients who had low baseline NT-proBNP levels (<1,078pg/ml) but high levels at 4 months had a similar mortality to those with constantly high NT-proBNP levels. In contrast, patients had better prognosis if initial high NT-proBNP levels decreased at a low level after 4 months.

Because natriuretic peptides are released from myocardium (atrial and ventricular) in all conditions of pressure overload, such as pulmonary embolism, pulmonary hypertension, valvular heart disease and AF, and their levels are affected in advancing age, renal dysfunction and obesity (lower BNP or NT-proBNP levels), they have high sensitivity but low specificity for HF. In other words, negative natriuretic peptides rule out HF [5, 35].

Natriuretic peptides have favorable renal and cardiovascular effects in HF. With respect to effects on kidneys, they stimulate natriuresis and diuresis, increase glomerular filtration rate and inhibit the secretion of renin, angiotensin II, and aldosterone. In cardiovascular system, they decrease blood pressure, suppress vasoconstriction and have lusitropic and antifibrotic effects on the heart. They also have central and peripheral sympathoinhibitory effects and decrease the release of catecholamines [36]. Because of these advantageous characteristics, there has been an effort to manipulate natriuretic peptides in the treatment of HF. Nesiritide, a human BNP, was tested in a clinical trial, exhibiting dyspnea improvement in acute HF patients, although no mortality reduction was observed [37]. Recently, the Prospective Comparison of Angiotensin Receptor – Neprilysin Inhibitor (ARNI) with Angiotensin – Converting – Enzyme Inhibitor (ACEI) to Determine Impact on Global Mortality and Morbidity in Heart Failure Trial (PARADIGM-HF) showed that LCZ696 is superior to enalapril in reducing the risks of death and hospitalization [38]. LCZ696 is a combination of sacubitril and the angiotensin receptor inhibitor (ARB) valsartan. Sacubitril is an inhibitor of neprilysin, which is a neutral endopeptidase that degrades natriuretic peptides.

Consequently, in current European Society of Cardiology (ESC) guidelines for the diagnosis and treatment of acute and chronic HF, the measurement of natriuretic peptides [BNP, NT-proBNP, mid-regional pro atrial natriuretic peptide (MR-proANP)] levels is a class IIa indication, in order to exclude alternative causes of dyspnoea in patients with suspected HF, or to obtain prognostic information in patients with established HF. In fact, echocardiography is not necessary in an untreated patient with suspected HF and negative natriuretic peptide measurement at the emergency department [5]. Recently, Maisel *et al.* demonstrated the feasibility of home BNP monitoring with a finger-stick test, in order to detect pulmonary congestion before symptoms occurrence, and accordingly tailor treatment [39].

Cholesterol and Lipids

It is well known that patients with advanced HF and reduced LVEF have low levels of total cholesterol (TC), low density lipoproteins (LDL), high density lipoproteins (HDL) and triglycerides (TG) [40]. Actually, higher levels of lipids predispose to better survival in these patients. Therefore, they constitute prognostic markers of HF. We have recently shown that in patients with severely (<35%) impaired LVEF, HDL predicted well their functional status, assessed by the 6 minute walking test (6MWT) (Fig. **1**) [41]. A protective role of serum cholesterol has been implied in HF, since it may act as a buffer for endotoxin (lipopolysaccharide - LPS), which is present in HF patients, leading to reduced LPS bioactivity and immune activation [42]. Furthermore, chronic HF is an energy consuming condition, where catabolism prevails over anabolism [43]. Szabó T *et al.* have also found that ANP has lipid-mobilizing (in adipose tissue) and lipid-oxidizing properties [44]. This fact may partly explain the metabolic alterations which occur in HF.

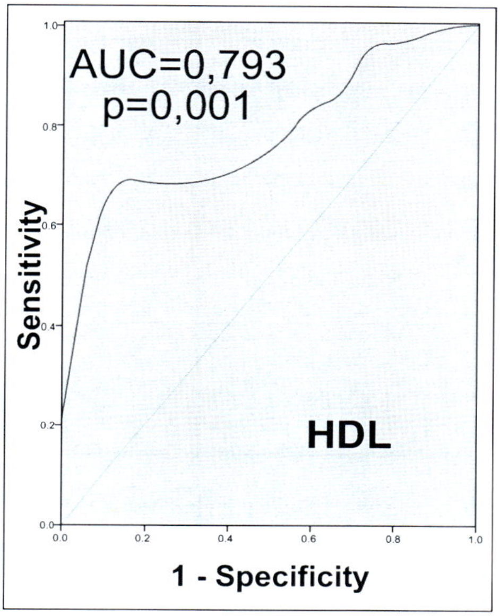

Fig. (1). High density lipoprotein (HDL) predicted well the functional status (as assessed by the 6 minute walking test – 6MWT) in patients with severely (<35%) impaired left ventricular ejection fraction (LVEF). The 6MWT Category refers to whether patients walked more or less than 80% of the predicted lower limit of the normal range achieved by healthy adults with the same anthropometric variables. Reprinted from ref [41]. with kind permission from John Wiley and Sons.
AUC: area under the curve; p: level of statistical significance.

C-Reacting Protein (CRP)

CRP is a protein synthesized by the liver and upregulated by inflammatory stimuli, like cytokines (mainly tumor necrosis factor – TNF and interleukin 6 – IL6). Subsequently, CRP activates the immune system *via* the classic complement pathway and opsonization [45]. In the Val-HeFT study, serum CRP was evaluated in more than 5,000 patients with congestive HF. Investigators found that patients with higher CRP levels had more severe HF, lower LVEF, more frequently atrial fibrillation and worse quality of life and neurohormonal profile [46]. CRP significantly predicted mortality in these patients; therefore it has been established as an important biomarker in HF. These findings were not associated with BNP levels or the cause (ischemic or non-ischemic) of HF, conveying a role independent of atherosclerosis. Our team has also demonstrated in a smaller group of patients with severe HF that serum CRP levels were significantly correlated with the functional status (Fig. **2**) [41]. Valsartan was proved to lower CRP levels, which meant less inflammatory process. More recently, Choi *et al.* demonstrated in more than 6,800 asymptomatic individuals without previous history of heart disease enrolled in the Multi-Ethnic Study of Atherosclerosis (MESA) that elevated high sensitive CRP levels (hs-CRP) were significantly related to regional myocardial functional deterioration, independent of coronary artery disease [47]. In summary, CRP is a robust prognostic biomarker, not only in HF patients, but also in asymptomatic adult individuals without history of prior heart disease.

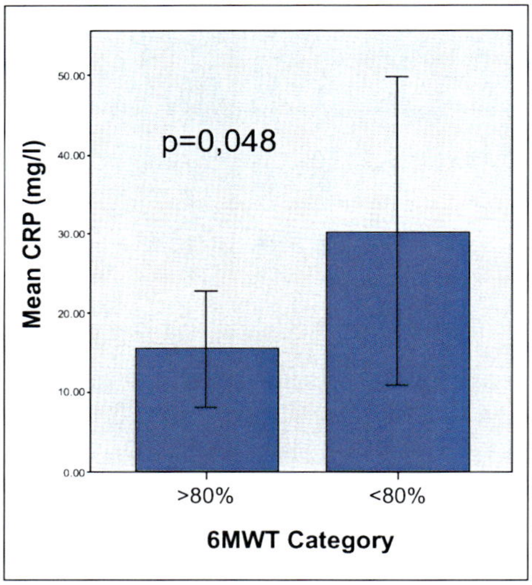

Fig. (2). Level of serum C-reactive protein (CRP) was significantly higher in heart failure patients with worse functional status (as assessed by the 6 minute walking test – 6MWT). The 6MWT Category refers to whether patients walked more or less than 80% of the predicted lower limit of the normal range achieved by healthy adults with the same anthropometric variables. Error bars represent 95% confidence intervals. Reprinted from ref [41]. with kind permission from John Wiley and Sons.
p: level of statistical significance.

Thyroid Hormones

The relationship between the thyroid gland and the heart has been reported in the medical literature for more than 80 years [48]. Congestive heart failure and atrial fibrillation were then reported to be linked with thyroid dysfunction. Manowitz *et al.* described in 1996 that a "low T3 state" was significantly prevalent in patients with moderate-to-severe congestive HF [49]. This state was regarded as an adaptive mechanism, so as to decrease energy consumption, therefore not necessitating any treatment. Nowadays, it is proved that there is a strong and independent relationship between lower levels of serum T3 hormone and mortality in HF patients [50]. In addition, Pantos *et al.* showed that total T3 is an independent predictor of LVEF and functional status of HF patients, as this is assessed by cardiopulmonary exercise testing (VO_{2max}) (Fig. **3**) [51]. More recently, subclinical hypothyroidism or hyperthyroidism was found to raise the risk of HF events in the Thyroid Studies Collaboration, which reviewed data from 25,390 participants [52]. In molecular level, the thyroid hormone receptor α1 (TRα1), which is predominantly expressed in the myocardium, seems to play a role of utmost importance, depending on thyroid hormone availability. Hence, it seems that TRα1 receptor functions as a "switch" between fetal and adult cardiomyocyte phenotype. If TRα1 is unliganded, a fetal cardiac phenotype prevails. Then, TRα1 liganded with triiodothyronine (T3) promotes an adult phenotype in cardiomyocytes [53]. This fact obtains significant clinical relevance, considering the "low T3 state" that exists in HF. Additionally, TRα1 receptor seems to play an important role in cell differentiation [54].

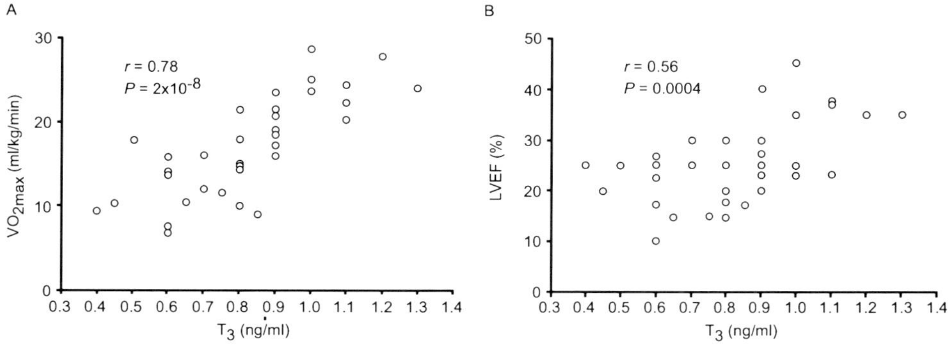

Fig. (3). Scatterplots showing correlation of T3 with VO_{2max} (A) and LVEF% (B) in patients with dilated cardiomyopathy. Reprinted from ref [51]. with kind permission from BioScientifica Ltd.
T3: triiodothyronine; VO_{2max}: maximal oxygen consumption; LVEF: left ventricular ejection fraction.

All the above and other similar findings have led to clinical studies of thyroid hormone replacement therapy in HF and in acute coronary syndromes, with promising results in albeit small patient samples and for short term thyroid hormone administration [55, 56]. The acute and long-term effects of Thyroid Hormone Replacement therapy in patients with ST-Elevation Myocardial Infarction (STEMI) and borderline/reduced triiodothyronine levels (The THiRST) study examines the safety of L-T3 replacement therapy in patients after acute myocardial infarction (AMI). This study also investigates the effect of L-T3 replacement therapy on chamber diameter / non-infarct wall thickness and its correlations with major (cardiac and non-cardiac death, re-infarction) and minor (angina, coronary revascularization, hospitalization) adverse cardiac events. Secondary end-points will be the effects of L-T3 replacement therapy on infarct size, wall motion abnormalities, systolic and diastolic myocardial function, neuroendocrine imbalance, quality of life, patients' functional capacity and cognitive and behavioral status. Preliminary results have demonstrated the safety of L-T3 administration, a significant improvement in LV wall motion score index and a non-significant trend of LVEF improvement [57]. The final results are eagerly anticipated. Lastly, in a very recent study, T4 replacement therapy in rats after provoked AMI attenuated atrial remodeling and reduced AF inducibility [58]. In the most current ESC guidelines for the diagnosis and treatment of acute and chronic heart failure, monitoring of the thyroid function is a class IC indication for the detection of reversible causes of HF and for prognostic reasons [5]. Hypo- or hyper-thyroidism should be treated accordingly. Last but not least, T3 has been recently proved to be associated with specific microRNAs, which primarily suppress pathological hypertrophy [59].

NOVEL BIOMARKERS

A common question that has been raised by the medical community during the last years is: "Why do we need new biomarkers?". We know that already used biomarkers, such as BNP, are affected by several factors. Many of these factors are extra-cardiac, like age, sex, body weight, hypertension and LV hypertrophy, AF, pulmonary embolism, right ventricular overload, myocardial ischemia, renal dysfunction, metabolic syndrome, liver cirrhosis, infection and sepsis [5]. Interestingly, as the understanding of the pathophysiology of HF goes deeper, the discovery of novel biomarkers leads to better diagnostic, prognostic and finally treatment tools. This trend can be explained by the fact that many of these novel biomarkers constitute treatment targets *per se*.

Suppression of Tumorgenicity 2 (ST2)

The ST2 gene and its protein were discovered in 1989 as an orphan receptor of the interleukin-1 (IL-1) receptor family [60]. ST2 was then associated with a number of diseases, such as asthma, pulmonary fibrosis, collagen vascular diseases, rheumatoid arthritis and sepsis [61 - 65]. In 2005, the IL-33 was discovered as a ST2 ligand with significant immunomodulatory functions [66]. Specifically, IL-33 led to the activation of T helper type 2 (Th2) lymphocytes to produce cytokines (IL-4, IL-5 and IL-13) and increased serum immunoglobulin levels, a pathway that involves the activation of nuclear factor-Kb (NF-κB) and mitogen-activated protein (MAP) kinase. These responses can potentially balance ongoing inflammation produced by Th1 cells. Four isoforms are transcripted by the ST2 gene, two of which are the most important: IL1RL1-b or ST2L, which is a membrane receptor of the interleukin-1 receptor family and IL1RL1-a or sST2a, which is a soluble receptor and lacks the transmembrane and intracellular domains. Therefore, the sST2 travels freely in the serum and can be measured [67]. It seems that IL-33 is released by cytoplasmic cell-vesicles, after mechanical stretch. Furthermore, cardiomyocytes and cardiac fibroblasts increase the release of ST2L and sST2 after biomechanical strain [68]. IL-33 has been found to decrease the hypertrophic and fibrotic effect of angiotensin II and phenylephrine on myocardium [69]. The interaction between IL-33 and ST2L is inhibited by the sST2, which binds IL-33 in bloodstream [69]. Hence, the cardioprotective action of IL-33 is attenuated. sST2 has been regarded as a marker of (adverse) prognosis, not only in acute, but also in chronic HF [70, 71]. Moreover, IL-33 and their receptors (ST2L and sST2) seem to constitute a new system which can be targeted for the treatment of HF, either by enhancing the protective action of IL-33, or by inhibiting sST2 [72]. Interestingly, in a very recent study, Bayes-Genis *et al.* showed that sST2 was a better mortality predictor than galectin-3, which is also a fibrosis marker [73]. Lastly, we have also demonstrated that higher levels of sST2 were associated with higher levels of galectin-3 and cTnT and lower incidence of AF in patients with HF and severely impaired LVEF [74].

Galectin-3

Galectin-3 is a β-galactoside-binding protein of the lectins' family, which were firstly described in 1972 in lower animals [75]. Two years later, a mammalian hepatic lectin was described, which agglutinated human and rabbit erythrocytes [76]. Teichberg *et al.* noticed that β-galactoside-specific hemagglutinin activity existed ubiquitously in several tissues and organs, such as lung, heart, liver, kidney, brain, thymus, spleen and muscles [77]. Human lung lectin was isolated in 1980 by Powell [78]. It was then speculated that lectins were involved in synaptogenesis and in adhesion of myoblasts. In the following years, lectins were estimated to interact in several pathophysiologic processes, including leukocyte adhesion, microbial opsonization, cell growth regulation, apoptosis, inflammation and more interestingly in cancer metastasis. Therefore, the potential to manipulate galectin activity for the treatment of a variety of human diseases was recognized [79]. Sharma *et al.* in their pioneering study proved that galectin-3 was overexpressed in hypertrophied rat hearts, long before they develop HF [80]. In the same study, galectin-3 was found to be produced by macrophages and to bind to cardiac fibroblasts. Its effects include the induction of fibroblast proliferation (through upregulation of cyclin D1) and the production of collagen I. Intrapericardial infusion of galectin-3 in healthy rats by the same investigators led to LV dysfunction and increased collagen I/III ratio. The fact that galectin-3 mRNA expression was higher in human hypertrophied hearts with relatively impaired LVEF than in those with normal LVEF resulted in the hypothesis that galectin-3 is a culprit biomarker that could be targeted before overt HF occurs [80]. In fact, Liu *et al.* demonstrated that N-acetyl-seryl-aspartyl-lysyl-proline (Ac-SDKP) actually prevented cardiac inflammation, fibrosis, hypertrophy, and dysfunction produced by intrapericardial infusion of galectin-3 [81]. More recently, higher levels of galectin-3 were significantly correlated with higher NYHA class, worse functional status, higher NT-proBNP and all-cause hospitalization or all-cause mortality, in ambulatory HF patients enrolled in the HF-ACTION study, the largest analysis for galectin-3 and outcomes to date [82]. Moreover, data from CORONA and COACH trials revealed the prognostic significance of fluctuations of galectin-3 levels over time [83]. Patients who had increasing galectin-3 levels (>15% from baseline or >17.8ng/ml) over time had higher morbidity and mortality in comparison with those with constant or decreasing galectin-3 levels. Furthermore, galectin-3, characterized as a marker for myocardial fibrosis, proved to be a determinant for LV reverse remodeling, independently of volume unloading [84, 85]. Very recently, inhibition of galectin-3 by citrus pectin or by genetic disruption was demonstrated to prevent cardiac dysfunction and fibrosis in rats treated with aldosterone [86]. Finally, galectin-3 levels may someday identify those HF patients who will mostly benefit from statin treatment, or cardiac resynchronization therapy (CRT) [87, 88].

Osteopontin (OPN)

OPN is a sialoprotein, which was firstly identified in bone tissue, and then proved to exist in cardiac fibroblasts and macrophages in necrotic cardiac tissue. Interestingly, it is produced by cardiac myocytes in idiopathic or ICM [89, 90]. Moreover, it is confirmed that the angiotensin II effects in cardiac remodeling that occur in HF, including hypertrophy, fibroblast proliferation and extracellular matrix (ECM) production, are achieved through OPN [91]. In fact, the same investigators showed that blocking OPN or β_3 integrin (a ligand of OPN on cell surface of cardiac fibroblasts) by antibodies, completely inhibited fibroblast proliferation. This also explains the antifibrotic action mechanism of the angiotensin converting enzyme (ACE) inhibitors or the ARBs [91]. OPN also inhibits matrix metalloproteinases (MMPs) [92]. Additionally, OPN participates in remodeling of the vasculature and in repair process of multiple systems of the human body [93 - 95]. Stawowy *et al.* have showed an upregulation of cardiac myocyte OPN in patients with dilated cardiomyopathy (DCM). Interestingly, OPN was significantly correlated with impaired LVEF and right ventricular ejection fraction (RVEF), heart dilation and higher LV end-diastolic pressure [96]. In a more recent study, Rosenberg *et al.* demonstrated that OPN levels in HF [ischemic cardiomyopathy (ICM) or DCM] discriminated patients with mild symptoms from those with more severe HF (NYHA III/IV) [97]. Moreover, OPN was a significant predictor of 4-year mortality in the same study, independently of NT-proBNP levels. Thus, OPN is a biomarker for advanced HF and adds significant information in risk stratification of these patients. In another recent study enrolling end-stage HF patients, OPN plasma levels significantly decreased after heart transplantation, but not after LVAD support, a fact that underscores the active role of OPN in HF sustainment and progression [98]. Finally, it has been demonstrated recently that OPN facilitates the formation of cross-linked insoluble collagen type I through up regulation of lysyl-oxidase in human cardiac and dermal fibroblasts, leading to increased cardiac stiffness [99].

Cytokines

It is well established that cytokines have a direct negative inotropic effect on the myocardium, which is mediated through a nitric oxide synthase [100]. Nowadays, we know that cytokines influence more the contractile mechanisms of the cardiomyocyte, including β-adrenergic receptors, nuclear factor-κB, phospholamban and the sarcoplasmic/endoplasmic reticulum Ca2+-ATPase (SERCA) [101]. Furthermore, Ikonomidis *et al.* have demonstrated that IL-6 levels are increased in patients with coronary artery disease and ischemic response during dobutamine stress echocardiography. Interestingly, increase was greater in patients with more dysfunctional myocardial segments and for longer recovery times [102].

In an Analysis of the Cytokine Database from the Vesnarinone Trial (VEST), which included 1,200 patients with advanced HF from 189 centers in North America, the independent prognostic value of high plasma levels of tumor necrosis factor (TNF) and IL-6 for mortality was established [103]. Moreover, soluble TNF receptors 1 and 2, and IL-6 were significantly higher in NYHA IV patients than those in NYHA III. In the same study, ICM was associated with consistently higher cytokine levels than DCM. Deliargyris *et al.* have also shown that the source of elevated plasma IL-6 in HF is not the myocardium, like in acute coronary syndromes (ACS), but peripheral organs [104]. Nevertheless, Vanderheyden *et al.* have reported a significant increase in myocardial gene expression of IL-1β, IL-6 and TNFα in patients with DCM compared to healthy subjects [105].

All these published data led to a great interest in blocking “harmful” cytokines, such as TNF or IL-1β, in ACS and HF, aiming to an improvement in myocardial function and a respective decrease in patients morbidity and. Two major trials, the Research into Etanercept CytOkine antagonism in VEntriculaR dysfunction

(RECOVER) and the Randomized Etanercept North AmerIcan Strategy to Study AntagoNism of CytokinEs (RENAISSANCE), and an analysis of the two studies on long-term outcome, the Randomized EtaNErcept Worldwide evALuation (RENEWAL), examined the effects of etanercept, a recombinant human TNF receptor antagonist, on morbidity/mortality of HF patients in NYHA II to IV class. All three trials were terminated prematurely, due to lack of benefit and more adverse events, especially infections [106]. Notwithstanding, Ikonomidis *et al.* have demonstrated that IL-1 inhibition with anakinra, a human recombinant interleukin-1a receptor antagonist, improved LV function in patients with rheumatoid arthritis and reduced oxidative stress and inflammation after a short term period of 30 days drug administration [107]. In the Virginia Commonwealth University-Anakinra Remodeling Trial (2) (VCU-ART2) pilot study, anakinra was tested in patients with re-perfused ST-segment elevation myocardial infarction, and was found to decrease the incidence of post-infarction HF [108]. Recently, it was demonstrated that injection of plasma from HF patients in healthy mice provoked a phenotype of systolic dysfunction. Most surprisingly, pretreatment of mice with anakinra prevented this effect, pointing out the significant role of cytokines in development and worsening of HF [109]. Finally, the Canakinumab Anti-inflammatory Thrombosis Outcomes Study (CANTOS) will evaluate canakinumab, a human monoclonal antibody that neutralizes IL-1β, in 17,200 stable post-infarction patients with persistent elevation of hs-CRP, for recurrent vascular events (*i.e.* nonfatal myocardial infarction, nonfatal stroke, cardiovascular death) and mortality/morbidity [110]. It is anticipated to end in 2017.

Prolactin (PRL)

PRL, a hormone produced by the anterior pituitary gland, was discovered in animals in 1935 and in humans in 1970 [111, 112]. Its main action is the stimulation of mammary glands to produce milk [113]. Furthermore, PRL is closely related with immune system and seems to play a role in pathogenesis of autoimmune diseases [114], as well as angiogenesis [115]. A great interest has been raised for PRL as a causative factor of postpartum cardiomyopathy (PPCM), after the pioneering study of Hilfiker-Kleiner *et al.* [116]. Thus, a cleaved 16kDa form of PRL, generated by cardiac cathepsin D, with pro-apoptotic and antiangiogenic properties, was found to be the culprit factor leading to PPCM. Bromocriptine, an inhibitor of PRL secretion, was then regarded as a potential medication for the treatment of PPCM. Many studies have investigated the role of hyperprolactinemia that is observed in HF [117]. Parissis *et al.* studied 180 patients with chronic HF and concluded that PRL levels were significantly associated with LVEF, NYHA class, 6MWT, BNP, soluble FAS, TNF, and that PRL levels independently predicted prognosis [118]. In contrast, Landberg *et al.* disputed any relation of prolactin with biochemical markers or mortality, in 462 elderly patients [119]. Finally, a very recent study, with a small number of patients, failed to demonstrate any relationship between PRL and NT-proBNP, hs-CRP, 6MWT or morbidity/mortality [120]. Hence, although the causative role of PRL in PPCM is established, there are conflicting results about the role of prolactin in HF. The EURObservational Research Programme will include 1,000 patients with HF from more than 20 countries, and perhaps will give new insights into pathophysiology and incidence of PPCM [121].

Neutrophil Gelatinase-Associated Lipocalin (NGAL)

NGAL is an acute phase protein of the lipocalin family. It is produced by neutrophils, macrophages and other immune cells, and also epithelial cells and cardiomyocytes [122 - 124]. Although NGAL has been proposed as an early and robust biomarker for acute kidney injury, it is also regarded to play a crucial role in atherosclerosis by protecting MMP [123]. It forms a stable dimeric complex that cannot be easily inactivated by the tissue inhibitor of metalloproteinase (TIMP) [125]. In this way the fibrous cap becomes less stable and consequently atherosclerotic plaques more susceptible to erosion. Moreover, NGAL was found to be a powerful predictor of 30 days outcome in the NGAL EvaLuation Along with B-type NaTriuretic Peptide in acutely decompensated HF (GALLANT) trial [126]. Surprisingly, NGAL was a better predictor of HF re-hospitalizations or (and) all-cause mortality than BNP, in the same study. Plasma NGAL was also proven to be an independent prognostic marker of cardiovascular mortality, all-cause mortality, and cardiovascular disease (CVD) in the very large community-dwelling Rancho Bernardo Study, which included 1,393 participants who were followed-up for 11 years [127]. Most interestingly, NGAL levels contributed to the prognostic model, independently of GFR, body mass index (BMI), age, sex or traditional CVD risk factors. What is more, NGAL significantly improved the predictive value of NT-proBNP and CRP in the same study. Nevertheless, in 1,415 patients with HF of ischemic etiology enrolled in the Controlled Rosuvastatin Multinational Trial in Heart Failure (CORONA), serum NGAL did not add any significant information to NT-proBNP and GFR [128]. This was the largest study of NGAL in chronic HF patients of only ischemic etiology though, and therefore similar conclusions cannot be extrapolated for DCM. In contrast, in the GISSI-HF trial, urinary NGAL was an independent and significant predictor of all-cause mortality and HF hospitalizations, even when GFR was normal and other clinical risk factors were adjusted [129]. Therefore, urinary NGAL may be a more robust prognostic biomarker than serum NGAL in chronic HF patients. Finally, the Acute Kidney Injury Neutrophil Gelatinase-Associated Lipocalin (N-GAL) Evaluation of Symptomatic Heart Failure Study (AKINESIS) will assess the value of plasma and urine NGAL to predict worsening renal function in acute HF patients treated with diuretics [130]. Its results are expected soon.

Cystatin-C (CyC)

CyC is a cysteine protease inhibitor produced in mammals at a constant rate by all nucleated cells [131]. CyC has a small size (13kDa), therefore it is freely filtered by the glomerulus. Moreover, it is not secreted, reabsorbed or catabolized in the proximal tubules, hence proposed as a more accurate estimate of GRF than serum creatinine [132]. CyC, as a protease inhibitor, inhibits cathepsin B which is an enzyme that degrades ECM proteins directly or indirectly, through activation of urokinase plasminogen activator or MMPs [133]. In this way CyC plays a crucial role in ECM remodeling by accumulation of ECM proteins. High CyC expression has been found in ischemic myocardium (protective mechanism), while low CyC expression is consistent with more severe atherosclerotic and aneurysmal lesions [134]. Moreover, it is well proven that higher CyC levels are significantly associated with worse prognosis, not only in chronic, but also in acute HF, even when creatinine levels are within normal range, independently of traditional risk factors and BNP [135 - 139]. Interestingly, CyC levels and GFR estimated by CyC, when combined with NT-proBNP, provided additional prognostic value in these studies.

Adiponectin (APN)

APN is a cytokine, which was firstly discovered to be produced by adipose tissue [140]. However, it is also synthesized in the failing myocardium [141]. Adiponectin has insulin-sensitizing, anti-atherogenic and anti-inflammatory actions [142, 143]. More specifically, hypoadiponectinemia was independently related with higher incidence of insulin resistance, diabetes type II and myocardial infarction. Unexpectedly, higher levels of APN have been associated with higher BNP levels and increased mortality in HF patients [144 - 146]. High APN levels are related to low functional capacity [147]. This phenomenon has been reported as "functional APN resistance", and is attributed to a decrease in density of AdipoR1 receptor on cardiomyocytes of failing hearts [148, 149]. Another potential explanation of this paradox may be that greater APN levels act as a compensatory mechanism in more severe HF [150]. Interestingly, in a relatively recent study, administration of a β-blocker (carvedilol) in patients with chronic HF resulted in drop of APN levels, which was correlated with LVEF improvement [151]. Similarly, exercise training is proven to reverse APN resistance and normalize APN levels in chronic HF patients [152]. Therefore, APN and its receptors constitute a novel biomarker for HF and a potential treatment target.

Other Experimental Biomarkers

There is a variety of other novel biomarkers associated with HF, under investigation. A very promising candidate biomarker is the pro-apoptotic protein, apoptosis-stimulating fragment (FAS) and its soluble ligand (sFAS), which is found to be an independent predictor of risk in advanced HF [153]. The soluble TNF-related apoptosis-inducing ligand (sTRAIL) is also regarded as a strongly protective agent for HF patients [153]. Osteoprotegerin (OPG) is a member of the TNF receptor superfamily that has attracted much attention during last years. In the GISSI-HF trial, in which 1,229 HF patients were included, OPG levels significantly predicted mortality, independently of conventional CVD risk factors [154]. Another peptide, adrenomedullin, which has many favorable actions in cardiovascular system, such as vasodilatation, increase in cardiac output, inhibition of secretion of endothelin-1, angiotensin II, aldosterone and catecholamines, diuresis and natriuresis, seems to be a robust predictor of mortality in mild/moderate HF patients [155]. Furthermore, urinary kidney injury molecule 1 (KIM-1), a transmembrane protein which indicates acute renal injury, was found to significantly predict worse outcome in chronic HF, independently of GFR [156]. Last but not least, another important biomarker is the growth differentiation factor-15 (GDF-15), which is a member of the transforming growth factor-β cytokine superfamily, expressed by activated macrophages [157]. In the Prospective Investigation of the Vasculature in Uppsala Seniors (PIVUS) Study, GDF-15 was found to be independently associated with reduced LVEF and NT-proBNP levels [158]. Finally, GDF-15 is reported to be a prognostic biomarker for mortality in chronic HF patients [159].

Micro-RNAs

Micro-RNAs (miRs) are noncoding single-stranded RNAs, approximately 22 nucleotides long, and were firstly discovered in the nematode worm in 1993 [160, 161]. They have attracted great interest because of their ability to regulate post-transcriptional gene expression, by binding to complementary sequences of messenger RNAs (mRNAs), inhibiting in this way their translation or leading to their degradation [162]. Until today, more than 1400 miR genes have been identified in humans [163], and their malfunction is associated with a number of diseases, such as cancer, diabetes, autoimmune diseases and HF [164]. Table **2** shows miRs with distinct role in HF.

Table 2. Characteristic micro-RNAs with distinct functions, involved in heart failure.

	Micro-RNA		
Functions in the cardiovascular system	**Increased**	**Decreased**	**ref.**
Induced in endothelial cells by shear stress; modulates apoptosis and the activity of eNOS; regulates the function of vascular smooth muscle cells; leads to fibroblast proliferation and fibrosis	**miR-21**		[168] [169] [170]
Downregulation of connective tissue growth factor; its decrease in HF contributes to fibrosis of myocardium		**miR-30**	[171]
Angiogenesis blockade		**miR-92**	[172]
Repression of the adult genes of α-myocin heavy chain and SERCA, isoproterenol induced up-regulation of fetal genes ANP and β-myocin heavy chain	**miR-100**		[173]

(Table 2) contd.....

	Micro-RNA		
Functions in the cardiovascular system	**Increased**	**Decreased**	**ref.**
Induction of cellular hypertrophy and fetal gene program	**miR-129**		[174]
Downregulation of connective tissue growth factor; its decrease in HF contributes to fibrosis of myocardium		**miR-133**	[171]
Antiapoptotic factor		**miR-182e**	[175]
Upregulation by hypoxia; increases endothelial cell migration and tubulogenesis	**miR-210**		[176] [177]
Induction of cell growth; maintenance epithelial barrier function	**miR-211**		[178] [179]
Induction of cellular hypertrophy and fetal gene program	**miR-212**		[174]
Predicts heart failure	**miR-423**		[180]
Increased in myocardial infarction	**miR-499**		[181]

ANP: atrial natriuretic peptide; HF: heart failure; eNOS: endothelial nitric oxide synthase; SERCA: sarco/endoplasmic reticulum Ca2+-ATPase.

The implication of miRs in clinical practice is predictable. MiRs can be used for diagnosis and prognosis of diseases, especially when these are circulating in the bloodstream [165]. Dysregulation of miRs which occurs in diseases such as HF, may be reversed by silencing those miRs, when they are overexpressed, or by replacing those that are decreased [162]. For this reason, the so called antagomiRs have been produced, which are single-stranded, anti-sense to miRs, oligonucleotides that inhibit the upregulated miRs. In contrast, artificially introduced miRs (miR mimics) may possibly replace the downregulated miRs [162]. However, things are not as simple as may seem, because most miRs are involved in multiple pathophysiological mechanisms and diseases, such as asthma, autoimmune diseases, cancer and cardiovascular diseases [164]. Nevertheless, some experimental studies are quite promising in this field. For example, Montgomery *et al.* have demonstrated that subcutaneous delivery of antimiR-208a prevented cardiac remodeling and improved cardiac function in Dahl hypertensive rats [166]. Additionally, Wang *et al.* reversed cardiac hypertrophy in rats and improved cardiac function by administering a double stranded miR mimic for miR-9 [167]. Hence, miRs have brought about a completely new era in diagnosis, prognosis and treatment of HF.

CONCLUDING REMARKS

During last years, we have approached HF from multiple pathophysiological aspects, such as inflammation, injury, apoptosis, remodeling, neurohormonal activation and renal dysfunction. This tendency of a multi-marker approach to HF patients for diagnosis, prognosis and therapy is of utmost importance, reflecting the multifactorial nuance of HF [182]. As a result, an integrated view of the HF patient can be succeeded.

CONFLICT OF INTEREST

The authors confirm that they have no conflict of interest to declare for this publication.

ACKNOWLEDGEMENTS

Declared none.

REFERENCES

[1] Braunwald E. Biomarkers in heart failure. N Engl J Med 2008; 358(20): 2148-59. [http://dx.doi.org/10.1056/NEJMra0800239] [PMID: 18480207]

[2] Morrow DA, de Lemos JA. Benchmarks for the assessment of novel cardiovascular biomarkers. Circulation 2007; 115(8): 949-52. [http://dx.doi.org/10.1161/CIRCULATIONAHA.106.683110] [PMID: 17325253]

[3] Biomarkers and surrogate endpoints: preferred definitions and conceptual framework. Clin Pharmacol Ther 2001; 69(3): 89-95. [http://dx.doi.org/10.1067/mcp.2001.113989] [PMID: 11240971]

[4] Smith JG, Newton-Cheh C, Almgren P, *et al.* Assessment of conventional cardiovascular risk factors and multiple biomarkers for the prediction of incident heart failure and atrial fibrillation. J Am Coll Cardiol 2010; 56(21): 1712-9. [http://dx.doi.org/10.1016/j.jacc.2010.05.049] [PMID: 21070922]

[5] McMurray JJ, Adamopoulos S, Anker SD, *et al.* ESC guidelines for the diagnosis and treatment of acute and chronic heart failure 2012: The Task Force for the Diagnosis and Treatment of Acute and Chronic Heart Failure 2012 of the European Society of Cardiology. Developed in collaboration with the Heart Failure Association (HFA) of the ESC. Eur J Heart Fail 2012; 14(8): 803-69. [http://dx.doi.org/10.1093/eurjhf/hfs105] [PMID: 22828712]

[6] Swedberg K, Young JB, Anand IS, *et al.* Treatment of anemia with darbepoetin alfa in systolic heart failure. N Engl J Med 2013; 368(13): 1210-9. [http://dx.doi.org/10.1056/NEJMoa1214865] [PMID: 23473338]

[7] Anker SD, Comin Colet J, Filippatos G, *et al.* Ferric carboxymaltose in patients with heart failure and iron deficiency. N Engl J Med 2009; 361(25): 2436-48. [http://dx.doi.org/10.1056/NEJMoa0908355] [PMID: 19920054]

[8] Ponikowski P, van Veldhuisen DJ, Comin-Colet J, *et al.* Beneficial effects of long-term intravenous iron therapy with ferric carboxymaltose in patients with symptomatic heart failure and iron deficiency. Eur Heart J 2014. [Epub ahead of print].

[9] Allen LA, Felker GM, Mehra MR, *et al.* Validation and potential mechanisms of red cell distribution width as a prognostic marker in heart failure. J Card Fail 2010; 16(3): 230-8. [http://dx.doi.org/10.1016/j.cardfail.2009.11.003] [PMID: 20206898]

[10] Taal MW, Brenner BM. Adaptation to nephrons loss and mechanisms of progression in chronic kidney disease. In: Skorecki K, Chertow GM, Marsden PA, Eds. Brenner and Rector's The Kidney. Philadelphia: Elsevier/Saunders 2012; pp. 1918-71.

[11] Tang WH, Mullens W. Cardiorenal syndrome in decompensated heart failure. Heart 2010; 96(4): 255-60. [http://dx.doi.org/10.1136/hrt.2009.166256] [PMID: 19401280]

[12] Ronco C, Haapio M, House AA, Anavekar N, Bellomo R. Cardiorenal syndrome. J Am Coll Cardiol 2008; 52(19): 1527-39. [http://dx.doi.org/10.1016/j.jacc.2008.07.051] [PMID: 19007588]

[13] Maggioni AP, Dahlström U, Filippatos G, *et al.* EURObservational Research Programme: regional differences and 1-year follow-up results of the Heart Failure Pilot Survey (ESC-HF Pilot). Eur J Heart Fail 2013; 15(7): 808-17. [http://dx.doi.org/10.1093/eurjhf/hft050] [PMID: 23537547]

[14] Verbrugge FH, Steels P, Grieten L, Nijst P, Tang WH, Mullens W. Hyponatremia in acute decompensated heart failure: depletion *versus* dilution. J Am Coll Cardiol 2015; 65(5): 480-92. [http://dx.doi.org/10.1016/j.jacc.2014.12.010] [PMID: 25660927]

[15] Gheorghiade M, Konstam MA, Burnett JC Jr, *et al.* Short-term clinical effects of tolvaptan, an oral vasopressin antagonist, in patients hospitalized for heart failure: the EVEREST Clinical Status Trials. JAMA 2007; 297(12): 1332-43. [http://dx.doi.org/10.1001/jama.297.12.1332] [PMID: 17384438]

[16] Bielecka-Dabrowa A, Mikhailidis DP, Jones L, Rysz J, Aronow WS, Banach M. The meaning of hypokalemia in heart failure. Int J Cardiol 2012; 158(1): 12-7. [http://dx.doi.org/10.1016/j.ijcard.2011.06.121] [PMID: 21775000]

[17] Samsky MD, Patel CB, DeWald TA, *et al.* Cardiohepatic interactions in heart failure: an overview and clinical implications. J Am Coll Cardiol 2013; 61(24): 2397-405. [http://dx.doi.org/10.1016/j.jacc.2013.03.042] [PMID: 23603231]

[18] Henrion J. Hypoxic hepatitis. Liver Int 2012; 32(7): 1039-52. [http://dx.doi.org/10.1111/j.1478-3231.2011.02655.x] [PMID: 22098491]

[19] Sherlock S. The liver in heart failure; relation of anatomical, functional, and circulatory changes. Br Heart J 1951; 13(3): 273-93. [http://dx.doi.org/10.1136/hrt.13.3.273] [PMID: 14848381]

[20] Cassidy WM, Reynolds TB. Serum lactic dehydrogenase in the differential diagnosis of acute hepatocellular injury. J Clin Gastroenterol 1994; 19(2): 118-21.
[http://dx.doi.org/10.1097/00004836-199409000-00008] [PMID: 7963356]

[21] Nikolaou M, Parissis J, Yilmaz MB, *et al.* Liver function abnormalities, clinical profile, and outcome in acute decompensated heart failure. Eur Heart J 2013; 34(10): 742-9.
[http://dx.doi.org/10.1093/eurheartj/ehs332] [PMID: 23091203]

[22] Allen LA, Felker GM, Pocock S, *et al.* Liver function abnormalities and outcome in patients with chronic heart failure: data from the Candesartan in Heart Failure: Assessment of Reduction in Mortality and Morbidity (CHARM) program. Eur J Heart Fail 2009; 11(2): 170-7.
[http://dx.doi.org/10.1093/eurjhf/hfn031] [PMID: 19168515]

[23] Poelzl G, Eberl C, Achrainer H, *et al.* Prevalence and prognostic significance of elevated gamma-glutamyltransferase in chronic heart failure. Circ Heart Fail 2009; 2(4): 294-302.
[http://dx.doi.org/10.1161/CIRCHEARTFAILURE.108.826735] [PMID: 19808352]

[24] Anker SD, Doehner W, Rauchhaus M, *et al.* Uric acid and survival in chronic heart failure: validation and application in metabolic, functional, and hemodynamic staging. Circulation 2003; 107(15): 1991-7.
[http://dx.doi.org/10.1161/01.CIR.0000065637.10517.A0] [PMID: 12707250]

[25] Kittleson MM, St John ME, Bead V, *et al.* Increased levels of uric acid predict haemodynamic compromise in patients with heart failure independently of B-type natriuretic peptide levels. Heart 2007; 93(3): 365-7.
[http://dx.doi.org/10.1136/hrt.2006.090845] [PMID: 17322514]

[26] Gotsman I, Keren A, Lotan C, Zwas DR. Changes in uric acid levels and allopurinol use in chronic heart failure: association with improved survival. J Card Fail 2012; 18(9): 694-701.
[http://dx.doi.org/10.1016/j.cardfail.2012.06.528] [PMID: 22939038]

[27] Givertz MM, Mann DL, Lee KL, *et al.* Xanthine oxidase inhibition for hyperuricemic heart failure patients: design and rationale of the EXACT-HF study. Circ Heart Fail 2013; 6(4): 862-8.
[http://dx.doi.org/10.1161/CIRCHEARTFAILURE.113.000394] [PMID: 23861505]

[28] Missov E, Mair J. A novel biochemical approach to congestive heart failure: cardiac troponin T. Am Heart J 1999; 138(1 Pt 1): 95-9.
[http://dx.doi.org/10.1016/S0002-8703(99)70252-8] [PMID: 10385770]

[29] Latini R, Masson S, Anand IS, *et al.* Prognostic value of very low plasma concentrations of troponin T in patients with stable chronic heart failure. Circulation 2007; 116(11): 1242-9.
[http://dx.doi.org/10.1161/CIRCULATIONAHA.106.655076] [PMID: 17698733]

[30] Masson S, Anand I, Favero C, *et al.* Serial measurement of cardiac troponin T using a highly sensitive assay in patients with chronic heart failure: data from 2 large randomized clinical trials. Circulation 2012; 125(2): 280-8.
[http://dx.doi.org/10.1161/CIRCULATIONAHA.111.044149] [PMID: 22139751]

[31] Sudoh T, Kangawa K, Minamino N, Matsuo H. A new natriuretic peptide in porcine brain. Nature 1988; 332(6159): 78-81.
[http://dx.doi.org/10.1038/332078a0] [PMID: 2964562]

[32] Hunt PJ, Yandle TG, Nicholls MG, Richards AM, Espiner EA. The amino-terminal portion of pro-brain natriuretic peptide (Pro-BNP) circulates in human plasma. Biochem Biophys Res Commun 1995; 214(3): 1175-83.
[http://dx.doi.org/10.1006/bbrc.1995.2410] [PMID: 7575527]

[33] Januzzi JL Jr, Sakhuja R, O'donoghue M, *et al.* Utility of amino-terminal pro-brain natriuretic peptide testing for prediction of 1-year mortality in patients with dyspnea treated in the emergency department. Arch Intern Med 2006; 166(3): 315-20.
[http://dx.doi.org/10.1001/archinte.166.3.315] [PMID: 16476871]

[34] Masson S, Latini R, Anand IS, *et al.* Prognostic value of changes in N-terminal pro-brain natriuretic peptide in Val-HeFT (Valsartan Heart Failure Trial). J Am Coll Cardiol 2008; 52(12): 997-1003.
[http://dx.doi.org/10.1016/j.jacc.2008.04.069] [PMID: 18786480]

[35] Kim HN, Januzzi JL Jr. Natriuretic peptide testing in heart failure. Circulation 2011; 123(18): 2015-9.
[http://dx.doi.org/10.1161/CIRCULATIONAHA.110.979500] [PMID: 21555724]

[36] Vanderheyden M, Bartunek J, Goethals M. Brain and other natriuretic peptides: molecular aspects. Eur J Heart Fail 2004; 6(3): 261-8.
[http://dx.doi.org/10.1016/j.ejheart.2004.01.004] [PMID: 14987574]

[37] O'Connor CM, Starling RC, Hernandez AF, *et al.* Effect of nesiritide in patients with acute decompensated heart failure. N Engl J Med 2011; 365(1): 32-43.
[http://dx.doi.org/10.1056/NEJMoa1100171] [PMID: 21732835]

[38] McMurray JJ, Packer M, Desai AS, *et al.* Angiotensin-neprilysin inhibition *versus* enalapril in heart failure. N Engl J Med 2014; 371(11): 993-1004.
[http://dx.doi.org/10.1056/NEJMoa1409077] [PMID: 25176015]

[39] Maisel A, Barnard D, Jaski B, *et al.* Primary results of the HABIT Trial (heart failure assessment with BNP in the home). J Am Coll Cardiol 2013; 61(16): 1726-35.
[http://dx.doi.org/10.1016/j.jacc.2013.01.052] [PMID: 23500322]

[40] Horwich TB, Hamilton MA, Maclellan WR, Fonarow GC. Low serum total cholesterol is associated with marked increase in mortality in advanced heart failure. J Card Fail 2002; 8(4): 216-24.
[http://dx.doi.org/10.1054/jcaf.2002.0804216] [PMID: 12397569]

[41] Zivlas C, Stefanidis A, Triposkiadis F, *et al.* Predictive biomarkers for functional status and quality of life in heart failure patients with severely impaired left ventricular systolic function. Eur J Heart Fail 2014; 16 (Suppl. 2): 172-3.

[42] Rauchhaus M, Clark AL, Doehner W, *et al.* The relationship between cholesterol and survival in patients with chronic heart failure. J Am Coll Cardiol 2003; 42(11): 1933-40.
[http://dx.doi.org/10.1016/j.jacc.2003.07.016] [PMID: 14662255]

[43] Anker SD, Chua TP, Ponikowski P, *et al.* Hormonal changes and catabolic/anabolic imbalance in chronic heart failure and their importance for cardiac cachexia. Circulation 1997; 96(2): 526-34.
[http://dx.doi.org/10.1161/01.CIR.96.2.526] [PMID: 9244221]

[44] Szabó T, Postrach E, Mähler A, *et al.* Increased catabolic activity in adipose tissue of patients with chronic heart failure. Eur J Heart Fail 2013; 15(10): 1131-7.
[http://dx.doi.org/10.1093/eurjhf/hft067] [PMID: 23696611]

[45] Mendall MA, Patel P, Asante M, *et al.* Relation of serum cytokine concentrations to cardiovascular risk factors and coronary heart disease. Heart 1997; 78(3): 273-7.
[http://dx.doi.org/10.1136/hrt.78.3.273] [PMID: 9391290]

[46] Anand IS, Latini R, Florea VG, *et al.* C-reactive protein in heart failure: prognostic value and the effect of valsartan. Circulation 2005; 112(10): 1428-34.
[http://dx.doi.org/10.1161/CIRCULATIONAHA.104.508465] [PMID: 16129801]

[47] Choi EY, Yan RT, Fernandes VR, *et al.* High-sensitivity C-reactive protein as an independent predictor of progressive myocardial functional deterioration: the multiethnic study of atherosclerosis. Am Heart J 2012; 164(2): 251-8.
[http://dx.doi.org/10.1016/j.ahj.2012.05.010] [PMID: 22877812]

[48] Hatfield WH. The Thyroid Heart. Can Med Assoc J 1933; 28(5): 546-8.
[PMID: 20319118]

[49] Manowitz NR, Mayor GH, Klepper MJ, DeGroot LJ. Subclinical Hypothyroidism and Euthyroid Sick Syndrome in Patients with Moderate-to-Severe Congestive Heart Failure. Am J Ther 1996; 3(12): 797-801.
[http://dx.doi.org/10.1097/00045391-199612000-00002] [PMID: 11862240]

[50] Iervasi G, Pingitore A, Landi P, *et al.* Low-T3 syndrome: a strong prognostic predictor of death in patients with heart disease. Circulation 2003; 107(5): 708-13.
[http://dx.doi.org/10.1161/01.CIR.0000048124.64204.3F] [PMID: 12578873]

[51] Pantos C, Dritsas A, Mourouzis I, *et al.* Thyroid hormone is a critical determinant of myocardial performance in patients with heart failure: potential therapeutic implications. Eur J Endocrinol 2007; 157(4): 515-20.
[http://dx.doi.org/10.1530/EJE-07-0318] [PMID: 17893267]

[52] Gencer B, Collet TH, Virgini V, *et al.* Subclinical thyroid dysfunction and the risk of heart failure events: an individual participant data analysis from 6 prospective cohorts. Circulation 2012; 126(9): 1040-9.
[http://dx.doi.org/10.1161/CIRCULATIONAHA.112.096024] [PMID: 22821943]

[53] Pantos C, Xinaris C, Mourouzis I, *et al.* Thyroid hormone receptor alpha 1: a switch to cardiac cell "metamorphosis"? J Physiol Pharmacol 2008; 59(2): 253-69.
[PMID: 18622044]

[54] van der Putten HH, Joosten BJ, Klaren PH, Everts ME. Uptake of tri-iodothyronine and thyroxine in myoblasts and myotubes of the embryonic heart cell line H9c2(2-1). J Endocrinol 2002; 175(3): 587-96.
[http://dx.doi.org/10.1677/joe.0.1750587] [PMID: 12475370]

[55] Pingitore A, Galli E, Barison A, *et al.* Acute effects of triiodothyronine (T3) replacement therapy in patients with chronic heart failure and low-T3 syndrome: a randomized, placebo-controlled study. J Clin Endocrinol Metab 2008; 93(4): 1351-8.
[http://dx.doi.org/10.1210/jc.2007-2210] [PMID: 18171701]

[56] Hamilton MA, Stevenson LW, Fonarow GC, *et al.* Safety and hemodynamic effects of intravenous triiodothyronine in advanced congestive heart failure. Am J Cardiol 1998; 81(4): 443-7.

[http://dx.doi.org/10.1016/S0002-9149(97)00950-8] [PMID: 9485134]

[57] Forini F, Ucciferri N, Kusmic C, *et al.* Low T3 State Is Correlated with Cardiac Mitochondrial Impairments after Ischemia Reperfusion Injury: Evidence from a Proteomic Approach. Int J Mol Sci 2015; 16(11): 26687-705.
[http://dx.doi.org/10.3390/ijms161125973] [PMID: 26561807]

[58] Zhang Y, Dedkov EI, Lee B III, Li Y, Pun K, Gerdes AM. Thyroid hormone replacement therapy attenuates atrial remodeling and reduces atrial fibrillation inducibility in a rat myocardial infarction-heart failure model. J Card Fail 2014; 20(12): 1012-9.
[http://dx.doi.org/10.1016/j.cardfail.2014.10.003] [PMID: 25305503]

[59] Janssen R, Zuidwijk MJ, Kuster DW, Muller A, Simonides WS. Thyroid hormone-regulated cardiac microRNAs are predicted to suppress pathological hypertrophic signaling. Front Endocrinol (Lausanne) 2014; 5: 171.
[http://dx.doi.org/10.3389/fendo.2014.00171] [PMID: 25368602]

[60] Tominaga S. A putative protein of a growth specific cDNA from BALB/c-3T3 cells is highly similar to the extracellular portion of mouse interleukin 1 receptor. FEBS Lett 1989; 258(2): 301-4.
[http://dx.doi.org/10.1016/0014-5793(89)81679-5] [PMID: 2532153]

[61] Oshikawa K, Kuroiwa K, Tago K, *et al.* Elevated soluble ST2 protein levels in sera of patients with asthma with an acute exacerbation. Am J Respir Crit Care Med 2001; 164(2): 277-81.
[http://dx.doi.org/10.1164/ajrccm.164.2.2008120] [PMID: 11463601]

[62] Leung BP, Xu D, Culshaw S, McInnes IB, Liew FY. A novel therapy of murine collagen-induced arthritis with soluble T1/ST2. J Immunol 2004; 173(1): 145-50.
[http://dx.doi.org/10.4049/jimmunol.173.1.145] [PMID: 15210768]

[63] Kuroiwa K, Arai T, Okazaki H, Minota S, Tominaga S. Identification of human ST2 protein in the sera of patients with autoimmune diseases. Biochem Biophys Res Commun 2001; 284(5): 1104-8.
[http://dx.doi.org/10.1006/bbrc.2001.5090] [PMID: 11414697]

[64] Brunner M, Krenn C, Roth G, *et al.* Increased levels of soluble ST2 protein and IgG1 production in patients with sepsis and trauma. Intensive Care Med 2004; 30(7): 1468-73.
[http://dx.doi.org/10.1007/s00134-004-2184-x] [PMID: 14991091]

[65] Barksby HE, Lea SR, Preshaw PM, Taylor JJ. The expanding family of interleukin-1 cytokines and their role in destructive inflammatory disorders. Clin Exp Immunol 2007; 149(2): 217-25.
[http://dx.doi.org/10.1111/j.1365-2249.2007.03441.x] [PMID: 17590166]

[66] Schmitz J, Owyang A, Oldham E, *et al.* IL-33, an interleukin-1-like cytokine that signals *via* the IL-1 receptor-related protein ST2 and induces T helper type 2-associated cytokines. Immunity 2005; 23(5): 479-90.
[http://dx.doi.org/10.1016/j.immuni.2005.09.015] [PMID: 16286016]

[67] Ciccone MM, Cortese F, Gesualdo M, *et al.* A novel cardiac bio-marker: ST2: a review. Molecules 2013; 18(12): 15314-28.
[http://dx.doi.org/10.3390/molecules181215314] [PMID: 24335613]

[68] Weinberg EO, Shimpo M, De Keulenaer GW, *et al.* Expression and regulation of ST2, an interleukin-1 receptor family member, in cardiomyocytes and myocardial infarction. Circulation 2002; 106(23):

2961-6.
[http://dx.doi.org/10.1161/01.CIR.0000038705.69871.D9] [PMID: 12460879]

[69] Sanada S, Hakuno D, Higgins LJ, Schreiter ER, McKenzie AN, Lee RT. IL-33 and ST2 comprise a critical biomechanically induced and cardioprotective signaling system. J Clin Invest 2007; 117(6): 1538-49.
[http://dx.doi.org/10.1172/JCI30634] [PMID: 17492053]

[70] Rehman SU, Mueller T, Januzzi JL Jr. Characteristics of the novel interleukin family biomarker ST2 in patients with acute heart failure. J Am Coll Cardiol 2008; 52(18): 1458-65.
[http://dx.doi.org/10.1016/j.jacc.2008.07.042] [PMID: 19017513]

[71] Ky B, French B, McCloskey K, *et al.* High-sensitivity ST2 for prediction of adverse outcomes in chronic heart failure. Circ Heart Fail 2011; 4(2): 180-7.
[http://dx.doi.org/10.1161/CIRCHEARTFAILURE.110.958223] [PMID: 21178018]

[72] Seki K, Sanada S, Kudinova AY, *et al.* Interleukin-33 prevents apoptosis and improves survival after experimental myocardial infarction through ST2 signaling. Circ Heart Fail 2009; 2(6): 684-91.
[http://dx.doi.org/10.1161/CIRCHEARTFAILURE.109.873240] [PMID: 19919994]

[73] Bayes-Genis A, de Antonio M, Vila J, *et al.* Head-to-head comparison of 2 myocardial fibrosis biomarkers for long-term heart failure risk stratification: ST2 *versus* galectin-3. J Am Coll Cardiol 2014; 63(2): 158-66.
[http://dx.doi.org/10.1016/j.jacc.2013.07.087] [PMID: 24076531]

[74] Zivlas C, Triposkiadis F, Psarras S, *et al.* Novel biomarkers in heart failure patients with very low ejection fraction. Proceedings of the 16th Hellenic Congress of Heart Failure. 2015 Jan 30 – Feb 01; Athens, Greece. 2015.

[75] Sharon N, Lis H. Lectins: cell-agglutinating and sugar-specific proteins. Science 1972; 177(4053): 949-59.
[http://dx.doi.org/10.1126/science.177.4053.949] [PMID: 5055944]

[76] Stockert RJ, Morell AG, Scheinberg IH. Mammalian hepatic lectin. Science 1974; 186(4161): 365-6.
[http://dx.doi.org/10.1126/science.186.4161.365] [PMID: 4472191]

[77] Teichberg VI, Silman I, Beitsch DD, Resheff G. A beta-D-galactoside binding protein from electric organ tissue of Electrophorus electricus. Proc Natl Acad Sci USA 1975; 72(4): 1383-7.
[http://dx.doi.org/10.1073/pnas.72.4.1383] [PMID: 1055413]

[78] Powell JT. Purification and properties of lung lectin. Rat lung and human lung beta-galactosid--binding proteins. Biochem J 1980; 187(1): 123-9.
[http://dx.doi.org/10.1042/bj1870123] [PMID: 7406857]

[79] Perillo NL, Marcus ME, Baum LG. Galectins: versatile modulators of cell adhesion, cell proliferation, and cell death. J Mol Med 1998; 76(6): 402-12.
[http://dx.doi.org/10.1007/s001090050232] [PMID: 9625297]

[80] Sharma UC, Pokharel S, van Brakel TJ, *et al.* Galectin-3 marks activated macrophages in failure-prone hypertrophied hearts and contributes to cardiac dysfunction. Circulation 2004; 110(19): 3121-8.
[http://dx.doi.org/10.1161/01.CIR.0000147181.65298.4D] [PMID: 15520318]

[81] Liu YH, D'Ambrosio M, Liao TD, *et al.* N-acetyl-seryl-aspartyl-lysyl-proline prevents cardiac

remodeling and dysfunction induced by galectin-3, a mammalian adhesion/growth-regulatory lectin. Am J Physiol Heart Circ Physiol 2009; 296(2): H404-12. [http://dx.doi.org/10.1152/ajpheart.00747.2008] [PMID: 19098114]

[82] Felker GM, Fiuzat M, Shaw LK, *et al.* Galectin-3 in ambulatory patients with heart failure: results from the HF-ACTION study. Circ Heart Fail 2012; 5(1): 72-8. [http://dx.doi.org/10.1161/CIRCHEARTFAILURE.111.963637] [PMID: 22016505]

[83] van der Velde AR, Gullestad L, Ueland T, *et al.* Prognostic value of changes in galectin-3 levels over time in patients with heart failure: data from CORONA and COACH. Circ Heart Fail 2013; 6(2): 219-26. [http://dx.doi.org/10.1161/CIRCHEARTFAILURE.112.000129] [PMID: 23395934]

[84] Lok DJ, Lok SI, Bruggink-André de la Porte PW, *et al.* Galectin-3 is an independent marker for ventricular remodeling and mortality in patients with chronic heart failure. Clin Res Cardiol 2013; 102(2): 103-10. [http://dx.doi.org/10.1007/s00392-012-0500-y] [PMID: 22886030]

[85] Milting H, Ellinghaus P, Seewald M, *et al.* Plasma biomarkers of myocardial fibrosis and remodeling in terminal heart failure patients supported by mechanical circulatory support devices. J Heart Lung Transplant 2008; 27(6): 589-96. [http://dx.doi.org/10.1016/j.healun.2008.02.018] [PMID: 18503956]

[86] Calvier L, Martinez-Martinez E, Miana M, *et al.* The impact of galectin-3 inhibition on aldosterone-induced cardiac and renal injuries. JACC Heart Fail 2015; 3(1): 59-67. [http://dx.doi.org/10.1016/j.jchf.2014.08.002] [PMID: 25458174]

[87] Gullestad L, Ueland T, Kjekshus J, *et al.* Galectin-3 predicts response to statin therapy in the Controlled Rosuvastatin Multinational Trial in Heart Failure (CORONA). Eur Heart J 2012; 33(18): 2290-6. [http://dx.doi.org/10.1093/eurheartj/ehs077] [PMID: 22513778]

[88] Stolen CM, Adourian A, Meyer TE, Stein KM, Solomon SD. Plasma galectin-3 and heart failure outcomes in MADIT-CRT (multicenter automatic defibrillator implantation trial with cardiac resynchronization therapy). J Card Fail 2014; 20(11): 793-9. [http://dx.doi.org/10.1016/j.cardfail.2014.07.018] [PMID: 25106783]

[89] Oldberg A, Franzén A, Heinegård D. Cloning and sequence analysis of rat bone sialoprotein (osteopontin) cDNA reveals an Arg-Gly-Asp cell-binding sequence. Proc Natl Acad Sci USA 1986; 83(23): 8819-23. [http://dx.doi.org/10.1073/pnas.83.23.8819] [PMID: 3024151]

[90] Graf K, Do YS, Ashizawa N, *et al.* Myocardial osteopontin expression is associated with left ventricular hypertrophy. Circulation 1997; 96(9): 3063-71. [http://dx.doi.org/10.1161/01.CIR.96.9.3063] [PMID: 9386176]

[91] Ashizawa N, Graf K, Do YS, *et al.* Osteopontin is produced by rat cardiac fibroblasts and mediates A(II)-induced DNA synthesis and collagen gel contraction. J Clin Invest 1996; 98(10): 2218-27. [http://dx.doi.org/10.1172/JCI119031] [PMID: 8941637]

[92] Krishnamurthy P, Peterson JT, Subramanian V, Singh M, Singh K. Inhibition of matrix metalloproteinases improves left ventricular function in mice lacking osteopontin after myocardial

infarction. Mol Cell Biochem 2009; 322(1-2): 53-62. [http://dx.doi.org/10.1007/s11010-008-9939-6] [PMID: 18979185]

[93] Giachelli CM, Schwartz SM, Liaw L. Molecular and cellular biology of osteopontin Potential role in cardiovascular disease. Trends Cardiovasc Med 1995; 5(3): 88-95. [http://dx.doi.org/10.1016/1050-1738(95)00005-T] [PMID: 21232243]

[94] Brown LF, Berse B, Van de Water L, *et al.* Expression and distribution of osteopontin in human tissues: widespread association with luminal epithelial surfaces. Mol Biol Cell 1992; 3(10): 1169-80. [http://dx.doi.org/10.1091/mbc.3.10.1169] [PMID: 1421573]

[95] Harter LV, Hruska KA, Duncan RL. Human osteoblast-like cells respond to mechanical strain with increased bone matrix protein production independent of hormonal regulation. Endocrinology 1995; 136(2): 528-35. [PMID: 7530647]

[96] Stawowy P, Blaschke F, Pfautsch P, *et al.* Increased myocardial expression of osteopontin in patients with advanced heart failure. Eur J Heart Fail 2002; 4(2): 139-46. [http://dx.doi.org/10.1016/S1388-9842(01)00237-9] [PMID: 11959041]

[97] Rosenberg M, Zugck C, Nelles M, *et al.* Osteopontin, a new prognostic biomarker in patients with chronic heart failure. Circ Heart Fail 2008; 1(1): 43-9. [http://dx.doi.org/10.1161/CIRCHEARTFAILURE.107.746172] [PMID: 19808269]

[98] Schipper ME, Scheenstra MR, van Kuik J, *et al.* Osteopontin: a potential biomarker for heart failure and reverse remodeling after left ventricular assist device support. J Heart Lung Transplant 2011; 30(7): 805-10. [http://dx.doi.org/10.1016/j.healun.2011.03.015] [PMID: 21531579]

[99] López B, González A, Lindner D, *et al.* Osteopontin-mediated myocardial fibrosis in heart failure: a role for lysyl oxidase? Cardiovasc Res 2013; 99(1): 111-20. [http://dx.doi.org/10.1093/cvr/cvt100] [PMID: 23619422]

[100] Finkel MS, Oddis CV, Jacob TD, Watkins SC, Hattler BG, Simmons RL. Negative inotropic effects of cytokines on the heart mediated by nitric oxide. Science 1992; 257(5068): 387-9. [http://dx.doi.org/10.1126/science.1631560] [PMID: 1631560]

[101] Van Tassell BW, Toldo S, Mezzaroma E, Abbate A. Targeting interleukin-1 in heart disease. Circulation 2013; 128(17): 1910-23. [http://dx.doi.org/10.1161/CIRCULATIONAHA.113.003199] [PMID: 24146121]

[102] Ikonomidis I, Athanassopoulos G, Lekakis J, *et al.* Myocardial ischemia induces interleukin-6 and tissue factor production in patients with coronary artery disease: a dobutamine stress echocardiography study. Circulation 2005; 112(21): 3272-9. [http://dx.doi.org/10.1161/CIRCULATIONAHA.104.532259] [PMID: 16286589]

[103] Deswal A, Petersen NJ, Feldman AM, Young JB, White BG, Mann DL. Cytokines and cytokine receptors in advanced heart failure: an analysis of the cytokine database from the Vesnarinone trial (VEST). Circulation 2001; 103(16): 2055-9. [http://dx.doi.org/10.1161/01.CIR.103.16.2055] [PMID: 11319194]

[104] Deliargyris EN, Raymond RJ, Theoharides TC, Boucher WS, Tate DA, Dehmer GJ. Sites of

interleukin-6 release in patients with acute coronary syndromes and in patients with congestive heart failure. Am J Cardiol 2000; 86(9): 913-8.
[http://dx.doi.org/10.1016/S0002-9149(00)01121-8] [PMID: 11053698]

[105] Vanderheyden M, Paulus WJ, Voss M, *et al.* Myocardial cytokine gene expression is higher in aortic stenosis than in idiopathic dilated cardiomyopathy. Heart 2005; 91(7): 926-31.
[http://dx.doi.org/10.1136/hrt.2004.035733] [PMID: 15958363]

[106] Mann DL, McMurray JJ, Packer M, *et al.* Targeted anticytokine therapy in patients with chronic heart failure: results of the Randomized Etanercept Worldwide Evaluation (RENEWAL). Circulation 2004; 109(13): 1594-602.
[http://dx.doi.org/10.1161/01.CIR.0000124490.27666.B2] [PMID: 15023878]

[107] Ikonomidis I, Lekakis JP, Nikolaou M, *et al.* Inhibition of interleukin-1 by anakinra improves vascular and left ventricular function in patients with rheumatoid arthritis. Circulation 2008; 117(20): 2662-9.
[http://dx.doi.org/10.1161/CIRCULATIONAHA.107.731877] [PMID: 18474811]

[108] Abbate A, Van Tassell BW, Biondi-Zoccai G, *et al.* Effects of interleukin-1 blockade with anakinra on adverse cardiac remodeling and heart failure after acute myocardial infarction [from the Virginia Commonwealth University-Anakinra Remodeling Trial (2) (VCU-ART2) pilot study]. Am J Cardiol 2013; 111(10): 1394-400. [from the Virginia Commonwealth University-Anakinra Remodeling Trial (2) (VCU-ART2) pilot study].
[http://dx.doi.org/10.1016/j.amjcard.2013.01.287] [PMID: 23453459]

[109] Van Tassell BW, Arena RA, Toldo S, *et al.* Enhanced interleukin-1 activity contributes to exercise intolerance in patients with systolic heart failure. PLoS One 2012; 7(3): e33438.
[http://dx.doi.org/10.1371/journal.pone.0033438] [PMID: 22438931]

[110] Ridker PM, Thuren T, Zalewski A, Libby P. Interleukin-1β inhibition and the prevention of recurrent cardiovascular events: rationale and design of the Canakinumab Anti-inflammatory Thrombosis Outcomes Study (CANTOS). Am Heart J 2011; 162(4): 597-605.
[http://dx.doi.org/10.1016/j.ahj.2011.06.012] [PMID: 21982649]

[111] Bates RW, Riddle O. The preparation of prolactin. J Pharmacol Exp Ther 1935; 55(3): 365-71.

[112] Friesen H, Guyda H, Hardy J. The biosynthesis of human growth hormone and prolactin. J Clin Endocrinol Metab 1970; 31(6): 611-24.
[http://dx.doi.org/10.1210/jcem-31-6-611] [PMID: 5483096]

[113] Ganong WF. Physiology of reproduction in women. In: DeCherney AH, Nathan L, Eds. Current Obstetric and Gynecologic Diagnosis and Treatment. New York: McGraw-Hill 2003; pp. 130-53.

[114] Jara LJ, Medina G, Saavedra MA, Vera-Lastra O, Navarro C. Prolactin and autoimmunity. Clin Rev Allergy Immunol 2011; 40(1): 50-9.
[http://dx.doi.org/10.1007/s12016-009-8185-3] [PMID: 19911311]

[115] Corbacho AM, Martínez De La Escalera G, Clapp C. Roles of prolactin and related members of the prolactin/growth hormone/placental lactogen family in angiogenesis. J Endocrinol 2002; 173(2): 219-38.
[http://dx.doi.org/10.1677/joe.0.1730219] [PMID: 12010630]

[116] Hilfiker-Kleiner D, Kaminski K, Podewski E, *et al.* A cathepsin D-cleaved 16 kDa form of prolactin

mediates postpartum cardiomyopathy. Cell 2007; 128(3): 589-600.
[http://dx.doi.org/10.1016/j.cell.2006.12.036] [PMID: 17289576]

[117] Limas CJ, Kroupis C, Haidaroglou A, Cokkinos DV. Hyperprolactinaemia in patients with heart failure: clinical and immunogenetic correlations. Eur J Clin Invest 2002; 32(2): 74-8.
[http://dx.doi.org/10.1046/j.1365-2362.2002.00924.x] [PMID: 11895452]

[118] Parissis JT, Farmakis D, Fountoulaki K, *et al.* Clinical and neurohormonal correlates and prognostic value of serum prolactin levels in patients with chronic heart failure. Eur J Heart Fail 2013; 15(10): 1122-30.
[http://dx.doi.org/10.1093/eurjhf/hft070] [PMID: 23639781]

[119] Landberg E, Dahlström U, Alehagen U. Serum prolactin and macroprolactin in heart failure: no relation to established laboratory or clinical parameters. Ann Clin Biochem 2011; 48(Pt 1): 51-6.
[http://dx.doi.org/10.1258/acb.2010.010164] [PMID: 21115571]

[120] Naderi N, Bakhshandeh H, Ardeshiri M, *et al.* Hyper-Prolactinemia in Men With Idiopathic Dilated Cardiomyopathy: Does It Have any Prognostic Implications? Res Cardiovasc Med 2014; 3(3): e19321.
[http://dx.doi.org/10.5812/cardiovascmed.19321] [PMID: 25478544]

[121] Sliwa K, Hilfiker-Kleiner D, Mebazaa A, *et al.* EURObservational Research Programme: a worldwide registry on peripartum cardiomyopathy (PPCM) in conjunction with the Heart Failure Association of the European Society of Cardiology Working Group on PPCM. Eur J Heart Fail 2014; 16(5): 583-91.
[http://dx.doi.org/10.1002/ejhf.68] [PMID: 24591060]

[122] Liu Q, Nilsen-Hamilton M. Identification of a new acute phase protein. J Biol Chem 1995; 270(38): 22565-70.
[http://dx.doi.org/10.1074/jbc.270.38.22565] [PMID: 7545679]

[123] Devarajan P. Neutrophil gelatinase-associated lipocalin--an emerging troponin for kidney injury. Nephrol Dial Transplant 2008; 23(12): 3737-43.
[http://dx.doi.org/10.1093/ndt/gfn531] [PMID: 18809975]

[124] Ding L, Hanawa H, Ota Y, *et al.* Lipocalin-2/neutrophil gelatinase-B associated lipocalin is strongly induced in hearts of rats with autoimmune myocarditis and in human myocarditis. Circ J 2010; 74(3): 523-30.
[http://dx.doi.org/10.1253/circj.CJ-09-0485] [PMID: 20057160]

[125] Yan L, Borregaard N, Kjeldsen L, Moses MA. The high molecular weight urinary matrix metalloproteinase (MMP) activity is a complex of gelatinase B/MMP-9 and neutrophil gelatinase-associated lipocalin (NGAL). Modulation of MMP-9 activity by NGAL. J Biol Chem 2001; 276(40): 37258-65.
[http://dx.doi.org/10.1074/jbc.M106089200] [PMID: 11486009]

[126] Maisel AS, Mueller C, Fitzgerald R, *et al.* Prognostic utility of plasma neutrophil gelatinase-associated lipocalin in patients with acute heart failure: the NGAL EvaLuation Along with B-type NaTriuretic Peptide in acutely decompensated heart failure (GALLANT) trial. Eur J Heart Fail 2011; 13(8): 846-51.
[http://dx.doi.org/10.1093/eurjhf/hfr087] [PMID: 21791540]

[127] Daniels LB, Barrett-Connor E, Clopton P, Laughlin GA, Ix JH, Maisel AS. Plasma neutrophil gelatinase-associated lipocalin is independently associated with cardiovascular disease and mortality in

community-dwelling older adults: The Rancho Bernardo Study. J Am Coll Cardiol 2012; 59(12): 1101-9.
[http://dx.doi.org/10.1016/j.jacc.2011.11.046] [PMID: 22421304]

[128] Nymo SH, Ueland T, Askevold ET, *et al.* The association between neutrophil gelatinase-associated lipocalin and clinical outcome in chronic heart failure: results from CORONA*. J Intern Med 2012; 271(5): 436-43.
[http://dx.doi.org/10.1111/j.1365-2796.2011.02503.x] [PMID: 22211640]

[129] Damman K, Masson S, Hillege HL, *et al.* Clinical outcome of renal tubular damage in chronic heart failure. Eur Heart J 2011; 32(21): 2705-12.
[http://dx.doi.org/10.1093/eurheartj/ehr190] [PMID: 21666249]

[130] Angeletti S, Fogolari M, Morolla D, *et al.* Role of neutrophil gelatinase-associated lipocalin in the diagnosis and early treatment of acute kidney injury in a case series of patients with acute decompensated heart failure: A case series. Cardiol Res Pract 2016.
[http://dx.doi.org/10.1155/2016/3708210]

[131] Coll E, Botey A, Alvarez L, *et al.* Serum cystatin C as a new marker for noninvasive estimation of glomerular filtration rate and as a marker for early renal impairment. Am J Kidney Dis 2000; 36(1): 29-34.
[http://dx.doi.org/10.1053/ajkd.2000.8237] [PMID: 10873868]

[132] Stevens LA, Coresh J, Schmid CH, *et al.* Estimating GFR using serum cystatin C alone and in combination with serum creatinine: a pooled analysis of 3,418 individuals with CKD. Am J Kidney Dis 2008; 51(3): 395-406.
[http://dx.doi.org/10.1053/j.ajkd.2007.11.018] [PMID: 18295055]

[133] Xie L, Terrand J, Xu B, Tsaprailis G, Boyer J, Chen QM. Cystatin C increases in cardiac injury: a role in extracellular matrix protein modulation. Cardiovasc Res 2010; 87(4): 628-35.
[http://dx.doi.org/10.1093/cvr/cvq138] [PMID: 20489058]

[134] Shi GP, Sukhova GK, Grubb A, *et al.* Cystatin C deficiency in human atherosclerosis and aortic aneurysms. J Clin Invest 1999; 104(9): 1191-7.
[http://dx.doi.org/10.1172/JCI7709] [PMID: 10545518]

[135] Arimoto T, Takeishi Y, Niizeki T, *et al.* Cystatin C, a novel measure of renal function, is an independent predictor of cardiac events in patients with heart failure. J Card Fail 2005; 11(8): 595-601.
[http://dx.doi.org/10.1016/j.cardfail.2005.06.001] [PMID: 16230262]

[136] Tang WH, Van Lente F, Shrestha K, *et al.* Impact of myocardial function on cystatin C measurements in chronic systolic heart failure. J Card Fail 2008; 14(5): 394-9.
[http://dx.doi.org/10.1016/j.cardfail.2008.01.006] [PMID: 18514931]

[137] Manzano-Fernández S, Boronat-Garcia M, Albaladejo-Otón MD, *et al.* Complementary prognostic value of cystatin C, N-terminal pro-B-type natriuretic Peptide and cardiac troponin T in patients with acute heart failure. Am J Cardiol 2009; 103(12): 1753-9.
[http://dx.doi.org/10.1016/j.amjcard.2009.02.029] [PMID: 19539088]

[138] Flores-Blanco PJ, Manzano-Fernández S, Pérez-Calvo JI, *et al.* Cystatin C-based CKD-EPI equations and N-terminal pro-B-type natriuretic peptide for predicting outcomes in acutely decompensated heart failure. Clin Cardiol 2015; 38(2): 106-13.

[http://dx.doi.org/10.1002/clc.22362] [PMID: 25663560]

[139] Dupont M, Wu Y, Hazen SL, Tang WH. Cystatin C identifies patients with stable chronic heart failure at increased risk for adverse cardiovascular events. Circ Heart Fail 2012; 5(5): 602-9. [http://dx.doi.org/10.1161/CIRCHEARTFAILURE.112.966960] [PMID: 22899766]

[140] Nakano Y, Tobe T, Choi-Miura NH, Mazda T, Tomita M. Isolation and characterization of GBP28, a novel gelatin-binding protein purified from human plasma. J Biochem 1996; 120(4): 803-12. [http://dx.doi.org/10.1093/oxfordjournals.jbchem.a021483] [PMID: 8947845]

[141] Takano H, Obata JE, Kodama Y, *et al.* Adiponectin is released from the heart in patients with heart failure. Int J Cardiol 2009; 132(2): 221-6. [http://dx.doi.org/10.1016/j.ijcard.2007.11.040] [PMID: 18192035]

[142] Kadowaki T, Yamauchi T, Kubota N, Hara K, Ueki K, Tobe K. Adiponectin and adiponectin receptors in insulin resistance, diabetes, and the metabolic syndrome. J Clin Invest 2006; 116(7): 1784-92. [http://dx.doi.org/10.1172/JCI29126] [PMID: 16823476]

[143] Pischon T, Girman CJ, Hotamisligil GS, Rifai N, Hu FB, Rimm EB. Plasma adiponectin levels and risk of myocardial infarction in men. JAMA 2004; 291(14): 1730-7. [http://dx.doi.org/10.1001/jama.291.14.1730] [PMID: 15082700]

[144] Tsukamoto O, Fujita M, Kato M, *et al.* Natriuretic peptides enhance the production of adiponectin in human adipocytes and in patients with chronic heart failure. J Am Coll Cardiol 2009; 53(22): 2070-7. [http://dx.doi.org/10.1016/j.jacc.2009.02.038] [PMID: 19477358]

[145] Wannamethee SG, Whincup PH, Lennon L, Sattar N. Circulating adiponectin levels and mortality in elderly men with and without cardiovascular disease and heart failure. Arch Intern Med 2007; 167(14): 1510-7. [http://dx.doi.org/10.1001/archinte.167.14.1510] [PMID: 17646605]

[146] Kistorp C, Faber J, Galatius S, *et al.* Plasma adiponectin, body mass index, and mortality in patients with chronic heart failure. Circulation 2005; 112(12): 1756-62. [http://dx.doi.org/10.1161/CIRCULATIONAHA.104.530972] [PMID: 16157772]

[147] Laoutaris ID, Vasiliadis IK, Dritsas A, *et al.* High plasma adiponectin is related to low functional capacity in patients with chronic heart failure. Int J Cardiol 2010; 144(2): 230-1. [http://dx.doi.org/10.1016/j.ijcard.2008.12.126] [PMID: 19176260]

[148] Kintscher U. Does adiponectin resistance exist in chronic heart failure? Eur Heart J 2007; 28(14): 1676-7. [http://dx.doi.org/10.1093/eurheartj/ehm233] [PMID: 17591684]

[149] von Haehling S, Doehner W, Anker SD. Nutrition, metabolism, and the complex pathophysiology of cachexia in chronic heart failure. Cardiovasc Res 2007; 73(2): 298-309. [http://dx.doi.org/10.1016/j.cardiores.2006.08.018] [PMID: 17034772]

[150] Beatty AL, Zhang MH, Ku IA, Na B, Schiller NB, Whooley MA. Adiponectin is associated with increased mortality and heart failure in patients with stable ischemic heart disease: data from the Heart and Soul Study. Atherosclerosis 2012; 220(2): 587-92. [http://dx.doi.org/10.1016/j.atherosclerosis.2011.11.038] [PMID: 22196150]

[151] Yamaji M, Tsutamoto T, Tanaka T, *et al.* Effect of carvedilol on plasma adiponectin concentration in

patients with chronic heart failure. Circ J 2009; 73(6): 1067-73.
[http://dx.doi.org/10.1253/circj.CJ-08-1026] [PMID: 19367012]

[152] Van Berendoncks AM, Garnier A, Beckers P, *et al.* Exercise training reverses adiponectin resistance in skeletal muscle of patients with chronic heart failure. Heart 2011; 97(17): 1403-9.
[http://dx.doi.org/10.1136/hrt.2011.226373] [PMID: 21685184]

[153] Niessner A, Hohensinner PJ, Rychli K, *et al.* Prognostic value of apoptosis markers in advanced heart failure patients. Eur Heart J 2009; 30(7): 789-96.
[http://dx.doi.org/10.1093/eurheartj/ehp004] [PMID: 19196721]

[154] Røysland R, Masson S, Omland T, *et al.* Prognostic value of osteoprotegerin in chronic heart failure: The GISSI-HF trial. Am Heart J 2010; 160(2): 286-93.
[http://dx.doi.org/10.1016/j.ahj.2010.05.015] [PMID: 20691834]

[155] Adlbrecht C, Hülsmann M, Strunk G, *et al.* Prognostic value of plasma midregional pro-adrenomedullin and C-terminal-pro-endothelin-1 in chronic heart failure outpatients. Eur J Heart Fail 2009; 11(4): 361-6.
[http://dx.doi.org/10.1093/eurjhf/hfp004] [PMID: 19190023]

[156] Damman K, Van Veldhuisen DJ, Navis G, *et al.* Tubular damage in chronic systolic heart failure is associated with reduced survival independent of glomerular filtration rate. Heart 2010; 96(16): 1297-302.
[http://dx.doi.org/10.1136/hrt.2010.194878] [PMID: 20659949]

[157] Bootcov MR, Bauskin AR, Valenzuela SM, *et al.* MIC-1, a novel macrophage inhibitory cytokine, is a divergent member of the TGF-beta superfamily. Proc Natl Acad Sci USA 1997; 94(21): 11514-9.
[http://dx.doi.org/10.1073/pnas.94.21.11514] [PMID: 9326641]

[158] Lind L, Wallentin L, Kempf T, *et al.* Growth-differentiation factor-15 is an independent marker of cardiovascular dysfunction and disease in the elderly: results from the Prospective Investigation of the Vasculature in Uppsala Seniors (PIVUS) Study. Eur Heart J 2009; 30(19): 2346-53.
[http://dx.doi.org/10.1093/eurheartj/ehp261] [PMID: 19561023]

[159] Kempf T, von Haehling S, Peter T, *et al.* Prognostic utility of growth differentiation factor-15 in patients with chronic heart failure. J Am Coll Cardiol 2007; 50(11): 1054-60.
[http://dx.doi.org/10.1016/j.jacc.2007.04.091] [PMID: 17825714]

[160] Lee RC, Feinbaum RL, Ambros V. The C. elegans heterochronic gene lin-4 encodes small RNAs with antisense complementarity to lin-14. Cell 1993; 75(5): 843-54.
[http://dx.doi.org/10.1016/0092-8674(93)90529-Y] [PMID: 8252621]

[161] Wightman B, Ha I, Ruvkun G. Posttranscriptional regulation of the heterochronic gene lin-14 by lin-4 mediates temporal pattern formation in C. elegans. Cell 1993; 75(5): 855-62.
[http://dx.doi.org/10.1016/0092-8674(93)90530-4] [PMID: 8252622]

[162] Condorelli G, Latronico MV, Dorn GW II. microRNAs in heart disease: putative novel therapeutic targets? Eur Heart J 2010; 31(6): 649-58.
[http://dx.doi.org/10.1093/eurheartj/ehp573] [PMID: 20118173]

[163] Poller W, Tank J, Skurk C, Gast M. Cardiovascular RNA interference therapy: the broadening tool and target spectrum. Circ Res 2013; 113(5): 588-602.

[http://dx.doi.org/10.1161/CIRCRESAHA.113.301056] [PMID: 23948584]

[164] Manolis A, Manolis T. Micro RNAs: a revolutionary discovery in biology. Hospital Chronicles 2012; 7(1): 4-8.

[165] Kalozoumi G, Yacoub M, Sanoudou D. MicroRNAs in heart failure: Small molecules with major impact. Glob Cardiol Sci Pract 2014; 2014(2): 79-102.
[http://dx.doi.org/10.5339/gcsp.2014.30] [PMID: 25419522]

[166] Montgomery RL, Hullinger TG, Semus HM, *et al.* Therapeutic inhibition of miR-208a improves cardiac function and survival during heart failure. Circulation 2011; 124(14): 1537-47.
[http://dx.doi.org/10.1161/CIRCULATIONAHA.111.030932] [PMID: 21900086]

[167] Wang K, Long B, Zhou J, Li PF. miR-9 and NFATc3 regulate myocardin in cardiac hypertrophy. J Biol Chem 2010; 285(16): 11903-12.
[http://dx.doi.org/10.1074/jbc.M109.098004] [PMID: 20177053]

[168] Cheng Y, Zhang C. MicroRNA-21 in cardiovascular disease. J Cardiovasc Transl Res 2010; 3(3): 251-5.
[http://dx.doi.org/10.1007/s12265-010-9169-7] [PMID: 20560046]

[169] Wang M, Li W, Chang GQ, *et al.* MicroRNA-21 regulates vascular smooth muscle cell function *via* targeting tropomyosin 1 in arteriosclerosis obliterans of lower extremities. Arterioscler Thromb Vasc Biol 2011; 31(9): 2044-53.
[http://dx.doi.org/10.1161/ATVBAHA.111.229559] [PMID: 21817107]

[170] Weber M, Baker MB, Moore JP, Searles CD. MiR-21 is induced in endothelial cells by shear stress and modulates apoptosis and eNOS activity. Biochem Biophys Res Commun 2010; 393(4): 643-8.
[http://dx.doi.org/10.1016/j.bbrc.2010.02.045] [PMID: 20153722]

[171] Duisters RF, Tijsen AJ, Schroen B, *et al.* miR-133 and miR-30 regulate connective tissue growth factor: implications for a role of microRNAs in myocardial matrix remodeling. Circ Res 2009; 104(2): 170-178, 6p, 178.
[http://dx.doi.org/10.1161/CIRCRESAHA.108.182535] [PMID: 19096030]

[172] Bonauer A, Carmona G, Iwasaki M, *et al.* MicroRNA-92a controls angiogenesis and functional recovery of ischemic tissues in mice. Science 2009; 324(5935): 1710-3.
[http://dx.doi.org/10.1126/science.1174381] [PMID: 19460962]

[173] Sucharov C, Bristow MR, Port JD. miRNA expression in the failing human heart: functional correlates. J Mol Cell Cardiol 2008; 45(2): 185-92.
[http://dx.doi.org/10.1016/j.yjmcc.2008.04.014] [PMID: 18582896]

[174] Thum T, Galuppo P, Wolf C, *et al.* MicroRNAs in the human heart: a clue to fetal gene reprogramming in heart failure. Circulation 2007; 116(3): 258-67.
[http://dx.doi.org/10.1161/CIRCULATIONAHA.107.687947] [PMID: 17606841]

[175] Pineles BL, Romero R, Montenegro D, *et al.* Distinct subsets of microRNAs are expressed differentially in the human placentas of patients with preeclampsia. Am J Obstet Gynecol 2007; 196(3): 1-6.
[http://dx.doi.org/10.1016/j.ajog.2007.01.008]

[176] Endo K, Naito Y, Ji X, *et al.* MicroRNA 210 as a biomarker for congestive heart failure. Biol Pharm

Bull 2013; 36(1): 48-54.
[http://dx.doi.org/10.1248/bpb.b12-00578] [PMID: 23302636]

[177] Fasanaro P, D'Alessandra Y, Di Stefano V, *et al.* MicroRNA-210 modulates endothelial cell response to hypoxia and inhibits the receptor tyrosine kinase ligand Ephrin-A3. J Biol Chem 2008; 283(23): 15878-83.
[http://dx.doi.org/10.1074/jbc.M800731200] [PMID: 18417479]

[178] Cheng AM, Byrom MW, Shelton J, Ford LP. Antisense inhibition of human miRNAs and indications for an involvement of miRNA in cell growth and apoptosis. Nucleic Acids Res 2005; 33(4): 1290-7.
[http://dx.doi.org/10.1093/nar/gki200] [PMID: 15741182]

[179] Wang FE, Zhang C, Maminishkis A, *et al.* MicroRNA-204/211 alters epithelial physiology. FASEB J 2010; 24(5): 1552-71.
[http://dx.doi.org/10.1096/fj.08-125856] [PMID: 20056717]

[180] Tijsen AJ, Creemers EE, Moerland PD, *et al.* MiR423-5p as a circulating biomarker for heart failure. Circ Res 2010; 106(6): 1035-9.
[http://dx.doi.org/10.1161/CIRCRESAHA.110.218297] [PMID: 20185794]

[181] Adachi T, Nakanishi M, Otsuka Y, *et al.* Plasma microRNA 499 as a biomarker of acute myocardial infarction. Clin Chem 2010; 56(7): 1183-5.
[http://dx.doi.org/10.1373/clinchem.2010.144121] [PMID: 20395621]

[182] Sun RR, Lu L, Liu M, *et al.* Biomarkers and heart disease. Eur Rev Med Pharmacol Sci 2014; 18(19): 2927-35.
[PMID: 25339488]

Frontiers in Heart Failure, 2016, *Vol. 1*, 213-231

CHAPTER 7

Echocardiography in the Management of Patients with Heart Failure

Elias Tsougkos*

2nd Cardiology Clinic (Heart Failure and Preventive Cardiology Section) Henry Dunant Hospital Center Athens Greece

Abstract: Echocardiography is a valuable diagnostic tool for the management of heart failure (HF), by demonstrating structural and functional abnormalities in individuals characterized by increased risk of developing HF, patients with clinical features indicating HF, or cases of symptomatic HF. Echocardiography evaluates cardiac structural and functional parameters, having an important role in investigating the aetiology of heart conditions and providing prognostic information. During past years, two-dimensional echocardiography has been a valuable technique because of its ability to provide reliable diagnostic and prognostic information in HF patients. On the other hand, Doppler ultrasound, as a non-invasive tool, contributes to the identification of systolic and diastolic dysfunction. In clinical trials, the predictive value of ejection fraction has been consistently demonstrated; lower ejection fraction has been related to higher risk of cardiac death. Although a normal left ventricular function is observed in 40–50% of HF patients based on the results of recent clinical trials, the development of a global parameter, reflecting the remodelling process and functional abnormalities, is required. In this regard, recently developed three-dimensional volumetric measures of left ventricular anatomy and function seem very promising; however, more trials should be performed for further validation. Echocardiographic evaluation is considered as an essential part of HF management, despite the fact that no single examination meets all imaging requirements for HF investigation. Other modalities can provide additional evidence regarding specific questions, such as tissue characterization.

* **Corresponding author Elias Tsougkos:** 2nd Cardiology Clinic (Heart Failure and Preventive Cardiology Section) Henry Dunant Hospital Center Athens Greece; Tel: +30 217 722 1009; Fax: +30 210 697 2276; E-mail: Tsougkos@yahoo.com.

Panagiotis Georgoulias (Ed.)

Keywords: 2D echocardiography, 3D echocardiography, Cardiomyopathy, Diastolic function, Heart failure, Prognosis, Strain, Strain rate, Systolic function, Tissue Doppler imaging, Ventricle dysfunction.

INTRODUCTION

Heart failure (HF) is defined as "a complex clinical syndrome that can result from any structural or functional cardiac disorder that impairs the ability of ventricles to fill with or eject blood" [1]. In particular, it is a constellation of clinical signs and symptoms that are associated with impaired cardiac output in systolic HF (*e.g.*, fatigue, cardiac cachexia, hypotension), or the consequences of circulatory congestion in diastolic HF (*e.g.*, dyspnoea, hepatomegaly, ascites, dependent edema) [1].

Echocardiography represents the single most valuable examination in the diagnostic investigation and management of HF, given that morphological abnormalities, systolic dysfunction, diastolic dysfunction, or a combination of these aberrations need to be demonstrated in cases showing resting or/and exertional HF symptoms, for the establishment of a definitive diagnosis. Generally, echocardiography can contribute to the investigation of three principal clinical characteristics (Table **1**):

a. HF aetiology investigation.
b. Haemodynamic profile assessment.
c. Estimation of the short–medium-term risk in HF patients.

Table 1. Roles of echocardiography in heart failure management.

• Establishment of a definite diagnosis
• High-risk features identification
• Prognostic investigation
• Guiding therapeutic decisions

The role of echocardiography is valuable in clinical HF staging, differentiating reversible *versus* non-reversible causes of left ventricular (LV) dysfunction. In approximately two-third of HF cases, coronary artery disease (CAD) is considered as the underlying cause of the syndrome. Notably, systolic dysfunction is related to the presence of viable, or irreversibly damaged, myocardium [2]. Also, echocardiography can identify high-risk features, predict prognosis in HF patients and finally guide therapeutic interventions [3].

The assessment of LV function may be qualitative (normal function, mild, moderate, or severely impaired function) or quantitative.

BASIC PRINCIPLES OF LEFT VENTRICULAR IMAGING

Initial attempts evaluating LV function involved only linear measurements (*e.g.* LV internal dimension in diastolic and systolic phase). These measurements permit the assessment of a number of parameters, such as fractional shortening and velocity of circumferential shortening [4]. However, area measurements and their derived volume calculations became available only after the introduction of two-dimensional echocardiography.

Systolic LV dysfunction is linked to spherical LV dilation, reduced wall thickness, ejection fraction (EF) less than 45%, but most of them appear to have diastolic dysfunction too (Table **2**). They often have right ventricular dysfunction, segmental wall motion abnormalities, and marked valvular disease [5].

Table 2. Basic echocardiographic findings in HF patients.

• LV spherical dilation • Normal or reduced wall thickness • Poor wall thickening • Dyssynchrony movement	• Abnormal systolic parameters • Four chamber enlargement • LVEDV >112%, EF <45%

EF: ejection fraction; LV: left ventricular; LVED: LV end-diastolic volume.

Dimensions and Thickness

LV dimensions and thickness are measured in the parasternal long-axis (PLAX), or parasternal short-axis (PSAX) view, using two-dimensional (2D) or M-mode:

a. M-mode measurements should be made from leading edge to leading edge.
b. 2D echocardiographic measurements should be made from trailing edge to leading edge.
c. M-mode echocardiographic measurements are always slightly greater than 2D

measurements because of these conventions.

d. Measurement is made at the LV minor axis level, about at the mitral valve leaflet tips.

In males, end-diastolic and end-systolic diameters exhibit higher values, even after correction for body surface area [6].

Left Ventricular Mass

LV mass is measured by M-mode at PLAX view, or by 2D method at the mid - papillary muscle level in the short-axis (SAX) view. Either 2D images or 2D-targeted M-mode echocardiography can be used for these linear measurements [7, 8].

Volume Estimations

The biplane method of disks represents the most widely used 2D measurement for volume assessments. The reproducibility of measurements in suboptimal studies and their correlation with other imaging modalities are improved through the administration of left-sided contrast agents for endocardial border delineation [9, 10]. LV volumes are increased in systolic HF [11].

End-diastolic volume [EDV and end-systolic volume (ESV) are smaller in females, while EF is higher, even after correction for body surface area (BSA)]. Fractional area change is assessed from the PLAX view based on the M-mode or 2D method as:

$$(LVEDD - LVESD)/LVEDD \times 100$$

where LVEDD: left ventricular end-diastolic dimension; LVESD: left ventricular end-systolic dimension.

2D- and M-mode–derived EF according to Teichholz method is based on minor dimensions:

$$(EDV - ESV)/ESV$$

where $EDV = 7/(2.4 + LVEDD) \times LVEDD\ 3$ and $ESV = 7/(2.4 + LVESD) \times LVESD\ 3$.

The rotational component of cardiac contraction is important for the estimation of LV volume (Fig. **1**). In HF patients, the reversed apical rotation and loss of LV torsion are linked to advanced LV remodelling, disordered ventricular geometry, increased electrical dyssynchrony, decreased systolic function and elevated LV filling pressures. The LV untwisting rate has been reported to be associated with the peak twisting angle and the LV ESV, both in cases of reduced EF and in patients showing diastolic dysfunction [12].

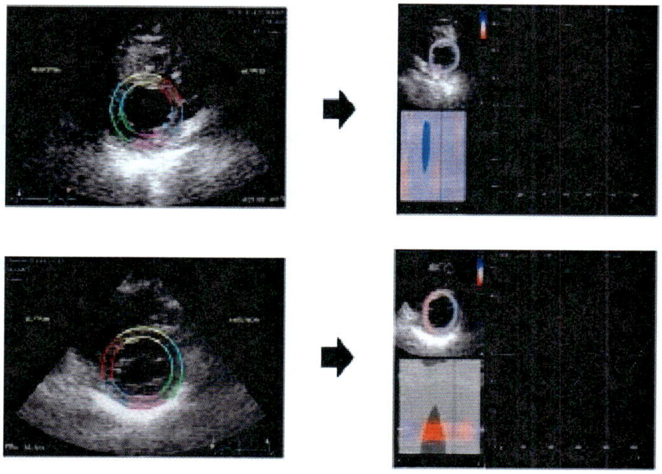

Fig. (1). Left ventricular torsion. When viewed from apex to base, the apex rotates in a counterclockwise direction and the base rotates in an overall clockwise direction.

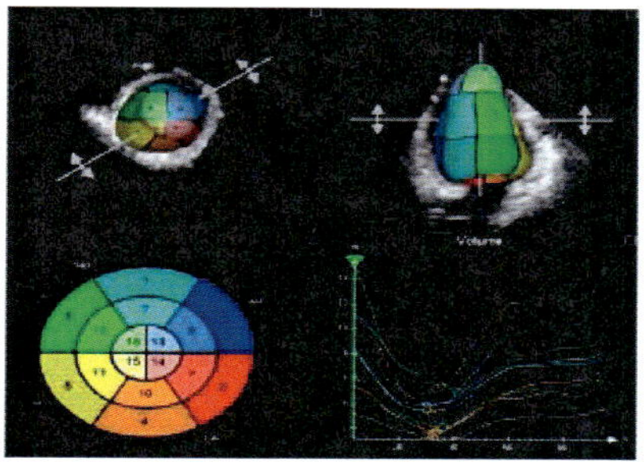

Fig. (2). 3-D echo16-segment model of time to minimal systolic volume for each of 16 left ventricular segments, normalized for heart rate.

Three-Dimensional (3D) Volumes and Ejection Fraction (EF)

3D echocardiography is a more accurate than 2D method for the assessment of LV volumes and EF since it overcomes the limitation of foreshortening (Fig. **2**). There is no need for geometric assumptions when calculating volumes based on 3D images. According to recently published results, 3D echocardiography provides reliable global and regional assessments of LV size and function in comparison to magnetic resonance imaging (MRI), which is considered as the gold standard [13]. Further, it is characterized by lower intra- and inter-observer variability compared to traditional techniques [13].

NON-INVASIVE HAEMODYNAMIC EVALUATION

Echocardiography represents a non-invasive modality for the estimation of the most useful haemodynamic parameters, including pulmonary capillary wedge pressure (PCWP) [14]. The classification of the transmitral flow velocity curve at pulsed Doppler into a restrictive or non-restrictive type is related to PCWP values in systolic HF patients [15]:

- Deceleration time (DT) of 120 ms (restrictive pattern) is highly predictive of PCWP value of approximately 20 mmHg.
- DT of 153 ms is highly predictive of PCWP value of about 12 mmHg.

The assessment of the transmitral flow pattern offers valuable prognostic evidence and its usefulness can be further increased through simple loading manipulations, or by evaluating its alterations after therapy optimization [15 - 19].

Another useful haemodynamic variable which can be assessed based on quantitative methods or through a simple categorization, according to dimensions and collapsibility of the inferior vena cava, is the right atrial pressure [20]. On the other hand, multivariable equations are required for the estimation of pulmonary vascular resistance [21].

An estimate of ventricular filling pressures can be obtained with fairly good accuracy using the ratio of the early mitral filling over the early diastolic tissue Doppler velocity of the mitral annulus (E/Ea) [22]. By providing information regarding ventricular filling pressures, Doppler echocardiography allows further characterization of diastolic function and can be used to refine further the treatment of patients with symptomatic HF (Fig. **3**).

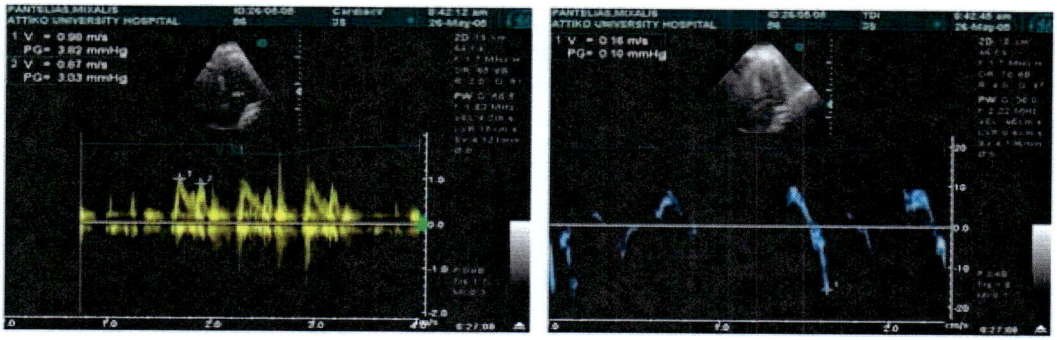

Fig. (3). Estimation of filling pressures and diastolic function by the ratio E/Ea.

AETIOLOGY AND CLINICAL STAGING OF HEART FAILURE (HF): ROLE OF ECHOCARDIOLOGY

Important evidence is obtained through echocardiographic studies for the clinical staging of HF patients. Echocardiography also contributes to the differentiation between reversible and non-reversible causes of LV dysfunction. A complete 2D and Doppler study at rest should be considered as the single most valuable diagnostic procedure to investigate HF aetiology in the initial patient management and, subsequently, to make therapeutic decisions and develop a follow-up plan.

Doppler echocardiography provides quantifications of valve disorders without serious difficulties. However, if a mild gradient through the aortic valve is related to advanced LV dysfunction, a stress echocardiography is required to evaluate the severity of aortic stenosis [23].

Other underlying conditions that may be involved in the development of HF and can be diagnosed or suspected through echocardiographic studies include hypertrophic cardiomyopathy, restrictive/infiltrative cardiomyopathy, and constrictive pericarditis [24, 25].

In patients with LV dilatation and decreased EF, the differential diagnosis should include primary dilated cardiomyopathy and ischaemic cardiomyopathy.

CAD is the underlying cause of HF in approximately two-third of patients. Segmental wall motion abnormalities are often present in systolic HF. We must take into consideration that the administration of contrast agents improves the assessment of wall motion abnormalities. In dilated ischaemic cardiomyopathy (ICM) there are hypokinetic segments, as well as akinetic segments, with or without thinning and increased echogenicity, suggesting scar formation. In dilated non-ischaemic cardiomyopathy (NICM), usually there is global hypokinesis and sometimes there are segments that may be akinetic, dyskinetic, or aneurysmal. Notably, echocardiography cannot replace invasive coronary angiography in the diagnostic investigation of HF patients.

A significant number of patients with symptomatic HF, particularly in the elderly, may have normal or mildly impaired LVEF. Therefore, diastolic HF has emerged as a discrete clinical entity during the last years. The establishment of diastolic HF diagnosis does not require echocardiographic demonstration of diastolic dysfunction [26 - 29].

In patients with dysfunctional, but viable, myocardium, there is an excellent opportunity to ameliorate HF through revascularization. Dobutamine stress echocardiography, or myocardial contrast echocardiography, in these patients provides useful information regarding the extent of viable myocardial and coronary microcirculatory reserve.

Quantification of Systolic Dysfunction

In general, LV systolic dysfunction defined as EF <50% occurs in approximately 50–60% of HF patients. The classification according to the presence of normal or impaired LV systolic performance, has therapeutic and prognostic significance.

2D echocardiography is associated with better spatial resolution for the investigation of LV size and function.

Several 2D echocardiographic views have been employed in order to provide evidence regarding ventricular systolic function. Some views are exclusively based on area measurements and others rely upon volume calculations from the two-dimensional image.

The most commonly used variable, for estimation of LV systolic function (*i.e.* EF) is "eyeball" estimation from 2D echocardiography, while M-mode echocardiography seems to be of limited accuracy [28].

A biplane determination of volume increases accuracy because EF can be calculated from these volumes. Once the diastolic and systolic volumes have been determined, the stroke volume can be calculated as the difference between these two volumes [28].

Doppler echocardiography, by permitting intra-cardiac blood flow assessment, offers useful data on systolic flow variables. Several available Doppler methodology-based algorithms, such as strain rate imaging, are significantly more sophisticated in terms of ventricular function determination. According to Tissue Doppler imaging (TDI), systolic and diastolic velocities can be obtained reliably in basal and mid-myocardial segments, by color-coded and pulsed wave (PW) Doppler techniques [30]. Velocity of motion, displacement and deformation can be evaluated in the longitudinal, radial, and circumferential planes.

2D strain echocardiography leads to better comprehension of pathophysiology, early diagnosis and more precise predictive estimation of heart diseases, *via* overall assessment of myocardial movement.

Another simple method, for estimation of LV systolic function, is the measurement of mitral E-point septal separation (E-PSS) [31]. Within the same cardiac cycle, E-PSS represents the minimal distance between the E point (most anterior motion of the anterior mitral leaflet during early diastole) and a line tangential to the most posterior interventricular septum excursion.

Quantification of Diastolic Dysfunction

Echocardiography has long been considered the best modality to assess diastolic dysfunction measuring relaxation intervals, while Doppler can detect filling abnormalities consistent with diastolic dysfunction. However, these measurements can vary substantially depending on loading conditions and heart rate. Aging also causes changes in Doppler filling patterns that are difficult to differentiate from impaired relaxation caused by specific diseases. With these limitations in mind, the following measurements are helpful [29].

Mitral Inflow Pulsed Wave (PW) Doppler

PW sample volume is placed between the tips of the mitral valve leaflets or at the level of the mitral annulus. Four major patterns of mitral inflow are seen with advancing diastolic dysfunction:

a. Grade I diastolic dysfunction: Mitral inflow filling shows an abnormal relaxation pattern with E/A ratio <1, a prolonged mitral inflow E-wave deceleration time (DT), and a prolonged isovolumic relaxation time (IVRT).
b. Grade II diastolic dysfunction: A pseudo-normal phase is seen on mitral inflow that looks like a normal inflow filling pattern. This usually reverses to an abnormal relaxation pattern upon Valsalva manoeuvre. Even in the presence of an abnormal relaxation pattern on mitral inflow, a reduction in E/A ratio of greater than 0.5 upon Valsalva manoeuvre indicates elevated left atrial preload and grade II diastolic dysfunction.
c. Grade III diastolic dysfunction: A markedly increased E-wave velocity appears with a small A-wave velocity and E/A ratio of greater than 2.0, while DT becomes short. This restrictive mitral inflow pattern is reversible upon preload reduction with the Valsalva manoeuvre or nitroglycerin or diuretic administration.
d. Grade IV diastolic dysfunction: Same findings with grade III, although no change in filling pattern occurs with preload-reducing manoeuvres. Advanced systolic dysfunction is often associated with grade IV diastolic dysfunction.

Tissue Doppler Imaging (TDI) of Mitral Annulus

The TDI PW Doppler sample volume is first placed at the medial (or septal) corner and then at the lateral corner of the mitral annulus, in the apical 4-chamber view. The myocardial early motion wave shows a progressive decline in amplitude with increasing stage of diastolic dysfunction. A markedly diminished early diastolic velocity (Ea) is observed in patients with advanced restrictive cardiomyopathy [32].

Color M-Mode Velocity Propagation

Color Doppler of LV inflow is obtained in the apical 4-chamber view. It is considered less load dependent than mitral inflow. Using the slope of the first aliasing contour, progressive LV diastolic dysfunction leads to progressive shortening of the slope. The normal value is considered to be greater than 50 cm/s. An averaged value from a few cardiac cycles should be obtained because of the physiologic beat-to-beat variability of the PW TDI data. Obtaining a reliable colour Doppler in M-mode, that extends 4 cm from the mitral annulus is technically difficult and requires significant initial training and frequent use.

DIASTOLIC HEART FAILURE – HEART FAILURE WITH PRESERVED EJECTION FRACTION (HF-PEF)

It is now well established that approximately 50% of HF patients show preserved systolic function, termed as HF with preserved EF (HF-PEF) [33]. Although initially regarded as a syndrome characterized by aberrations in diastolic function (relaxation and/or stiffness), subsequent studies revealed that, despite the presence of diastolic disorders in many patients, additional pathophysiologic mechanisms possibly result in the clinical features [34]. The diagnosis of HF-PEF is based upon the following criteria:

a. Evidence of normal systolic LV function, LVEF>50%.
b. Left ventricular end-diastolic volume index (LVEDVI) <97ml/m^2.
c. Diagnostic value of elevated LV filling pressures, E/Ea >14.
d. Elevated plasma natriuretic peptide levels [N-terminal pro - brain natriuretic peptide (NT- proBNP) >220 pg/ml].
e. Left atrial enlargement [left atrial volume index (LAVI) >40ml/m^2].
f. Pulmonary artery systolic pressure (PASP) >45mmHg.

Patients with HF-PEF exhibit reduced values of longitudinal and a slight decrease of radial strain, while circumferential strain is within normal values. Twist of left ventricle is increased in the early phase and later returns within normal limits, or even more is diminished. Rate of untwisting delays is decreased in the later period of this entity [34].

PROGNOSTIC STRATIFICATION

Several clinical, functional, haemodynamic, and biochemical factors have been suggested in previous studies for the evaluation of short- or medium-term risk in HF patients. Nevertheless, none of these factors can offer a prediction of mortality with adequate sensitivity and specificity. In fact, the decision for performing heart transplantation is still made mainly based on the presence of certain clinical features and poor therapeutic outcome, rather than on specific haemodynamic or functional parameters. Moreover, predictors of cardiac death due to refractory HF do not seem to be of high reliability regarding sudden death [35].

On the other hand, echocardiography information in terms of cardiac geometry, function and right heart haemodynamics, integrate the clinical information to develop a risk profile of the HF patient, leading to the most accurate prediction that can be obtained. Also the non-invasive character of echocardiographic studies allows monitoring of the haemodynamic and functional variables over time; in fact, it is well documented that alterations after therapy optimization (rather than baseline data) correlate better with prognosis [36].

LVEF seems to be the best marker at normality values. In the V-HeFT trial, patients with normal EF showed annual mortality rate of 8%, whereas this rate was 19% in patients with decreased EF [37]. In the CHARM programme, it was confirmed that EF is inversely related to mortality [38]. Given that EF of 30-35% indicates the presence of advanced LV dysfunction, another EF threshold is usually positioned at these levels. Implantation of defibrillators and biventricular pacemakers is recommended in these patients [39].

Prognostic stratification is also related to progressive changes in LV dimensions and function. Poorer prognosis is anticipated after reverse remodelling at 1 year, whereas a 5% increase in EF at 6 or 12 months should be regarded as an indicator of favourable clinical outcome [40].

A restrictive pattern of the transmitral pulsed Doppler flow velocity curve is a crucial factor of poor prognosis, reflecting an elevated PCWP. As previously stated, alterations of this pattern with simple loading manipulations, or after therapy optimization, improve its prognostic value [41].

Finally, in cases of advanced LV dysfunction with restrictive transmitral flow pattern, the right ventricular function should be evaluated. Pulmonary hypertension combined with decreased right ventricular function indicates end-stage patients.

The tricuspid annular plane systolic excursion (TAPSE) represents a simple echocardiographic parameter in the investigation of right ventricular function; TAPSE 14 mm is independently associated with poor prognosis in cases of advanced LV dysfunction.

NEW HORIZONS FOR ADVANCED ECHOCARDIOGRAPHIC TECHNIQUES IN HEART FAILURE (HF)

Significant improvements have been made regarding echocardiographic methods, which may be applicable to HF investigation. The development of new techniques for myocardial mechanics imaging can provide more accurate measurements, which are very helpful in therapeutic decision-making.

In HF patients, dyssynchrony investigation is one of the most common applications of tissue velocity, strain, and strain rate imaging. TDI techniques can offer a prediction of response to biventricular pacing in terms of clinical and echocardiographic parameters, with high sensitivity and specificity [42]. Moreover, the peak systolic myocardial velocity, reflective of longitudinal myocardial fibre shortening, has been employed in the evaluation of systolic function [43].

The rotational component of cardiac contraction affects significantly the LV ejection and relaxation, but its demonstration through most TDI techniques remains poor. Although there are no large studies validating the prognostic significance of abnormal ventricular torsion, available findings indicate that rotational motion may serve as a sensitive marker of myocardial ischaemia and cardiac loading conditions [44, 45]. It might also be useful in HF as a refined measure of LV dysfunction and as an evaluation tool of regional and global dyssynchrony [46].

Finally, 3D echocardiography provided reliable global and regional results regarding LV size and function in comparison to MRI as a gold standard, as well as less significant intra- and inter-observer variability compared to traditional techniques [47, 48]. Novel endocardial border detection techniques might permit direct LV volumes and EF measurements, resulting in even better reproducibility [49, 50].

CONCLUDING REMARKS

Nowadays, echocardiography / Doppler methods are the most frequently used techniques for diagnosis, characterization and management of HF patients. There is no other portable imaging technique that provides non-invasively detailed anatomic, pathologic and functional information. Also it is a safe and cost-effective method.

New techniques, such as 3-D echocardiography and tissue Doppler, are advancing rapidly offering better characterization of cardiac size and function. Therefore, echocardiography is the standard imaging tool for the diagnosis and management of HF patients.

CONFLICT OF INTEREST

The author confirms that author has no conflict of interest to declare for this publication.

ACKNOWLEDGEMENTS

Declared none.

REFERENCES

[1] Hunt S, Abraham WT, Chin MH, *et al.* American College of Cardiology; American Heart Association Task Force on Practice Guidelines; American College of Chest Physicians; International Society for Heart and Lung Transplantation; Heart Rhythm Society. ACC/AHA 2005 guideline update for the evaluation and management of chronic heart failure in the adult. A report of the American College of Cardiology/American Heart Association task force on practice guidelines. Developed in collaboration with the American College of Chest Physicians and the International Society for Heart and Lung Transplantation. Circulation 2005; 112: e154-235. [http://dx.doi.org/10.1161/CIRCULATIONAHA.105.167586] [PMID: 16160202]

[2] Swedberg K, Cleland J, Dargie H, *et al.* Task force for the diagnosis treatment of chronic heart failure of the european society of cardiology. Guidelines for the diagnosis and treatment of chronic heart

failure (update 2005): the task force for the diagnosis and treatment of chronic heart failure of the European Society of Cardiology. Eur Heart J 2005; 26: 1115-40.
[http://dx.doi.org/10.1093/eurheartj/ehi204] [PMID: 15901669]

[3] Lee DS, Austin PC, Rouleau JL, Liu PP, Naimark D, Tu JV. Predicting mortality among patients hospitalized for heart failure: derivation and validation of a clinical model. JAMA 2003; 290(19): 2581-7.
[http://dx.doi.org/10.1001/jama.290.19.2581] [PMID: 14625335]

[4] Ghio S, Gavazzi A, Campana C, *et al.* Independent and additive prognostic value of right ventricular systolic function and pulmonary artery pressure in patients with chronic heart failure. J Am Coll Cardiol 2001; 37(1): 183-8.
[http://dx.doi.org/10.1016/S0735-1097(00)01102-5] [PMID: 11153735]

[5] Mikkelsen KV, Møller JE, Bie P, Ryde H, Videbaek L, Haghfelt T. Tei index and neurohormonal activation in patients with incident heart failure: serial changes and prognostic value. Eur J Heart Fail 2006; 8(6): 599-608.
[http://dx.doi.org/10.1016/j.ejheart.2005.11.015] [PMID: 16469536]

[6] Yu EH, Sloggett CE, Iwanochko RM, Rakowski H, Siu SC. Feasibility and accuracy of left ventricular volumes and ejection fraction determination by fundamental, tissue harmonic, and intravenous contrast imaging in difficult-to-image patients. J Am Soc Echocardiogr 2000; 13(3): 216-24.
[http://dx.doi.org/10.1067/mje.2000.103597] [PMID: 10708470]

[7] Cooper RS, Simmons BE, Castaner A, Santhanam V, Ghali J, Mar M. Left ventricular hypertrophy is associated with worse survival independent of ventricular function and number of coronary arteries severely narrowed. Am J Cardiol 1990; 65(7): 441-5.
[http://dx.doi.org/10.1016/0002-9149(90)90807-D] [PMID: 2137665]

[8] Park SH, Shub C, Nobrega TP, Bailey KR, Seward JB. Two-dimensional echocardiographic calculation of left ventricular mass as recommended by the American Society of Echocardiography: correlation with autopsy and M-mode echocardiography. J Am Soc Echocardiogr 1996; 9(2): 119-28.
[http://dx.doi.org/10.1016/S0894-7317(96)90019-X] [PMID: 8849607]

[9] Lang RM, Bierig M, Devereux RB, *et al.* Recommendations for chamber quantification. J Am Soc Echocardiogr 2005; 18(12): 1440-63.
[http://dx.doi.org/10.1016/j.echo.2005.10.005] [PMID: 16376782]

[10] Lang RM, Mor-Avi V, Zoghbi WA, *et al.* The role of contrast enhancement in the echocardiographic assessment of the left ventricle. Am J Cardiol 2002; 90: 28-34.
[http://dx.doi.org/10.1016/S0002-9149(02)02945-4]

[11] Vasan RS, Larson MG, Benjamin EJ, Evans JC, Reiss CK, Levy D. Congestive heart failure in subjects with normal *versus* reduced left ventricular ejection fraction: prevalence and mortality in a population-based cohort. J Am Coll Cardiol 1999; 33(7): 1948-55.
[http://dx.doi.org/10.1016/S0735-1097(99)00118-7] [PMID: 10362198]

[12] Kim HK, Sohn DW, Lee SE, *et al.* Assessment of left ventricular rotation and torsion with two-dimensional speckle tracking echocardiography. J Am Soc Echocardiogr 2007; 20(1): 45-53.
[http://dx.doi.org/10.1016/j.echo.2006.07.007] [PMID: 17218201]

[13] Picano E, Pellikka PA. Stress echo applications beyond coronary artery disease. Eur Heart J 2014;

35(16): 1033-40.
[http://dx.doi.org/10.1093/eurheartj/eht350] [PMID: 24126880]

[14] Kircher BJ, Himelman RB, Schiller NB. Noninvasive estimation of right atrial pressure from the inspiratory collapse of the inferior vena cava. Am J Cardiol 1990; 66(4): 493-6.
[http://dx.doi.org/10.1016/0002-9149(90)90711-9] [PMID: 2386120]

[15] Giannuzzi P, Temporelli PL, Bosimini E, *et al.* Independent and incremental prognostic value of Doppler-derived mitral deceleration time of early filling in both symptomatic and asymptomatic patients with left ventricular dysfunction. J Am Coll Cardiol 1996; 28(2): 383-90.
[http://dx.doi.org/10.1016/0735-1097(96)00163-5] [PMID: 8800114]

[16] Temporelli PL, Corrà U, Imparato A, Bosimini E, Scapellato F, Giannuzzi P. Reversible restrictive left ventricular diastolic filling with optimized oral therapy predicts a more favorable prognosis in patients with chronic heart failure. J Am Coll Cardiol 1998; 31(7): 1591-7.
[http://dx.doi.org/10.1016/S0735-1097(98)00165-X] [PMID: 9626839]

[17] Traversi E, Pozzoli M, Cioffi G, *et al.* Mitral flow velocity changes after 6 months of optimized therapy provide important hemodynamic and prognostic information in patients with chronic heart failure. Am Heart J 1996; 132(4): 809-19.
[http://dx.doi.org/10.1016/S0002-8703(96)90316-6] [PMID: 8831371]

[18] Pinamonti B, Zecchin M, Di Lenarda A, Gregori D, Sinagra G, Camerini F. Persistence of restrictive left ventricular filling pattern in dilated cardiomyopathy: an ominous prognostic sign. J Am Coll Cardiol 1997; 29(3): 604-12.
[http://dx.doi.org/10.1016/S0735-1097(96)00539-6] [PMID: 9060900]

[19] Pozzoli M, Traversi E, Cioffi G, Stenner R, Sanarico M, Tavazzi L. Loading manipulations improve the prognostic value of Doppler evaluation of mitral flow in patients with chronic heart failure. Circulation 1997; 95(5): 1222-30.
[http://dx.doi.org/10.1161/01.CIR.95.5.1222] [PMID: 9054853]

[20] Pinamonti B, Di Lenarda A, Sinagra G, Camerini F. Restrictive left ventricular filling pattern in dilated cardiomyopathy assessed by Doppler echocardiography: clinical, echocardiographic and hemodynamic correlations and prognostic implications. J Am Coll Cardiol 1993; 22(3): 808-15.
[http://dx.doi.org/10.1016/0735-1097(93)90195-7] [PMID: 8354816]

[21] Scapellato F, Eleuteri E, Temporelli PL, Imparato A, Corrà U, Giannuzzi P. Doppler-derived acceleration rate of right ventricular early filling as a measurement of right atrial pressure in chronic heart failure secondary to ischemic or idiopathic dilated cardiomyopathy. Am J Cardiol 1998; 81(4): 513-5.
[http://dx.doi.org/10.1016/S0002-9149(97)00931-4] [PMID: 9485149]

[22] Casaclang-Verzosa G, Nkomo VT, Sarano ME, Malouf JF, Miller FA Jr, Oh JK. E/Ea is the major determinant of pulmonary artery pressure in moderate to severe aortic stenosis. J Am Soc Echocardiogr 2008; 21(7): 824-7.
[http://dx.doi.org/10.1016/j.echo.2007.12.002] [PMID: 18222635]

[23] Capomolla S, Ceresa M, Pinna G, *et al.* Echo-Doppler and clinical evaluations to define hemodynamic profile in patients with chronic heart failure: accuracy and influence on therapeutic management. Eur J Heart Fail 2005; 7(4): 624-30.

[http://dx.doi.org/10.1016/j.ejheart.2004.07.013] [PMID: 15921804]

[24] Jessup M, Brozena S. Heart failure. N Engl J Med 2003; 348(20): 2007-18. [http://dx.doi.org/10.1056/NEJMra021498] [PMID: 12748317]

[25] Dhir M, Nagueh SF. Echocardiography and prognosis of heart failure. Curr Opin Cardiol 2002; 17(3): 253-6. [http://dx.doi.org/10.1097/00001573-200205000-00007] [PMID: 12015474]

[26] Eichhorn EJ, Grayburn PA, Mayer SA, *et al.* Myocardial contractile reserve by dobutamine stress echocardiography predicts improvement in ejection fraction with beta-blockade in patients with heart failure: the Beta-Blocker Evaluation of Survival Trial (BEST). Circulation 2003; 108(19): 2336-41. [http://dx.doi.org/10.1161/01.CIR.0000097111.00170.7B] [PMID: 14597587]

[27] Devereux RB, Roman MJ, Palmieri V, *et al.* Prognostic implications of ejection fraction from linear echocardiographic dimensions: the Strong Heart Study. Am Heart J 2003; 146(3): 527-34. [http://dx.doi.org/10.1016/S0002-8703(03)00229-1] [PMID: 12947374]

[28] McGowan JH, Cleland JG. Reliability of reporting left ventricular systolic function by echocardiography: a systematic review of 3 methods. Am Heart J 2003; 146(3): 388-97. [http://dx.doi.org/10.1016/S0002-8703(03)00248-5] [PMID: 12947354]

[29] Vasan RS. Diastolic heart failure. BMJ 2003; 327(7425): 1181-2. [http://dx.doi.org/10.1136/bmj.327.7425.1181] [PMID: 14630731]

[30] Garcia MJ, Ares MA, Asher C, Rodriguez L, Vandervoort P, Thomas JD. An index of early left ventricular filling that combined with pulsed Doppler peak E velocity may estimate capillary wedge pressure. J Am Coll Cardiol 1997; 29(2): 448-54. [http://dx.doi.org/10.1016/S0735-1097(96)00496-2] [PMID: 9015003]

[31] Lehmann KG, Johnson AD, Goldberger AL. Mitral valve E point-septal separation as an index of left ventricular function with valvular heart disease. Chest 1983; 83(1): 102-8. [http://dx.doi.org/10.1378/chest.83.1.102] [PMID: 6848313]

[32] Redfield MM, Jacobsen SJ, Burnett JC Jr, Mahoney DW, Bailey KR, Rodeheffer RJ. Burden of systolic and diastolic ventricular dysfunction in the community: appreciating the scope of the heart failure epidemic. JAMA 2003; 289(2): 194-202. [http://dx.doi.org/10.1001/jama.289.2.194] [PMID: 12517230]

[33] Ommen SR, Nishimura RA. A clinical approach to the assessment of left ventricular diastolic function by Doppler echocardiography: update 2003. Heart 2003; 89 (Suppl. 3): iii18-23. [http://dx.doi.org/10.1136/heart.89.suppl_3.iii18] [PMID: 14594871]

[34] Naqvi TZ. Diastolic function assessment incorporating new techniques in Doppler echocardiography. Rev Cardiovasc Med 2003; 4(2): 81-99. [PMID: 12776017]

[35] Wan D, Tan YT, Al-Lawati K, *et al.* Progression of heart failure following biventricular pacing: Is there a sub-group of "Favorable Non-Responders". Heart Rhythm 2015.

[36] Smith GL, Masoudi FA, Vaccarino V, Radford MJ, Krumholz HM. Outcomes in heart failure patients with preserved ejection fraction: mortality, readmission, and functional decline. J Am Coll Cardiol 2003; 41(9): 1510-8.

[http://dx.doi.org/10.1016/S0735-1097(03)00185-2] [PMID: 12742291]

[37] Cohn JN. Vasodilators in heart failure. Conclusions from V-HeFT II and rationale for V-HeFT III. Drugs 1994; 47 (Suppl. 4): 47-57.
[http://dx.doi.org/10.2165/00003495-199400474-00008] [PMID: 7523062]

[38] Badar AA, Perez-Moreno AC, Hawkins NM, *et al.* Clinical characteristics and outcomes of patients with angina and heart failure in the CHARM (Candesartan in Heart Failure Assessment of Reduction in Mortality and Morbidity) Programme. Eur J Heart Fail 2015; 17(2): 196-204.
[http://dx.doi.org/10.1002/ejhf.221] [PMID: 25678097]

[39] Fonarow GC, Adams KF Jr, Abraham WT, Yancy CW, Boscardin WJ. Risk stratification for in-hospital mortality in acutely decompensated heart failure: classification and regression tree analysis. JAMA 2005; 293(5): 572-80.
[http://dx.doi.org/10.1001/jama.293.5.572] [PMID: 15687312]

[40] Tsutsui H, Tsuchihashi M, Takeshita A. Mortality and readmission of hospitalized patients with congestive heart failure and preserved *versus* depressed systolic function. Am J Cardiol 2001; 88(5): 530-3.
[http://dx.doi.org/10.1016/S0002-9149(01)01732-5] [PMID: 11524063]

[41] Helle-Valle T, Crosby J, Edvardsen T, *et al.* New noninvasive method for assessment of left ventricular rotation: speckle tracking echocardiography. Circulation 2005; 112(20): 3149-56.
[http://dx.doi.org/10.1161/CIRCULATIONAHA.104.531558] [PMID: 16286606]

[42] Notomi Y, Lysyansky P, Setser RM, *et al.* Measurement of ventricular torsion by two-dimensional ultrasound speckle tracking imaging. J Am Coll Cardiol 2005; 45(12): 2034-41.
[http://dx.doi.org/10.1016/j.jacc.2005.02.082] [PMID: 15963406]

[43] Knudtson ML, Galbraith PD, Hildebrand KL, Tyberg JV, Beyar R. Dynamics of left ventricular apex rotation during angioplasty: a sensitive index of ischemic dysfunction. Circulation 1997; 96(3): 801-8.
[http://dx.doi.org/10.1161/01.CIR.96.3.801] [PMID: 9264485]

[44] Stuber M, Scheidegger MB, Fischer SE, *et al.* Alterations in the local myocardial motion pattern in patients suffering from pressure overload due to aortic stenosis. Circulation 1999; 100(4): 361-8.
[http://dx.doi.org/10.1161/01.CIR.100.4.361] [PMID: 10421595]

[45] Vannan MA, Pedrizzetti G, Li P, *et al.* Effect of cardiac resynchronization therapy on longitudinal and circumferential left ventricular mechanics by velocity vector imaging: description and initial clinical application of a novel method using high-frame rate B-mode echocardiographic images. Echocardiography 2005; 22(10): 826-30.
[http://dx.doi.org/10.1111/j.1540-8175.2005.00172.x] [PMID: 16343165]

[46] Fuchs E, Müller MF, Oswald H, Thöny H, Mohacsi P, Hess OM. Cardiac rotation and relaxation in patients with chronic heart failure. Eur J Heart Fail 2004; 6(6): 715-22.
[http://dx.doi.org/10.1016/j.ejheart.2003.12.018] [PMID: 15542406]

[47] Sugeng L, Weinert L, Lang RM. Left ventricular assessment using real time three dimensional echocardiography. Heart 2003; 89 (Suppl. 3): iii29-36.
[http://dx.doi.org/10.1136/heart.89.suppl_3.iii29] [PMID: 14594873]

[48] Jenkins C, Bricknell K, Hanekom L, Marwick TH. Reproducibility and accuracy of echocardiographic

measurements of left ventricular parameters using real-time three-dimensional echocardiography. J Am Coll Cardiol 2004; 44(4): 878-86.
[http://dx.doi.org/10.1016/j.jacc.2004.05.050] [PMID: 15312875]

[49] Sugeng L, Mor-Avi V, Weinert L, *et al.* Quantitative assessment of left ventricular size and function: side-by-side comparison of real-time three-dimensional echocardiography and computed tomography with magnetic resonance reference. Circulation 2006; 114(7): 654-61.
[http://dx.doi.org/10.1161/CIRCULATIONAHA.106.626143] [PMID: 16894035]

[50] Corsi C, Lang RM, Veronesi F, *et al.* Volumetric quantification of global and regional left ventricular function from real-time three-dimensional echocardiographic images. Circulation 2005; 112(8): 1161-70.
[http://dx.doi.org/10.1161/CIRCULATIONAHA.104.513689] [PMID: 16103242]

CHAPTER 8

Medical Therapy of Heart Failure

Spyridon Katsanos and **John T. Parissis***

Heart Failure Unit, Attikon University Hospital, Athens, Greece

Abstract: Diuretics are first line drugs to improve symptoms of heart failure patients; however they do not increase their long term survival. Administration of medications blocking the neurohormonal activation, such as angiotensin converting enzyme(ACE) inhibitors (alternatively, angiotensin II receptor blockers in patients with intolerance to ACE inhibitors), mineralocorticoid receptor antagonists and beta blockers, lead to long term improvement of both symptoms and prognosis of chronic heart failure patients with reduced ejection fraction (EF<40%). Digoxin and ivabradine are also therapeutic options for heart failure patients in specific clinical scenarios. LCZ 696 is the new promising medication that improves more effectively cardiovascular outcomes in chronic heart failure cases in comparison to ACE inhibitors. In contrast, there are no available life prolonging medications for patients with preserved ejection fraction (EF>50%), and treatment remains empirical targeting only to symptomatic improvement. Treatment of comorbidities, including renal dysfunction, anemia and depression, may improve the well-being and quality of life in chronic heart failure patients, although evidence-based data are still limited.

Keywords: Angiotensin converting enzyme inhibitors, Angiotensin II receptor blockers, Beta blockers, Digoxin, Diuretics, Heart failure, Hydralazine, Isosorbide dinitrate, Ivabradine, Mineralocorticoid receptor antagonists.

INTRODUCTION

Heart failure (HF) syndrome affects almost 10% of the population > 60 years with expected mortality of 50% within 5 years of diagnosis [1]. Survival of HF has dramatically improved in the last decays; however, the prevalence of the synd-

* **Corresponding author John T Parissis:** Heart Failure Unit, Attikon University Hospital, Athens, Greece; Tel: +30 210 583 2355; Fax: +30 210 53 26520; E-mail: jparissis@yahoo.com.

Panagiotis Georgoulias (Ed.)

rome is paradoxically growing. Until the late 70s the therapeutic armamentarium of HF consisted of only two drugs, diuretics and digoxin, and focused on symptomatic patients' relief. Currently, the key element of the medical management of HF syndrome is the blockage of the neurohormonal stimulation that aims to prevent the vicious circle of the stimulation of renin-angiotensin-aldosterone axis and restrain the deleterious effects of catecholamines over-secretion. Accordingly, 3 new classes of drugs were introduced [angiotensin converting enzyme (ACE) inhibitor/angiotensin II receptor blockers (ARBs), mineralocorticoid receptor (MR) antagonists and beta blockers] which have improved the quality of life and life expectancy of these patients [2, 3]. Diuretics are still first-line drugs that relieve pulmonary congestion by reducing plasma volume and venous return (Fig. **1**). As such, they provide fast but temporary symptom relief; however, they have not shown to improve long term survival. Digoxin may still be used with caution in limited subgroups of HF patients. The advantages of medical therapies recommended for the management of chronic HF patients, as well as the pivotal trials that have supported the evidence for their clinical use, are summarized in this chapter. Additionally, therapeutic challenges and adjustments in different clinical scenarios and specific subgroups will be described.

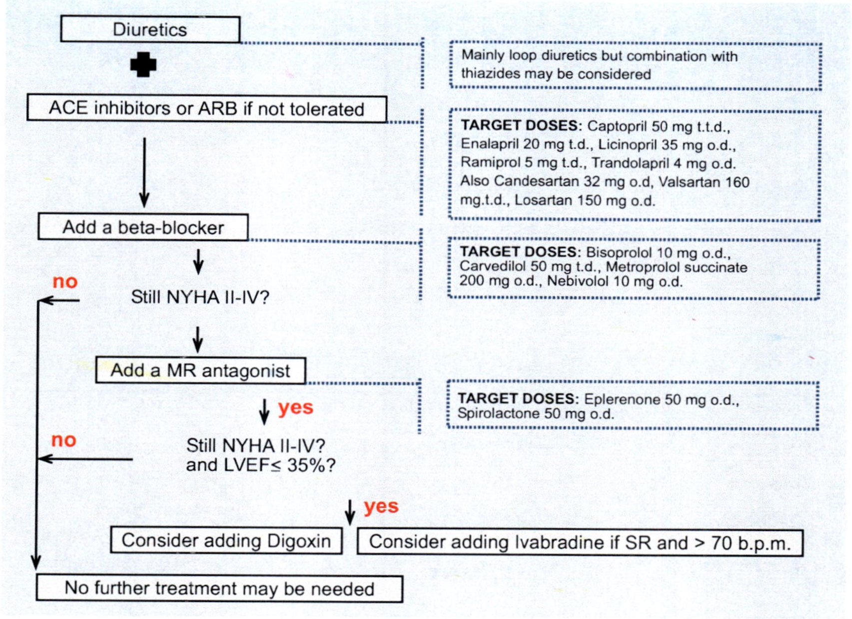

Fig. (1). Practical recommendations for the medical treatment of patients with chronic systolic heart failure. ACE: angiotensin converting enzyme; ARB: angiotensin II receptor blocker; b.p.m.: beats per minute; LVEF: left ventricular ejection fraction; MR; mineralocorticoid receptor; NYHA: New York Heart Association; o.d.: once daily; SR: sinus rhythm; t.d.: twice daily; t.t.d.: three times daily.

DIURETICS

Secreted from the proximal tubule, loop diuretics inhibit re-absorption of sodium and chloride ions at the thick ascending loop of Henle in the kidney. Their use is recommended in all HF patients with signs of fluid retention (Fig. **1**). Loop diuretics provide fast relief of edema, congestion and dyspnea and their dose may be adjusted to the clinical features of the patient. Complications of their excessive use include renal dysfunction, hypotension, dehydration, and serum electrolyte imbalances. It has been observed that higher doses of diuretics are linked to an increase in morality of HF patients, possibly related to HF syndrome deterioration. In the Diuretic Optimization Strategies Evaluation (DOSE) trial, enrolling patients with decompensated HF, bolus (every 12 hours) administration of furosemide as compared to continuous infusion did not affect clinical symptoms or creatinine level [4]. Similarly, high-dose (2.5 times the previous oral dose) *vs.* low-dose (patient's previous oral dose) strategy had only a weak effect on symptom reduction; however, at the expense of more frequent renal deterioration (23% in the high-dose compared to 14% in the low-dose group) [4]. Resistance to diuretics is prevalent in up to 35% of chronic HF patients and a few strategies may be recommended to overcome this problem: a) continuous intravenous (iv) infusion, b) alternative administration of bumetanide or torasemide instead of furosemide, c) combination of loop and thiazide diuretics (*e.g.* metolazone) and peripheral ultrafiltration.

ANGIOTENSIN CONVERTING ENZYME (ACE) INHIBITORS

Chronic overstimulation of the renin-angiotensin-aldosterone axis in HF syndrome leads to oxidative stress, inflammation, endothelial dysfunction, vascular smooth muscle proliferation, apoptosis and collagen formation. Inhibition of ACE results in decreased angiotensin II formation and inhibition of bradykinin breakdown. The hypothesis that ACE inhibitor administration could be beneficial for HF patients was first tested in the late 80s in the Cooperative North Scandinavian Enalapril Survival Study (CONSENSUS). Interestingly, enalapril (an ACE inhibitor) reduced mortality by 27% compared to placebo in severely symptomatic HF patients [5]. These findings were confirmed in the subsequent SOLVD trial in which enalapril reduced mortality of symptomatic HF patients with left ventricular ejection fraction (LVEF) ≤35% [6]. In the SOLVD-prevention trial, a similar benefit of enalapril administration was reported in asymptomatic HF patients with reduced LVEF [7]. Nonetheless, these trials were conducted before the widespread use of beta blockers in HF patients. In the ATLAS trial, higher doses of lisinopril (32.5 to 35 mg daily) as compared to lower doses (2.5 to 5.0 mg daily) were related to reduced risk of death or hospitalization at more than 3 years follow up, underlining the need for appropriate up titration of this medication [8]. Albeit ACE inhibitors are considered relatively safe drugs, cough (20%), rash and metallic taste may occur. Their use is also contradicted in patients with impaired renal function (creatinine ≥2.5 mg/dL or glomerular filtration rate ≤30 mL/min/1.73m^2), patients with previous severe adverse reactions (angioedema), borderline blood pressure, bilateral renal stenosis, serum potassium levels >5mEq/L and pregnancy (or planning of pregnancy). Currently, captopril, enalapril, lisinopril, ramipril, and trandolapril are approved medications for the treatment of HF patients (Fig. **1**) [2, 3].

ANGIOTENSIN II RECEPTOR BLOCKERS (ARBS)

For HF patients intolerant to ACE inhibitors, ARBs may be an alternative choice. ARBs block the renin-agiotensin-aldosterone axis by binding competitively to AT1 receptors. Recommendations for ARBs use are based on the results of at least two multi-center randomized trials. In the Valsartan Heart Failure Trial (Val-HeFT), the addition of valsartan to standard HF treatment led to increase in survival of patients not receiving ACE inhibitors or beta blockers, and was associated with improvement of functional class, quality of life and LVEF [9]. Also CHARM-Added trial found compelling evidence that addition of candesartan to ACE, in patients already receiving ACE inhibitors, led to reduction of the composite end point of cardiovascular death or hospitalization at 41 months follow up [10]. In a similar way with the ACE inhibitors, higher doses of ARBs had a better effect in reducing mortality and HF related hospitalizations. This was demonstrated in the HEAAL study, comparing losartan 150 mg to 50 mg dose daily in symptomatic patients with LVEF ≤40% [11]. At present, only evidence for candesartan, valsartan and losartan is adequate to justify guideline recommendation for HF patients (Fig. **1**) [2, 3].

BETA-BLOCKERS

Secretion of epinephrine (80%) and norepinephrine (20%) is basically a compensative mechanism to increase cardiac output in HF patients. This pathophysiology paradigm was responsible for considering HF as a contradiction for beta blocker administration in many previous decays. However, there were accumulating evidence that chronic catecholamin hyperactivity leads to oxidative stress, high oxygen demand, ischemia and peripheral vasoconstriction. Given these findings, the first trials evaluating beta blockers as a therapeutic tool in HF, were conducted. In the Cardiac Insufficiency Bisoprolol Study II (CIBIS-II), bisoprolol administration led to significant improvement of survival of New York Heart Association (NYHA) class III-IV patients with LVEF ≤35% [12]. Similarly, in the Metoprolol CR/XL Randomised Intervention Trial in Congestive Heart Failure (MERIT-HF) metoprolol controlled release/extended release (at once daily dose) improved survival of HF patients as compared to placebo treatment [13]. Additionally, administration of carvedilol to severely symptomatic patients with LVEF <25% led to reduction of the composite endpoint of mortality and HF related hospitalization, in the carvedilol prospective randomized cumulative survival (COPERNICUS) study [14].

It should be acknowledged that different beta blockers have variant adrenergic beta-receptors selectivity and variant effects on alpha-receptors. Also they may have heterogeneous vasoconstriction properties and may be related to varying cytokine inflammation production. Therefore, all beta blockers are not equally beneficial for HF patients. For example, bucindolol did not affect overall mortality while nebivolol reduced only HF related hospitalizations in well-designed randomized trials [15, 16]. Interestingly, only metoprolol controlled release/extended release but not short acting metoprolol titrate (tartrate), is a beta blocker of choice for HF patients. According to currently available data other beta blockers of choice for HF syndrome include carvedilol, bisoprolol and nebivolol. Symptomatic bradycardia or heart block, hypotension, fatigue and worsening of HF due to fluid retention, are potential adverse reactions related to this medication category. Beta blockers should be administered to HF patients even with mild symptoms and adequate dose up-titration should be attempted (Fig. **1**).

MINERALOCORTICOID RECEPTOR ANTAGONISTS

Aldosterone increase in HF is part of a pathophysiological mechanism retaining extracellular fluid volume through sodium and water re-absorption. Still, chronic stimulation of receptors for mineralocorticoid hormones in cardiac myocytes and fibroblasts may prompt inflammation, fibrosis and LV hypertrophy. Aldosterone blockade for prevention and treatment of HF has been evaluated in several randomized trials.

The Randomized Aldactone Evaluation Study (RALES) enrolled HF patients with LVEF <35% who were administered either placebo or aldactone [17]. Aldactone treated arm had a clear improvement in morbidity and survival, a benefit independent of ACE inhibitor administration. However there was a 10% breast enlargement in men (as opposed to 1% in the placebo arm). Compared to aldosterone, eplerenone has lower affinity for progesterone and androgen receptors, which could lead to fewer side effects. In the EMPHASIS-HF trial, mildly symptomatic patients with LVEF ≤30%, treated with the recommended or maximally tolerated dose of ACE inhibitor (or an ARB or both) and a beta blocker (unless contraindicated), were randomized to receive eplerenone or placebo [18]. At 21 months a clear reduction of mortality and hospitalization rates were observed in the eplerenone group in comparison to the placebo treated group [18]. The benefits of eplerenone were also confirmed for patients with left myocardial dysfunction following myocardial infarction, in the EPHESUS trial [19]. As expected, gynecomastia was a rare (<1%) side effect of eplerenone. Nonetheless, hyperkalaemia and renal function deterioration were potential adverse effects that cannot be underestimated. Patients with serum creatinine >2.5 mg/dL (or glomerular filtration rate <30 mL/min/1.73m2) should be precluded from MR antagonist treatment. MR antagonists are currently recommended for symptomatic (NYHA class II-IV) HF patients with reduced LVEF, on top of ACE inhibitor (or ARBs) and beta blocker treatment (Fig. **1**).

UP-TITRATION OF LIFE PROLONGING MEDICATION

Initiation and up-titration of ACE inhibitors/ARBs in chronic HF patients do not require hospitalization. A low starting dose of clinical-trial-proven ACE inhibitors/ARBs is recommended in cases with no contradictions to specific agents. Subsequently, dose could be uptitrated at 1-2 week intervals targeting maximum doses used in landmark trials. Clinical and laboratory monitor is needed before each up titration attempt (Fig. **1**). Also, laboratory tests should be repeated after optimal dosage. A small rise of creatinine and potassium levels does not require any special action. However, after a rise in creatinine levels >50% above baseline or >3 mg/dL, ACE/ARBs dose should be adjusted and cessation may be even considered (especially when creatinine >3.5 mg/dL and/or potassium >5.5 mmol/L). Patients must be alert for side effects of symptomatic hypotension. Calcium-channel blockers and other vasodilators may be reduced or even stopped if symptomatic hypotension manifests. Patients should be also reassured that initial dizziness may improve with time and that HF symptoms will also improve within the following weeks to a few months of treatment. Co-administration of ACE inhibitors / ARBs with non-steroidal anti-inflammatory drugs, trimethoprim / trimethoprim-sulfamethoxazole and K+ sparing diuretics (amiloride, triamterene) requires closer laboratory monitoring (Table **1**).

Table 1. Medical treatment NOT recommended in symptomatic heart failure patients.

Medical treatment	Reason to avoid in HF patients
Non-steroidal anti-inflammatory drugs and cyclooxygenase-2 inhibitors	Renal function deterioration, water retention, ischemia in CAD patients
Theazolidones (glitazones)	Water retention
Calcium channel blockers	Negative inotropic effect
Triple combination of angiotensin converting enzyme inhibitors + angiotensin II receptor blockers + mineralocorticoid receptor antagonists	Renal function deterioration, hyperkalaemia

CAD: coronary artery disease; HF: heart failure.

Similarly, administration of MR antagonists can start with a low initial dose followed by careful gradual increments in dose within 1-4 weeks and each 4 weeks thereafter (Fig. **1**). Again, special attention is warranted when there is a need for administration of non-steroidal anti-inflammatory drugs, trimethoprim/trimethoprim-sulfamethoxazole and K+ sparing diuretics. MR antagonists should be stopped if potassium rises to >6.0 mmol/L and/or creatinine rises >3.5 mg/dL. Because of the high risk of developing hyperkalaemia, combination of ACE inhibitors, ARBs and MR antagonists is not advised (Table **1**). The concomitant use of eplerenone with other CYP3A4 potent inhibitors, such as ketoconazole, itraconazole, nefazodone, telithromycin and clarithromycin, should be avoided.

Beta blockers should be administered after the first manifestation of HF symptoms and signs in all patients with LVEF <40%, even if they are on a low dose of ACE inhibitors/ARBs (Fig. **1**). Treatment can start with low doses under specialist guidance. Symptomatic hypotension is rare and in this case administration of other pressure lowering medication at a different time schedule may be helpful. Particular attention should be paid in cases with signs of congestion, where beta blockers should be prescribed with diuretics. Also co-administration with other bradycardia-inducing medication, such as verapamil, diltiazem and digoxin, should be avoided especially when heart rate is <60 beats per minute (bpm). Efforts for up-titration should be made every 1-2 weeks, taking under consideration that even minimum beta blocker dosage is better than no beta blocker administration. It should be emphasised that with careful monitoring and appropriate patient education (to weight themselves regularly and to adjust their diuretic dose), optimal dosage of beta blockers may be attained in almost 85% of HF patients (Fig. **1**).

DIGOXIN

Digoxin acts though the inhibition of the Na^+/K^+ ATPase pump which leads to an increase in myocardial intracellular sodium levels. This in turn leads to a reverse of the sodium-calcium exchange, increasing intracellular calcium levels. Digoxin prompts a positive inotropic effect without additional energy demands. Small studies have exhibited improvement of symptoms and quality of life for HF patients treated with digoxin. The only large trial so far was the DIG trial, conducted before the wide use of beta blockers for HF [20]. Patients at NYHA II-IV functional class with LVEF ≤45% treated with ACE inhibitors were administered either placebo or a daily dose of 0.25 mg of digoxin. At 3 years follow-up there was no difference in mortality, but only a 7.9% reduction of hospitalization rate in the digoxin treated arm. There are however many concerns regarding digoxin side effects, including atrioventricular block, atrial and ventricular arrhythmias, nausea, visual disturbances and confusion. Toxicity may be increased with concurrent impaired renal function, low lean body mass, hypokalemia, hypomagnesemia and co-administration of amiodarone, dronedarone, propafenone, verapamil, erythromycin and quinidine. It seems that low doses (0.125 mg daily) leading to 0.5 to 0.8 ng/mL serum concentrations are equally beneficial to higher doses, while they entail lower rates of side effects. Serum levels >2 ng/mL are potentially toxic.

It should be pointed out that digoxin is currently used as an adjunct to and not a substitute of neurohormonal blockage. Patients should be in NYHA class II-IV and already treated with ACE inhibitors/ARBs, MR antagonists and beta blockers (preferably on guideline-recommended doses), before digoxin administration is considered (Fig. **1**). Moreover, digoxin may be prescribed for heart rate reduction in HF patients with atrial fibrillation (AF) after optimum treatment with beta blockers, or in AF patients intolerant to beta blockers. Digitoxin does not have renal excretion (it is eliminated *via* the liver) and could conceptually have a better profile than digoxin; nevertheless, it has not been adequately studied in HF patients and specific recommendations are lacking.

IVABRADINE

Ivabradine inhibits the I_f channel in the sinus node and reduces the heart rate only in patients in sinus rhythm. The systolic HF treatment with the I_f inhibitor ivabradine randomized trial (SHIFT) has tested the effects of this drug in HF patients in sinus rhythm [21]. The trial concluded that at a median follow up of 2 years there was no significant improvement in mortality rate with the addition of this agent; however, there was a 26% reduction in hospitalization rate compared to placebo treatment [21]. It should be noted that only 26% of patients were on optimum beta blocker doses. Thus, there was no answer to the question of how effective this treatment would have been if patients were treated according to guidelines. Actually, in a subgroup treated with at least half of recommended beta blocker dose, benefits of ivabradine addition were dubious. Furthermore, administration of ivabradine in this trial was associated with symptomatic bradyarrhythmias requiring treatment cessation. Summing up, ivabradine use should be considered in chronic HF patients with sinus rhythm on optimal ACE inhibitors/ARBs, MR antagonist and beta blocker treatment, when there is still potential for additional heart rate reduction (>70 bpm) (Fig. **1**).

HYDRALAZINE AND ISOSORBIDE DINITRATE

The concept behind the use of this combined administration was the simultaneous reduction of preload with isosorbide dinitrate and afterload with hydralazine. Indeed, this combination seemed to affect vascular tone, myocardial hypertrophy and LV remodelling, while reducing oxidative stress. In initial studies it appeared superior to placebo, but unfortunately was inferior to ACE inhibitors in a head to head comparison in randomised trials. A meta-analysis showed that HF patients of the black race may have a better survival when treated with isosorbide dinitrate and hydralazine than with ACE inhibitors. These results led to the design of the African-American Heart Failure Trial (A-HeFT), enrolling HF patients self-identified as black race who were on optimal treatment with ACE inhibitors or ARBs, beta blockers and MR antagonists [22]. Patients receiving an optimal dose of 120 mg isosorbide dinitrate and 225 mg hydralazine (after appropriate up-titration) had an impressive 43% relative mortality benefit compared to placebo treatment. As expected, this trial fuelled a bioethical debate. Critics of this approach pointed out that after centuries of genetic merge there is hardly any "clean" race population, so racial categorization may be a poor distinction marker. However proponents insisted that based on the recruitment of this self-identified black population, results were too significant to ignore. Currently, this combination is recommended for self-described African Americans with NYHA II-IV class HF on optimal treatment with ACE inhibitors and beta blockers. Also combination of isosorbide dinitrate and hydralazine may be considered for HF patients at both sides of the racial divide who are intolerant to ACE inhibitors and ARBs [2, 3].

Nevertheless, only 7% of eligible patients are treated with this combination in everyday clinical practise. The side effects of headache, dizziness, nausea and a lupus-like syndrome, in combination with the need for frequent administration (three times daily) and careful up-titration, are partly responsible for the limited use of this medication. Although this therapeutical option has many restrictions and may even be considered obsolete, it was the first successful nitric oxide (NO)-modulating strategy. Decays later, a number of novel agents affecting different points in the NO-pathway are returning at the central stage of the industrial pharmaceutical research in HF.

ADJUSTMENTS IN MEDICAL THERAPY DUE TO HOSPITALIZATION

In the setting of acutely decompensated chronic HF, iv therapies such as diuretics, vasodilators or inotropes should be considered according to the clinical presentation (congestion and/or low output state), initial systolic blood pressure, renal function and underlying cause of HF worsening. Hospitalization for HF decompensation is not an uncommon clinical scenario for chronic HF patients, leading to modification of their routine medical treatment. It is now acknowledged that beta blockers should be maintained in case of acute HF deterioration even if their dose has to be reduced. Accordingly, when there is a need for inotropes -in cases of hypotension jeopardising organ function- milrinone may be preferred over beta agonists, because in this case discontinuation of beta blockers may not be needed. Another clinical concern is that extreme use of loop diuretics in the acute phase of decompensation may lead to symptomatic hypotension and quick deterioration of renal function. Discontinuation of ACE inhibitors, beta blockers, and MR antagonists may be required, or at least adequate up-titration of these life prolonging pharmaceutical agents may be restrained. It seems that the effort to up-titrate standard of care medication during hospitalization is crucial for these patients. After discharge, in order to achieve optimal guideline-directed doses, there is an absolute need for early (at 7-14 days) follow-up with clinical and laboratory evaluation and close collaboration with community physicians and/or specialist HF nurses.

ROLE OF COMMORBIDITIES IN EVIDENCE-BASED THERAPY

Cardiovascular (coronary artery disease, diabetes, hyperlipidemia, AF), and non cardiovascular comorbidities (chronic kidney disease, anaemia, depression, chronic obstructive pulmonary disease) increase mortality of HF patients.

Coronary artery disease and hyperlipidemia are treated according to the existing guidelines, as in other patient populations (routine administration of statins to all

HF patients does not improve outcomes of myocardial infarction, stroke and all cause mortality). Thiazolidinediones are contradicted in diabetic HF patients because they cause fluid retention, and there are also concerns for the use of metformin (Table **1**). AF is present in 4- 40% of HF patients according to their NYHA classification. In cases of suspected AF-associated HF, rhythm control is favoured; otherwise rhythm control strategy may not be superior to rate control. Anticoagulants should be administered to all HF patients and the decision for warfarin or one of the newer agents (dabigatran, rivaroxaban, apixaban) should be individualized. Beta blockers can be used for rate lowering and digoxin may also be prescribed; however, diltiazem and verapamil are contradicted. Kidney disease may prohibit up-titration of life prolonging medication or even pose a contradiction for their use (see also section above).

As part of an integrated approach, treatment of concurrent non cardiac comorbidities could seemingly improve survival and/or quality of life of HF patients. This hypothesis has been tested in HF patients with various comorbidities. Anemia (defined hemoglobin <13 g/dL in men and <12 g/dL in women) may be present in up to 40% of HF patients, leading to a 2-fold increase in mortality. There are indefinite results for the treatment of anemia with erythropoietin-stimulating agents; nevertheless iv administration of ferric carboxymaltose improved HF symptoms in patients with and without anemia [23]. Currently, routine treatment of anemia remains questionable in HF patients [2, 3]. Depression has been reported in up to 63% of hospitalized HF patients. Selective serotonin re-uptake inhibitors are the drugs of choice for depression in HF patients and tricyclic antidepressants should not be administered as they may cause arrhythmias. Although the current evidence is insufficient, it seems that depressive patients with better functional capacity may benefit most from treatment whereas, in terminal stage, HF somatic symptoms perpetuate depressive symptoms and this may be an unsurpassable obstacle.

Patients with chronic obstructive pulmonary disease are less likely to be treated with evidence-based pharmacological therapy compared to patients free of this comorbidity [24]. Beta blockers recommended for HF syndrome (bisoprolol, metoprolol succinate, nebibolol) are beta -1 adrenorecepto selective and are not contradicted for these patients. Albeit obesity is a risk factor for HF development, mild obesity (BMI between 30-35 kg/m2) paradoxically portends better long term survival in patients already diagnosed with HF. Currently there are no specific weight lowering guidelines for obese HF patients. The prevalence of obesity, AF and anemia is higher among HF patients with preserved EF (HFpEF) compared to HF patients with reduced EF (HFrEF).

THERAPEUTIC LIMITATIONS IN HEART FAILURE PATIENTS WITH PRESERVED EJECTION FRACTION (HFPEF)

HFrEF and HFpEF are no longer considered overlapping syndromes, although the mere existence of HFpEF as a different syndrome had been questioned in the past. A wealth of evidence is currently supporting HFpEF as a separate entity. Firstly, the acknowledgment of signs and symptoms of HF syndrome in patients with preserved LVEF has been constantly confirmed in HF clinical trials and registries; almost half of the included patients have normal or near normal LVEF. Secondly, neurohormonal activation has been documented in HFpEF patients and a high mortality has been confirmed, although there is rare evolution from preserved to reduced LVEF in this group. Thirdly, there are distinct structural changes (concentric left ventricular remodelling in HFpEF as opposed to eccentric remodelling in HFrEF patients) and distinct differences in myocardial cellular and interstitial characteristics. Most importantly, there is an ambiguous benefit of classical life prolonging medication used in HFrEF patients when prescribed in the HFpEF group.

Indeed, routine administration of ACE inhibitors and ARBs has not shown any clear benefit for HFpEF patients. In the Perindopril for Elderly Patients with Chronic HF (PEP-CHF) trial no reduction in all-cause mortality was observed in patients with LVEF >40% treated with placebo or perindopril [25]. In the Irbesartan in HF with preserved systolic function (I-PRESERVE) trial there was no difference in hard endpoints in patients with LVEF >45% treated either with placebo or irbesartan [26]. Treatment with nebivolol did not reduce symptoms in HFpEF patients in the ELANDD study [27]. Some HF registries have also shown that HFpEF patients benefit less with beta blockers when compared with their HFrEF counterparts. To date, there is also no robust evidence supporting the administration of heart rate lowering calcium channel blockers in HFpEF patients.

Furthermore, in randomized trials, aldosterone did not influence long term mortality of these patients, although it had a modest favourable effect in re-hospitalization rates. Likewise, prescription of digoxin in HFpEF patients does not influence long term mortality or re-hospitalization rates. Disappointing results of these trials have been attributed to the high rate of non-cardiac causes of death among HFpEF patients, but also to the heterogeneous patterns of pathophysiology of this syndrome. It is a fact that while many patients have predominantly left ventricular diastolic dysfunction, in others subclinical contractile dysfunction, left atrial dysfunction, pulmonary hypertension or volume overload may be prominent. This emphasizes the need for the design of trials in specific subgroups that may benefit most. However, there are promising results for HFpEF patients treated with a number of novel pharmaceutical agents, including soluble guanylate cyclase stimulators (BAY1021189), ARB plus neprilysin inhibitors (LCZ696) and calcium-cycling modulators (ryanodine stabilizers). These preliminary encouraging results have not been confirmed so far in well-designed trials.

Current guidelines recommendations for HFpEF patients include diuretics for symptomatic relief and adequate treatment of hypertension (ACE or ARBs, beta blockers, amlodipine, MR antagonists). Notwithstanding, diltiazem and verapamil should be administered with caution because of their negative inotropic effect. In patients with AF, beta blockers or heart rate lowering calcium channel blockers are still an option for heart rate control [2, 3].

MEDICAL TREATMENT IN END-STAGE HEART FAILURE (HF)

In terminal HF stage, new clinical problems may arise. Renal failure and hypotension may preclude optimal doses of ACE inhibitors/ARBs and MR antagonists. Also, fluid retention may be an additional parameter restricting high doses of beta blockers. Renal failure and hyperkalaemia may require discontinuation of digoxin. Resistance to diuretics may be more common and difficult to deal with in clinical practice. Continuous inotropic circulatory support (dopamine, dobutamine, milrinone) may only be a temporary solution, causing malignant ventricular arrhythmias and local infections. Community physicians should be able to recognize when HF patients become intolerant to first line medications and refer them for invasive treatment options: cardiac resynchronization therapy, implantable cardioverter-defibrillator and mechanical circulatory support (LV assist device or bi-ventricular assist device). Finally, there may be an inescapable terminal HF stage where palliative treatment strategy is a one way option. Practically, continuous or periodic inotropic support, aggressive diuresis and opioids may be used to improve the quality of the patients' remaining life.

EMERGING ROLE OF ANGIOTENSIN – NEPRILYSIN INHIBITION

Angiotensin - neprilysin inhibition (LCZ696) is currently the most promising advance in pharmaceutical treatment of HF. It acts by enhancing the activity of endogenous compensatory mechanisms mediated though the secretion of endogenous peptides. These peptides are eliminated mainly though the neprilysin enzyme and therefore inhibition of neprilysin practically leads to increase of their serum levels. This in turn reduces fibrosis, while prompting vasodilator effects and renal protective effects. The fusion of angiotensin and neprilysin inhibitors in a single molecular complex was introduced to overcome the unacceptably high rates of angioedema caused by synchronous separate administration of these two agents.

In PARADIGM-HF trial, 8442 HF participants (NYHA II-IV) were randomly assigned to either receive 200mg of LCZ696 twice daily (t.d.) or 10mg of enalapril t.d. At 27-month follow-up the trial showed an outstanding reduction in death from cardiovascular causes, HF hospitalizations and all-cause mortality in the LCX696 treated arm as compared to the enalapril treated arm (by 20%, 21% and 16%, respectively). Patients receiving LCZ696 had higher incidence of symptomatic hypotension albeit this did not often lead to cessation of treatment [28]. These results are implicitly stating that ACE inhibitors, a long standing first line treatment for HF, may soon have to be substituted by an agent combining both angiotensin and neprilysin inhibition. This drug is currently recommended for patients with HFrEF, and there is anticipation of more phase III trials, for its use in HFpEF patients.

CONCLUDING REMARKS

Diuretics provide quick symptom amelioration, while administration of ACE inhibitors/ARBs, beta blockers and MR antagonists leads to long term improvement of symptoms and survival of HFrEF patients. In contrast, there are no effective medications in order to improve survival of HFpEF patients. A multi-disciplinary team approach in the management of chronic HF should guide effective strategies targeting to optimization of life prolonging medications and education of HF patients

CONFLICT OF INTEREST

The authors confirm that they have no conflict of interest to declare for this publication.

ACKNOWLEDGEMENTS

Declared none.

REFERENCES

[1] Braunwald E. Heart failure. JACC Heart Fail 2013; 1(1): 1-20. [http://dx.doi.org/10.1016/j.jchf.2012.10.002] [PMID: 24621794]

[2] McMurray JJ, Adamopoulos S, Anker SD, *et al.* ESC Guidelines for the diagnosis and treatment of acute and chronic heart failure 2012: The Task Force for the Diagnosis and Treatment of Acute and Chronic Heart Failure 2012 of the European Society of Cardiology. Developed in collaboration with the Heart Failure Association (HFA) of the ESC. Eur Heart J 2012; 33(14): 1787-847. [http://dx.doi.org/10.1093/eurheartj/ehs104] [PMID: 22611136]

[3] Yancy CW, Jessup M, Bozkurt B, *et al.* 2013 ACCF/AHA guideline for the management of heart failure: a report of the American College of Cardiology Foundation/American Heart Association Task Force on practice guidelines. Circulation 2013; 128: 240-327. [http://dx.doi.org/10.1161/CIR.0b013e31829e8807]

[4] Felker GM, Lee KL, Bull DA, *et al.* Diuretic strategies in patients with acute decompensated heart failure. N Engl J Med 2011; 364(9): 797-805. [http://dx.doi.org/10.1056/NEJMoa1005419] [PMID: 21366472]

[5] Effects of enalapril on mortality in severe congestive heart failure. Results of the Cooperative North Scandinavian Enalapril Survival Study (CONSENSUS). N Engl J Med 1987; 316(23): 1429-35. [http://dx.doi.org/10.1056/NEJM198706043162301] [PMID: 2883575]

[6] Effect of enalapril on survival in patients with reduced left ventricular ejection fractions and congestive heart failure. N Engl J Med 1991; 325(5): 293-302. [http://dx.doi.org/10.1056/NEJM199108013250501] [PMID: 2057034]

[7] Effect of enalapril on mortality and the development of heart failure in asymptomatic patients with reduced left ventricular ejection fractions. The SOLVD Investigattors. N Engl J Med 1992; 327(10):

685-91.
[http://dx.doi.org/10.1056/NEJM199209033271003] [PMID: 1463530]

[8] Packer M, Poole-Wilson PA, Armstrong PW, *et al.* Comparative effects of low and high doses of the angiotensin-converting enzyme inhibitor, lisinopril, on morbidity and mortality in chronic heart failure. Circulation 1999; 100(23): 2312-8.
[http://dx.doi.org/10.1161/01.CIR.100.23.2312] [PMID: 10587334]

[9] Cohn JN, Tognoni G. A randomized trial of the angiotensin-receptor blocker valsartan in chronic heart failure. N Engl J Med 2001; 345(23): 1667-75.
[http://dx.doi.org/10.1056/NEJMoa010713] [PMID: 11759645]

[10] McMurray JJ, Ostergren J, Swedberg K, *et al.* Effects of candesartan in patients with chronic heart failure and reduced left-ventricular systolic function taking angiotensin-converting-enzyme inhibitors: the CHARM-Added trial. Lancet 2003; 362(9386): 767-71.
[http://dx.doi.org/10.1016/S0140-6736(03)14283-3] [PMID: 13678869]

[11] Konstam MA, Neaton JD, Dickstein K, *et al.* Effects of high-dose *versus* low-dose losartan on clinical outcomes in patients with heart failure (HEAAL study): a randomised, double-blind trial. Lancet 2009; 374(9704): 1840-8.
[http://dx.doi.org/10.1016/S0140-6736(09)61913-9] [PMID: 19922995]

[12] The Cardiac Insufficiency Bisoprolol Study II (CIBIS-II): a randomised trial. Lancet 1999; 353(9146): 9-13.
[http://dx.doi.org/10.1016/S0140-6736(98)11181-9] [PMID: 10023943]

[13] Effect of metoprolol CR/XL in chronic heart failure: Metoprolol CR/XL Randomised Intervention Trial in Congestive Heart Failure (MERIT-HF). Lancet 1999; 353(9169): 2001-7.
[http://dx.doi.org/10.1016/S0140-6736(99)04440-2] [PMID: 10376614]

[14] Packer M, Fowler MB, Roecker EB, *et al.* Effect of carvedilol on the morbidity of patients with severe chronic heart failure: results of the carvedilol prospective randomized cumulative survival (COPERNICUS) study. Circulation 2002; 106(17): 2194-9.
[http://dx.doi.org/10.1161/01.CIR.0000035653.72855.BF] [PMID: 12390947]

[15] A trial of the beta-blocker bucindolol in patients with advanced chronic heart failure. N Engl J Med 2001; 344(22): 1659-67.
[http://dx.doi.org/10.1056/NEJM200105313442202] [PMID: 11386264]

[16] Flather MD, Shibata MC, Coats AJ, *et al.* Randomized trial to determine the effect of nebivolol on mortality and cardiovascular hospital admission in elderly patients with heart failure (SENIORS). Eur Heart J 2005; 26(3): 215-25.
[http://dx.doi.org/10.1093/eurheartj/ehi115] [PMID: 15642700]

[17] Pitt B, Zannad F, Remme WJ, *et al.* The effect of spironolactone on morbidity and mortality in patients with severe heart failure. N Engl J Med 1999; 341(10): 709-17.
[http://dx.doi.org/10.1056/NEJM199909023411001] [PMID: 10471456]

[18] Zannad F, McMurray JJ, Krum H, *et al.* Eplerenone in patients with systolic heart failure and mild symptoms. N Engl J Med 2011; 364(1): 11-21.
[http://dx.doi.org/10.1056/NEJMoa1009492] [PMID: 21073363]

[19] Pitt B, Remme W, Zannad F, *et al.* Eplerenone, a selective aldosterone blocker, in patients with left ventricular dysfunction after myocardial infarction. N Engl J Med 2003; 348(14): 1309-21. [http://dx.doi.org/10.1056/NEJMoa030207] [PMID: 12668699]

[20] The effect of digoxin on mortality and morbidity in patients with heart failure. N Engl J Med 1997; 336(8): 525-33. [http://dx.doi.org/10.1056/NEJM199702203360801] [PMID: 9036306]

[21] Swedberg K, Komajda M, Böhm M, *et al.* Ivabradine and outcomes in chronic heart failure (SHIFT): a randomised placebo-controlled study. Lancet 2010; 376(9744): 875-85. [http://dx.doi.org/10.1016/S0140-6736(10)61198-1] [PMID: 20801500]

[22] Taylor AL, Ziesche S, Yancy C, *et al.* Combination of isosorbide dinitrate and hydralazine in blacks with heart failure. N Engl J Med 2004; 351(20): 2049-57. [http://dx.doi.org/10.1056/NEJMoa042934] [PMID: 15533851]

[23] Anker SD, Comin Colet J, Filippatos G, *et al.* Ferric carboxymaltose in patients with heart failure and iron deficiency. N Engl J Med 2009; 361(25): 2436-48. [http://dx.doi.org/10.1056/NEJMoa0908355] [PMID: 19920054]

[24] Parissis JT, Andreoli C, Kadoglou N, *et al.* Differences in clinical characteristics, management and short-term outcome between acute heart failure patients chronic obstructive pulmonary disease and those without this co-morbidity. Clin Res Cardiol 2014; 103(9): 733-41. [http://dx.doi.org/10.1007/s00392-014-0708-0] [PMID: 24718849]

[25] Cleland JG, Tendera M, Adamus J, Freemantle N, Polonski L, Taylor J. The perindopril in elderly people with chronic heart failure (PEP-CHF) study. Eur Heart J 2006; 27(19): 2338-45. [http://dx.doi.org/10.1093/eurheartj/ehl250] [PMID: 16963472]

[26] Massie BM, Carson PE, McMurray JJ, *et al.* Irbesartan in patients with heart failure and preserved ejection fraction. N Engl J Med 2008; 359(23): 2456-67. [http://dx.doi.org/10.1056/NEJMoa0805450] [PMID: 19001508]

[27] Conraads VM, Metra M, Kamp O, *et al.* Effects of the long-term administration of nebivolol on the clinical symptoms, exercise capacity, and left ventricular function of patients with diastolic dysfunction: results of the ELANDD study. Eur J Heart Fail 2012; 14(2): 219-25. [http://dx.doi.org/10.1093/eurjhf/hfr161] [PMID: 22147202]

[28] McMurray JJ, Packer M, Desai AS, *et al.* Angiotensin-neprilysin inhibition versus enalapril in heart failure. N Engl J Med 2014; 371(11): 993-1004. [http://dx.doi.org/10.1056/NEJMoa1409077] [PMID: 25176015]

CHAPTER 9

Interventional Therapy and Device Therapy

Polychronis Antonitsis[1,*], **Chrysovalantou Nikolaidou**[2] and **Antonios Ziakas**[2]

[1] *Cardiothoracic Department, AHEPA University Hospital, Thessaloniki, Greece*

[2] *1st Department of Cardiology, AHEPA University Hospital, Thessaloniki, Greece*

Abstract: Despite therapeutic advances in the medical treatment of HF patients, the prognosis remains poor. Coronary revascularization in patients with ischaemic cardiomyopathy is associated with amelioration of symptoms and survival benefit. Percutaneous coronary intervention with stenting is associated with excellent outcome, high procedural success rate, low event rates, and can be safely performed in patients with ischaemic cardiomyopathy. Patients with complex coronary artery disease require surgical revascularization (Coronary Artery Bypass Grafting - CABG). Cardiac resynchronization therapy (CRT) aims to re-establishing synchronous contraction between the left ventricular free wall and the interventricular septum, resulting in an increase in stroke volume. In clinical terms, this is translated in functional class improvement. This generally involves biventricular pacing (pacing of the left and right ventricle through separate leads). Surgical strategy for the management of patients with end-stage ischaemic heart disease includes "conventional" techniques (surgical revascularization, the most common surgical procedure, surgical ventricular restoration in patient with a dyskinetic part in the left ventricle and mitral valve surgery for mitral regurgitation). Mechanical circulatory support aims to restore blood flow and pressure, and thus end-organ function, in patients with profound cardiogenic shock or in end-stage patients (stage D) with advanced NYHA III-IV symptoms as a bridge to transplantation or as lifelong support (destination therapy). Heart transplantation is associated with excellent long-term results in terms of symptomatic relief and prognostic benefit under strict criteria involving the recipient and the donor. In the face of evolving technology, lifetime mechanical support provides a realistic alternative to heart transplantation.

Keywords: Cardiac resynchronization therapy, Coronary artery bypass grafting,

* **Corresponding author Polychronis Antonitsis:** Cardiothoracic Department, AHEPA University Hospital, Thessaloniki, Greece; Tel: +30 2310 99 4871; Fax: +30 2310 99 4814; E-mail: antonits@auth.gr.

Panagiotis Georgoulias (Ed.)

Coronary heart disease, Extracorporeal life support, Heart transplantation, Implantable cardioverter defibrillator, Ischeamic heart failure, Left ventricular assist device, Mechanical circulatory support, Percutaneous coronary intervention, Surgical ventricular restoration.

INTRODUCTION

Coronary artery disease (CAD) constitutes a major cause of mortality, morbidity and disability worldwide and imposes a significant financial burden on global healthcare systems. The number of patients afflicted worldwide makes CAD a global epidemic. In 2008, epidemiological data from the United States showed that heart disease was the predominant cause of death for those aged 65 years and older, and second leading cause for those aged 45 - 64 years with an estimated total prevalence of 16,300,000 people [1]. In Europe CAD is responsible for almost 1.8 million deaths annually (20% of all deaths) [2]. Although the abovementioned mortality rates have shown striking improvement during the last decades in developed countries, the prevalence of the multifaceted symptoms and the various clinical presentations of CAD remains high due to the improved survival of patients after acute myocardial infarction, and the ageing world population [3].

Currently, CAD represents the most common underlying cause of heart failure (HF) in developed countries, and is referred to as ischaemic cardiomyopathy (ICM). In the United States the estimated prevalence of HF for the year 2008 was 5,700,000 people. CAD accounts for almost half to two thirds of all cases of HF worldwide [4 - 6]. The prognosis of ischaemic HF is poor. The annual mortality is 10 to 15 times higher than age-matched controls for patients with systolic heart failure [HF with reduced ejection fraction (EF)], and 5 to 8 times higher for patients with diastolic HF (HF with preserved EF) [7].

The term ICM is used to describe severe myocardial dysfunction caused by CAD, with clinical manifestations and symptoms that resemble those of primary dilated cardiomyopathy. ICM is characterized by a combination of myocardial dysfunction and hibernation, diffuse fibrosis, or multiple infarctions. In the early stages of chronic CAD, angina may be the main clinical feature. When HF becomes more prominent, dyspnea predominates. Other patients with silent ischaemia finally develop ICM, with no history of angina or myocardial infarction [8].

PATHOPHYSIOLOGY OF ISHAEMIC MYOCARDIAL DYSFUNCTION

CAD can lead to impaired ventricular function and HF through different mechanisms (Fig. **1**). After an acute ischaemic event, such as a myocardial infarction, there is a loss of functioning myocytes, which leads to myocardial fibrosis and dilatation of the left ventricle (LV). The ensuing neurohormonal activation and LV remodeling result in progressive deterioration of the remaining viable myocardium. This LV remodeling may occur even after the achieved patency of the infarct-related artery with revascularization. Acute ischaemia also causes impaired regional LV function, presenting with hypokinesia or dyskinesia, and impaired LV relaxation, resulting in elevated filling pressures [9].

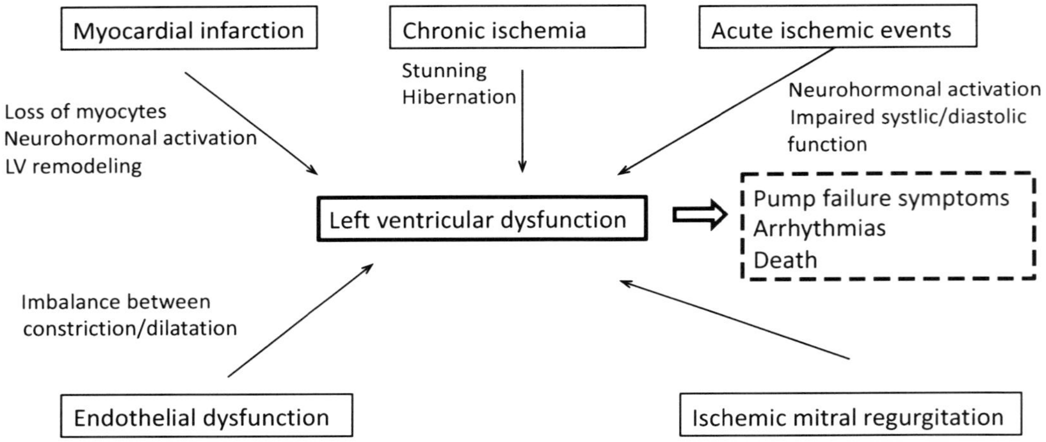

Fig. (1). Mechanisms of ischaemic heart failure and its consequences [9].

Chronic ischaemia results in hibernation and/or stunning of the myocardium, with further decline in LV function. Stunned myocardium refers to dysfunction in viable myocardium associated with transient ischaemia, such as demand-induced ischaemia, with normal resting blood flow. Thus, there is a dissociation of the usual close relationship between subendocardial flow and function. Repeated reversible ischaemia results in persistent dysfunction or chronic "repetitive" stunning. Hibernating myocardium is chronically dysfunctional tissue associated with inadequate coronary blood flow or coronary flow reserve. There is usually a progression from stunned to hibernating myocardium. In hibernation, regional cellular mechanisms downregulate contractile and metabolic function of the heart so as to protect it from irreversible injury. As a result many patients with hibernating myocardium present with LV dysfunction rather than symptomatic ischemia. The hibernating myocardium is functionally non-contractile, though metabolically active, and thus potentially viable after the restoration of blood flow [10 - 12]. It has been reported that approximately two-thirds of patients with ICM show viable myocardium [13].

Myocardial ischaemia is also associated with an altered nitric oxide (NO)-dependent relaxation of coronary arteries and increased endothelin concentrations, which along with the neurohormonal activation and the massive increase in the concentration of endogenous catecholamines, lead to myocardial apoptosis and fibrosis and contribute to the progression of LV dysfunction [14, 15]. Mitral regurgitation is another complication of myocardial infarction or ischaemia, caused by LV global or regional pathological remodelling and LV dysfunction, resulting in increased tethering on the mitral valve. Volume overload resulting from mitral regurgitation creates a vicious circle. Progression of LV remodeling increases the severity of mitral regurgitation, which leads to further LV dilatation, worsened LV function and thus, severe mitral regurgitation [16].

HF with preserved EF can be another presentation of ischaemic heart disease. Transient episodes of ischaemia impair LV relaxation, lead to elevation of LV filling pressures and can finally cause pulmonary congestion. The prevalence of CAD in patients with HF with preserved EF varies from 14% to 100% [9].

ROLE OF PERCUTANEOUS CORONARY INTERVENTION (PCI) IN PATIENTS WITH HEART FAILURE (HF)

Despite therapeutic advances in the medical treatment of patients with HF, the prognosis remains poor. Coronary revascularization can have a role in the amelioration of symptoms and possibly on survival.

The Significance of Viable Myocardium

Areas of stunned myocardium after a myocardial infarction, and short-term chronic hibernating myocardium as a result of post-ischaemic stunning, can coexist with irreversibly injured myocardium. Viable dysfunctional myocardium can be defined as any region that directionally improves contractile function after coronary revascularization [10]. Viable myocardium can be detected by identification of preserved metabolism by positron emission tomography (PET), cell membrane integrity by single-photon emission computed tomography (SPECT), contractility by dobutamine stress echocardiography or magnetic resonance imaging (MRI), and strain rate echocardiography imaging [12]. Cardiac MRI is an emerging non-invasive imaging technique which can provide assessment of cardiac morphology, function as well as myocardial perfusion and contractile function [17].

Evaluating the extent of viable myocardium and the presence of contractile reserve may be important to predict functional recovery after revascularization in patients with ischaemic HF. When PET is used, >10% viability of hibernating myocardium identifies the patients who will be benefited [18]. Patients with asyngergic myocardial segments on SPECT showing preserved radiotracer (thallium-201, 99mTc-sestamibi/tetrofosmin) uptake based on quantitative rest scintigraphy (≥50% or ≥ 60% peak uptake) demonstrate subsequent improvement in systolic LV function after revascularization [19]. On cardiac MRI, a greater transmural extent of infarction, for example hyperenhancement involving >50% of the wall thickness, can predict regions that are less likely to show functional improvement after therapy [20]. According to the European Society of Cardiology Guidelines on Acute and Chronic Heart Failure, patients with >10% of dysfunctional but viable LV myocardium (documented by any non-invasive test) may be more likely to benefit from myocardial revascularization [21]. Revascularization provides long-term benefits, even in patients without LV contractile reserve, by preventing further functional deterioration, progression of LV dilatation, recurrence of ischaemia and sudden cardiac death.

Several meta-analyses have demonstrated improved survival in patients with documented viability in the setting of ischaemic dysfunction, who subsequently underwent revascularization [11]. On the contrary, medically treated patients with viability (based on non-invasive tests) have the lowest survival rate. In the STICH trial which included mainly patients with 2 or 3 vessel disease amenable to coronary artery bypass grafting (CABG), the presence of viable myocardium (defined by SPECT or dobutamine stress echocardiography) was linked to improved survival in patients with ICM [22]. The presence of hibernating myocardium also predicts improvement in regional and global LV function, as well as in the severity of HF symptoms and exercise capacity after revascularization [23].

Percutaneous Coronary Intervention (PCI) in Patients with Ischaemic Heart Failure (HF)

Percutaneous coronary intervention (PCI) with stenting can be safely performed in patients with HF and is associated with excellent outcome, high procedural success rate and low adverse event rates [24, 25].

Revascularization with PCI in patients with ischaemic HF can improve overall myocardial contractility, wall motion abnormalities, LV function and symptoms. Moreover, it protects from further deterioration of LV function due to new ischaemic events. Additional mechanisms of benefit include a reduction of LV remodeling, diminished ventricular instability and arrhythmias, and maintenance of collateral circulation in the event of further coronary artery occlusion [12].

In the GRACE Registry, patients who presented with HF on admission for an acute coronary syndrome or developed HF, had 3- to 4-fold higher in-hospital mortality rates, longer hospital stay, higher readmission rates, and increased mortality up to six months after discharge. Revascularization significantly reduced post-discharge six-month mortality rates [26]. Revascularization has been also been associated with improved survival in patients with HF post acute myocardial infarction or in cardiogenic shock [27, 28]. In non-ST-elevation acute coronary syndromes, randomized trials have provided consistent evidence of the benefit of early revascularization, regardless of the presence of HF [26]. Further to systolic function, revascularization also improves LV diastolic filling in patients with ICM. The improvement of diastolic dysfunction is related to the amount of viable myocardium [29].

Existing data regarding revascularization in patients with ICM caused by complex CAD, are more robust for CABG than for PCI, and CABG has been the main type of revascularization used in most studies. Some studies have proven benefit of CABG over PCI, but were conducted before the introduction of contemporary drug eluting stents [30]. In the BARI trial the five-year survival rates for all patients with ICM and for those without treated diabetes, were slightly higher in patients who underwent CABG compared to patients revascularized with PCI. The figures were the same for the seven-year survival rates, but the differences were not statistically significant [31, 32]. In the AWESOME trial patients with ICM (LVEF <35%) showed worse overall survival at three years, with better results in patients assigned to CABG compared to PCI, while in the overall study population, PCI group showed improved survival [33]. When patients with ischaemic HF underwent revascularization exclusively with drug eluting stent implantation, the long term mortality and major cardiac adverse events (MACCE) rates were comparable to the mortality and event rates of patients assigned to CABG [34]. Overall, results from large multicenter randomized studies provide inconclusive evidence of the comparative efficacy for PCI and CABG in patients with depressed LV function. Optimization of PCI strategies and the use of new medications and new generation drug eluting stents could increase the efficacy of PCI in patients with ischaemic HF.

Guidelines

According to the European Society of Cardiology Guidelines, coronary angiography should be considered in HF patients and angina pectoris or a history of cardiac arrest if the patient is otherwise suitable for coronary revascularization. Non-invasive evaluation of myocardial viability may also be performed before angiography as some observational data show that coronary angiography may be of little, if any, benefit and may confer considerable risk, in the absence of significant viability. Coronary angiography may also be required, urgently, in selected patients with acute failure of the LV (cardiogenic shock or acute pulmonary oedema) or the right ventricle (RV), particularly in those with an associated acute coronary syndrome [21].

Coronary revascularization (percutaneous or surgical) is indicated for the symptomatic relief of angina pectoris in HF patients with either reduced or preserved EF. Patients with >10% of dysfunctional but viable LV myocardium may be more likely to benefit from myocardial revascularization, while the benefit – risk balance in patients without angina/ischaemia or without viable myocardium remains less clear. According both to the European Society of Cardiology and the American College of Cardiology Foundation/American Heart Association/Society for Cardiovascular Angiography and Interventions Guidelines, the choice between PCI and CABG should be made by the Heart Team, including a heart failure specialist, and be based on a careful evaluation of the patient's clinical status and coronary anatomy, including SYNTAX score, expected completeness of revascularization, associated valvular disease and the presence of co-morbidities, such as diabetes mellitus. Patient preference should be also taken into account (Table **1**) [21, 35, 36].

Table 1. Recommendations for myocardial revascularization in patients with chronic HF and reduced EF (≤35%). Class stands for Class of recommendation, Level for Level of evidence.

Recommendations	Class	Level	ref.
CABG is recommended for patients with angina and significant left main stenosis, who are otherwise suitable for surgery and expected to survive >1 year with good functional status, to reduce the risk of premature death	I	C	21
CABG is recommended for patients with angina and two- or three-vessel CAD, including a left anterior descending stenosis, who are otherwise suitable for surgery and expected to survive >1 year with good functional status, to reduce the risk of hospitalization for cardiovascular causes and the risk of premature death from cardiovascular causes	I	B	21
Alternative to CABG: PCI may be considered as an alternative to CABG in the above categories of patients unsuitable for surgery	IIb	C	21
Myocardial revascularization should be considered in the presence of viable myocardium	IIb	B	35
CABG or PCI is indicated for HF patients on guideline-directed medical therapy and angina and suitable coronary anatomy, especially significant left main stenosis or left main equivalent	I	C	37
CABG and PCI are NOT recommended in patients without angina AND without viable myocardium	III	C	21
Emergency PCI is indicated for patients with cardiogenic shock due to STEMI or NSTE-ACS if coronary anatomy is amenable	I	B	35

(Table 1) contd.....

Recommendations	Class	Level	ref.
Emergency CABG is recommended for patients with cardiogenic shock if the coronary anatomy is not amenable to PCI	I	B	35

Classes of Recommendation:
Class I: Evidence and/or general agreement that a given treatment or procedure is beneficial, useful, effective.
Class IIa: Weight of evidence/opinion is in favor of usefulness/efficacy.
Class IIb: Usefulness/efficacy is less well established by evidence/opinion.
Class III: Evidence or general agreement that the given treatment or procedure is not useful/effective, and in some cases may be harmful.
Levels of evidence:
A: Data derived from multiple randomized clinical trials or meta-analyses.
B: Data derived from a single randomized clinical trial or large non-randomized studies.
C: Consensus of opinion of the experts and/or small studies, retrospective studies, registries.
CABG: coronary artery bypass grafting; EF: ejection fraction; HF: heart failure; NSTE-ACS: non ST elevated acute coronary syndrome; PCI: percutaneous coronary intervention; STEMI: ST elevated myocardial infarction.

CARDIAC RESYNCHRONIZATION THERAPY (CRT)

Association of QRS Duration and Morphology with Mechanical Dyssynchrony

A QRS duration of greater than 120 ms, which is most commonly recorded as left bundle-branch block (LBBB), is evident in approximately one third of patients with systolic HF. In the Italian Network on Congestive Heart Failure registry, 25% of patients had complete LBBB, 6% had complete right bundle-branch block (RBBB) and 6% had other types of intraventricular conduction delay. The risk of developing LBBB is estimated at 10% in ambulatory patients with chronic HF per year [38, 39]. Patients with a broad QRS complex have a worse prognosis than patients with a narrow QRS complex. More specifically LBBB is associated with an increased one-year mortality rate from any cause, even after adjustment for other variables such as age, HF severity and concomitant drug therapy [40]. But even patients with RBBB or other intraventricular conduction delay have an unfavorable prognosis. As shown in the Multicenter Automatic Defibrillator Trial (MADIT) CRT study, 3-year mortality rates for patients with LBBB, RBBB, or other intraventricular conduction delay were 8%, 7% and 4% respectively [41].

In LBBB, the LV is activated through the interventricular septum from the right His bundle, resulting in a significant delay between the onset of LV and RV contraction. Contraction starts at the anterior septum, then follows the inferoseptal wall, while the inferior and lateral aspects of the LV are being activated latest. The abnormal ventricular septal motion, and the asynchronous contraction of LV wall regions (ventricular dyssynchrony), result in impaired cardiac systolic function, reduced stroke volume and systolic blood pressure, and abnormal pressure gradient between the LV and RV [38, 39, 42]. Mechanical dyssynchrony also results in prolongation of the isovolumic contraction and isovolumic relaxation periods and a significant decrease in LV filling time [43]. All the above further deteriorate the LV systolic function and the symptoms of HF patients.

A prolonged QRS duration has been shown to be a marker for atrioventricular, interventricular and intraleft ventricular dyssynchronies [43]. Prolongation of the atrioventricular interval results in a delay of systolic contraction, which might then encroach on early diastolic filling. In such circumstance, LV diastolic pressure rises above left atrial pressure leading to development of mitral regurgitation. Moreover, functional systolic mitral regurgitation may be caused or aggravated by poorly coordinated papillary muscle function due to LV dyssynchrony and systolic dysfunction [39]. Ventricular dyssynchrony due to LBBB is also associated with significantly delayed aortic opening and aortic valve closure, which results in a relative decrease in the duration of LV filling, and thus stroke volume [42].

The Role of Cardiac Resynchronization Therapy (RCT)

CRT aims to re-establishing synchronous contraction between the LV free wall and ventricular septum in order to improve LVEF. This may translate in clinical terms into improvement in NYHA functional class (Table **2**). This generally involves biventricular pacing, that is pacing of the LV and RV through separate leads (Fig. **2**) [44]. Mechanism of the benefit of implanted CRT devices is heterogeneous and is likely to vary between patients and within an individual patient over time. CRT may stimulate both ventricles almost simultaneously, thereby improving the coordination of ventricular contraction and reducing the severity of mitral regurgitation. This effect also prolongs the time available for myocardial perfusion [38, 45].

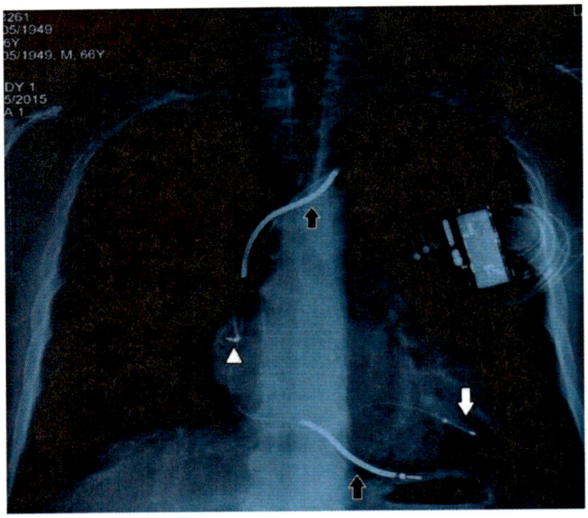

Fig. (2). Chest X-ray of a patient with a cardiac resynchronization therapy (CRT-Defibrillator). The LV lead placed on the surface of the LV (transvenously through the coronary sinus) is shown with the white arrow, the right ventricular lead and defibrillator coils are shown with the black arrows, and the right atrial lead is shown with the white arrowhead.
CRT: cardiac resynchronization therapy; LV: left ventricle.

Table 2. Recommendations for cardiac resynchronization therapy (CRT) in patients in sinus rhythm (SR) [39, 57]. Class stands for Class of recommendation, Level for Level of evidence and NA for not applicable.

	ESC 2013		**ACCF/AHA/HRS 2012**	
Recommendations	**Class**	**Level**	**Class**	**Level**
LBBB with SR and QRS duration >150 msec: CRT is recommended in chronic HF patients and LVEF ≤35% who remain in NYHA functional class III and ambulatory IV despite adequate medical treatment.	I	A	I	A
LBBB with SR and QRS duration ≥150 msec: CRT is indicated for HF patients and LVEF ≤35% and NYHA II class on guideline-directed medical therapy.	I	A	I	B
LBBB with sinus rhythm (SR) and QRS duration ≥150 msec: CRT may be considered for patients who have LVEF ≤30%, ischaemic etiology of HF and NYHA class I symptoms on guideline-directed medical therapy.	NA	NA	IIb	C
LBBB with SR and QRS duration 120–150 msec: CRT is recommended in chronic HF patients and LVEF ≤35% who remain in NYHA functional class II, III and ambulatory IV despite adequate medical treatment.	I	B	IIa	B

(Table 2) contd.....

	ESC 2013		ACCF/AHA/ HRS 2012	
Recommendations	**Class**	**Level**	**Class**	**Level**
Non-LBBB with SR and QRS duration >150 msec: CRT should be considered in chronic HF patients and LVEF ≤35% who remain in NYHA functional III and ambulatory IV despite adequate medical treatment.	**IIa**	**B**	**IIa**	**A**
Non-LBBB with SR and QRS duration >150 msec: CRT should be considered in chronic HF patients and LVEF ≤35% who remain in NYHA functional class II despite adequate medical treatment.	**IIa**	**B**	**IIb**	**B**
Non-LBBB with SR and QRS duration 120–150 msec: CRT may be considered in chronic HF patients and LVEF ≤35% who remain in NYHA functional class II (ESC only), III and ambulatory IV despite adequate medical treatment.	**IIb**	**B**	**IIb**	**B**
CRT in patients with chronic HF with QRS duration <120 ms is not recommended.	**III**	**B**	**NA**	**NA**
CRT is not recommended in patients with NYHA class I or II symptoms and non-LBBB pattern with QRS duration less than 150 msec.	**NA**	**NA**	**III**	**B**
CRT is not indicated for patients whose comorbidities and/or frailty limit survival with good functional capacity to less than 1 year.	**NA**	**NA**	**III**	**C**

ACCF/AHA/HRS: American College of Cardiology Foundation/American Heart Association/Heart Rhythm Society; ESC: European Society of Cardiology; HF: heart failure; LBBB: left bundle-branch block; LVEF: left ventricular ejection fraction; NYHA: New York Heart Association.

As evidenced from many randomized control studies, CRT helps to restore atrioventricular, inter- and intra-ventricular synchrony, and improves LV function and structure, reduces functional mitral regurgitation and induces LV reverse remodeling [39]. CRT, added to optimal medical therapy, results in significant decrease in patient mortality, increased survival, reduction in the number of hospitalizations for worsening HF, reversal of LV remodeling, and improved quality of life and exercise capacity [46]. In a meta-analysis of 14 randomized controlled trials including 4420 patients with LVEF ≤35% and prolonged QRS duration, CRT therapy improved LVEF, functional status and quality of life, and decreased HF hospitalizations by 37% and all-cause mortality by 22% [47].

The beneficial effects of CRT on morbidity, mortality and LV function may be greater in females, patients with non-ischaemic cardiomyopathy and patients with QRS duration >150 msec (Fig. **3**). These patients show important clinical improvement. However, a significant proportion, up to 30% of patients receiving CRT, does not have a positive response and are called "non-responders". Of course, this may reflect the natural history of the disease rather than the effect of CRT. On the other hand, in patients who show the most important clinical improvement and LV reverse remodeling, anatomy and function approach normal state ("super-responders" to CRT). These patients are expected to have the best outcome after CRT [39, 48].

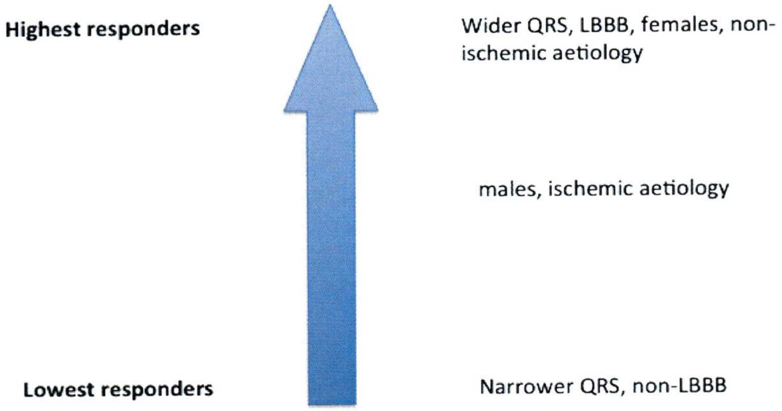

Fig. (3). Clinical factors influencing the magnitude of benefit to cardiac resynchronization therapy [39]. LBBB: left bundle-branch block.

CRT has proven benefit in HF patients with severely reduced EF (≤35%). Mainly, the beneficial effect is achieved in New York Heart Association (NYHA) class II-IV patients showing sinus rhythm and LBBB morphology (≥120msec QRS duration). Recently, CRT was reported to improve survival even in patients with mild HF [49]. Notably, patients with RBBB or non-LBBB morphology are a high-risk HF subgroup that is less likely to respond to CRT therapy [50]. No benefit from CRT has been evidenced in patients with QRS duration <120 msec; on the contrary it may be harmful [51]. Patients with atrial fibrillation (AF) pose a therapeutic challenge to the use of CRT, as the goal to achieve biventricular pacing as close to 100% as possible is difficult to be achieved. AF is a major determinant of loss of biventricular pacing, as the patients show no atrioventricular synchrony, and thus no coordinated atrioventricular pacing. Tachycardia and irregular conduction may interfere with adequate biventricular pacing delivery. Also, the presence of spontaneous, fusion or pseudo-fusion beats may reduce the rate of real biventricular capture [52]. In a meta-analysis of twenty-three observational studies, patients with AF had an increased risk of non-response to CRT and all-cause mortality. The presence of AF was also associated with less improvement in quality of life, exercise capacity, and LV end-systolic dimension [53]. The subgroup of patients with a biventricular pacing of at least >85% were shown improvement with the use of CRT [54]. The solution to the problem of low rate biventricular pacing in HF patients with AF involves atrioventricular (AV) junction ablation, which was found to confer improvements in LVEF, functional capacity and exercise capacity, and to achieve a reverse remodeling effect, similar to that observed in patients with sinus rhythm [55]. Moreover, the addition of AV junction ablation to CRT is associated with a substantial reduction in cardiovascular and all-cause mortality and with improvement in NYHA functional class, compared to the combination of CRT and medical therapy, without AV junction ablation [56]. Therefore, there is a strong recommendation (Class IIa) of adding AV junction ablation to CRT therapy in the Guidelines (Table **3**), although the evidence does not stem from large randomized trials.

Table 3. Recommendations for cardiac resynchronization therapy (CRT) in patients with permanent atrial fibrillation (AF) and patients requiring or already having a pacemaker or implantable cardioverter-defibrillator [39, 57]. Class stands for Class of recommendation, Level for Level of evidence and NA for not applicable.

	ESC (2013)		ACCF/AHA/ HRS (2012)	
Recommendations	**Class**	**Level**	**Class**	**Level**
Patients with AF, wide QRS and reduced LVEF: CRT should be considered in chronic HF patients, intrinsic QRS ≥120 ms and LVEF ≤35% who remain in NYHA functional class III and ambulatory IV despite adequate medical treatment, provided that a biventricular pacing as close to 100% as possible can be achieved.	**IIa**	**B**	**IIa**	**B**
Patients with AF, wide QRS and reduced LVEF: AV junction ablation should be added in case of incomplete biventricular pacing.	**IIa**	**B**	**IIa**	**B**
Patients with AF with uncontrolled heart rate who are candidates for AV junction ablation: CRT should be considered in patients with reduced LVEF who are candidates for AV junction ablation for rate control.	**IIa**	**B**	**NA**	**NA**

(Table 3) contd.....

	ESC (2013)		ACCF/AHA/ HRS (2012)	
Recommendations	**Class**	**Level**	**Class**	**Level**
Patients with an indication for pacemaker: CRT can be useful in patients with LVEF ≤35% on guideline-directed medical therapy if the patient requires ventricular pacing, with anticipated requirement for significant (>40%) ventricular pacing.	**IIa**	**B**	**IIa**	**C**
Upgrade from conventional pacemaker or implantable cardioverter-defibrillator: CRT is indicated in HF patients with LVEF <35% and high percentage of ventricular pacing who remain in NYHA class III and ambulatory IV despite adequate medical treatment.	**I**	**B**	**NA**	**NA**

AV: atrioventricular; HF: heart failure; LVEF: left ventricular ejection fraction; NYHA: New York Heart Association.

Implantable Cardioverter Defibrillators (ICDs)

Approximately half of the deaths in HF patients, particularly in those presenting with milder symptoms, occur suddenly and unexpectedly, and are linked to ventricular arrhythmias. Ventricular arrhythmias in patients with LV dysfunction are associated with altered cardiac morphology, neurohormonal activation and presence of scarred myocardium. Prevention of sudden death is therefore a crucial goal in HF, a goal that cannot be achieved solely with antiarrhythmic drugs, which may be the cause of life-threatening arrhythmias because of their pro-arrhythmic action [21, 58]. ICDs reduce the risk of ventricular arrhythmia-related sudden death in HF patients, at an acceptable cost-effectiveness profile [59]. The benefit of ICD therapy usually becomes apparent a year after implantation of the device [46].

An ICD consists of two main components: the pulse generator and the lead with the defibrillator shock coils. The proximal shock coil usually lies in the superior vena cava and the distal shock coil in the RV (Fig. **2**). Defibrillator leads transmit electrical signals from the heart to the pulse generator for analysis, and deliver pacing and shocking pulses to the myocardium. All ICD systems have four essential functions: arrhythmia detection, arrhythmia treatment, bradycardia pacing and episode-data storage [60]. An ICD is indicated for secondary prevention, after an unprovoked episode of ventricular fibrillation or in cases of sustained ventricular tachycardia, irrespectively of LVEF. For primary prevention,

ICD indication includes NYHA functional class II or III patients with EF persistently 35% or less. The above indications apply only to patients receiving optimal medical therapy for at least 3 months, who are expected to survive for at least 1 year with a reasonable quality of life and functional status [21, 61].

The benefit of ICD therapy in reducing mortality has been shown in patients with both ischaemic (>40 days after an acute myocardial infarction), and non-ischaemic HF aetiology, whereas amiodarone presented a similar risk of death when compared to placebo [62 - 64]. The current criteria and recommendations of the European Society of Cardiology and the American College of Cardiology Foundation/American Heart Association/Heart Rhythm Society for the use of ICD therapy are shown in Table **4**.

Table 4. Recommendations for the use of Implantable Cardioverter Defibrillators (ICDs) in patients with heart failure (HF). Class stands for Class of recommendation, Level for Level of evidence and NA for not applicable [21, 61].

	ESC (2012)		ACCF/AHA/ HRS (2012)	
Recommendations	**Class**	**Level**	**Class**	**Level**
Secondary prevention: An ICD is recommended in a patient with a ventricular arrhythmia causing haemodynamic instability, who is expected to survive for >1 year with good functional status, to reduce the risk of sudden death.	I	A	I	A
Primary prevention: An ICD is recommended in a patient with symptomatic HF (NYHA class II-III) and an LVEF ≤35% despite ≥3 months of treatment with optimal pharmacological therapy, who is expected to survive for >1 year with good functional status, to reduce the risk of sudden death • Ischaemic aetiology and >40 days after acute myocardial infarction.	I	A	I	A
• Non-ischaemic aetiology.	I	B	I	B
Patients with LVEF <40% and prior myocardial infarction: CRT is indicated with inducible VF or sustained VT at the electrophysiological study.	NA	NA	I	B
HF patients with syncope of undetermined origin with clinically relevant, haemodynamically significant sustained VT or VF induced at electrophysiological study.	NA	NA	I	B

ACCF/AHA/HRS: American College of Cardiology Foundation/American Heart Association/Heart Rhythm Society; CRT: cardiac resynchronization therapy; ESC: European Society of Cardiology; HF: heart failure; LVEF: left ventricular ejection fraction; NYHA: New York Heart Association; VF: ventricular fibrillation; VT: ventricular tachycardia.

THE ROLE OF SURGERY IN HEART FAILURE (HF)

Current and emerging surgical strategies for HF focus on patients with: a) a LVEF <30%, b) mean pulmonary artery pressure >25mm Hg, c) an akinetic or dyskinetic portion of the LV that exceeds 60% and d) LV end-diastolic volume (LVEDV) >250ml (LVEDV index (LVEDVI) >140ml/m^2). Most of these patients receive medical treatment and are classified as NYHA functional class III or IV [65]. In CAD, mortality is related to infarct size. Based on the STICHES study, ten year event-free survival for patients with LVEF <35% was 41.1% with surgery and 33.9% with medical treatment [66]. In patients with dilated cardiomyopathy, mortality is also directly associated with the severity of LV dysfunction. Increased LVEDVI and the presence of mitral regurgitation are indicators of worse prognosis. Mitral regurgitation occurs in HF patients secondary to annular dilatation, LV remodeling or papillary muscle dysfunction. It leads to volume overload which creates progressive LV and annular dilatation, which subsequently worsen mitral regurgitation. Surgical options in end-stage ischaemic heart disease are summarized in Table **5**. Surgical revascularization represents the most conventional operation in HF patients, as discussed in previous section.

Table 5. Surgical options in ischaemic heart failure patients.

Conditions	Interventions
Reversible ischaemia, LVESVI <60 ml/m2	CABG
Reversible ischaemia, dyskinetic area in LV, LVESVI > 60 ml/m2	Surgical ventricular restoration ± CABG
Grade III/IV mitral regurgitation	Mitral repair ± CABG
No reversible ischaemia, biventricular failure	LVAD or transplantation

CABG: Coronary Artery Bypass Grafting; LVAD: Left Ventricular Assist Device; LVESVI: Left ventricular end-systolic volume index.

Surgical Ventricular Restoration

The goal of surgical ventricular restoration (SVR) is to reverse LV remodeling and exclude the infarcted part of interventricular septum and LV free wall, in an attempt to reshape the LV (from globular to elliptical), without critically decreasing ventricular volume. This strategy discontinues progression of LV failure and improves global LVEF. Moderate to severe mitral regurgitation could be addressed during the same procedure. In the Dor procedure (circular endoventricular patch plasty), the LV is opened through scar. The boundary between the normal endocardium and dyskinetic scar is identified. A circumferential endoventricular (Fontan) circular suture is passed approximately 1-2 cm outside the limit of healthy myocardium (Fig. **4**). This circular suture is tied to constrict the size of the LV around a balloon inflated within the cavity to a diastolic volume of 50-70 ml/m^2. The residual myocardial defect is then closed after removing the balloon. This technique restores an elliptical LV shape (Fig. **5**) which shows improved contractile properties compared to a globular LV. This procedure is associated with a significant decrease in LVEDV and LV end-systolic volume (LVESV) resulting in an improvement in LVEF. Dor procedure is associated with a hospital mortality of 12-18% in patients with extremely low LVEF (< 20%) and pulmonary hypertension, as compared to 3% mortality for those with EF > 30%. Most patients show clinical improvement. However, approximately 10% of survivors show no signs of clinical improvement and about 25% have persistent pulmonary hypertension due to diastolic LV failure. Surgical ventricular restoration also improves myocardial function through reduction in wall tension.

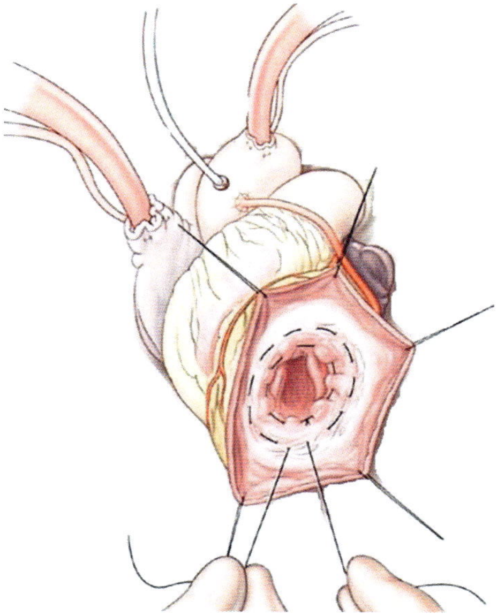

Fig. (4). Surgical ventricular restoration. The circular (Fontan) stich is passed at the border between the scar tissue and the working myocardium (Adapted from CTSNet, http://www.ctsnet.org).

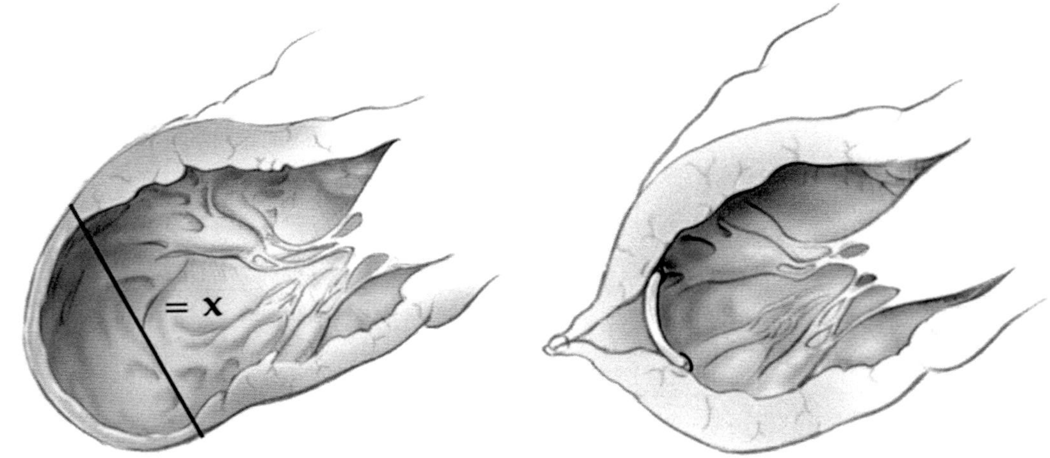

Fig. (5). Geometric restoration of a dilated failing LV from a circular to an elliptical shape after a Dor procedure.
LV: left ventricular.

A large amount of data derived mainly from registries and large cohort single-institutional studies have shown that SVR is relatively safe and effective with a favorable 5-year outcome [67]. However, controversy rose with the results from the STICH trial, which questioned the additional benefit of the SVR. According to the Hypothesis 2 STICH trial there was no difference in clinical outcome by adding SVR to CABG [68]. SVR combined with CABG produced a significant decrease in LVESVI (16 ml/m^2, a proportional reduction of 19%). A lot of criticism was focused on the observation that this percentage was significantly lower than the percentage of reduction found in previous observational series, which ranged from 30 to 50%. It should be emphasized that in STICH trial, the postoperative LVESVI remained unacceptably large (>60 ml/m^2) in both arms. This finding raised concerns on the extent of the SVR procedure that was applied by STICH surgeons. The role of LVESVI in ICM related LV remodeling is critical. According to White *et al.* patients with LVESVI >60 ml/m^2 after reperfusion for a myocardial infarction had approximately 5 times higher mortality compared with those with preserved LVESVI [69]. This was also confirmed by GUSTO-I trial [70]. A landmark study by Di Donato *et al.* showed that LVESVI following SVR affects mortality, being significantly higher in patients with a postoperative LVESVI of ≥60 ml/m^2 [71]. In the light of this evidence, the lack of survival benefit observed in the STICH trial might be related to inadequate LV volume reduction [72]. Further analysis of the STICH trial data showed that SVR combined with CABG conferred a survival benefit in the subgroup of patients with a postoperative LVESVI $\leq$70 ml/m^2 [73]. The Task Force on Myocardial Revascularization of the European Society of Cardiology (ESC) and the European Association for Cardio-Thoracic Surgery (EACTS) suggest SVR as a surgical option combined with CABG in selected HF patients with a scar in the LAD territory and a baseline LVESVI $\geq$60 ml/ m^2 (Class of Recommendation IIb; Level of evidence B) [74].

Management of Mitral Regurgitation

As the failing LV dilates, the papillary muscles are displaced resulting in decreased coaptation of the mitral valve leaflets and, thus, development of a central jet of mitral regurgitation. This results in volume overload of the already dilated LV. Traditional reports noted that the failing ventricle deteriorates further, if the "blow off" into the left atrium is removed. However, results from studies performed in the early 1990s showed that mitral valve repair (or replacement) with preservation of the subvalvar apparatus is associated with symptomatic improvement and satisfactory medium-term survival bearing a low perioperative mortality [75]. Mitral valve repair with or without revascularization in HF patients has the following indications:

a. Ischaemia manifested by angina and/or dyspnoea at rest, or pulmonary oedema accompanied with moderate to severe mitral regurgitation.
b. Acute myocardial ischaemia or infarction located at the inferobasal wall (caused by occlusion of the right coronary artery or dominant circumflex), which causes posteromedial papillary muscle dysfunction and mitral regurgitation.
c. Papillary muscle rupture post acute inferobasal myocardial infarction.
d. Chronic progressive dyspnoea (NYHA III or IV) related to previous myocardial infarction. The enlarged dysfunctional LV is accompanied by varying degrees of pulmonary hypertension. This comprises the largest group of patients.
e. Patients with idiopathic dilated cardiomyopathy and moderate to severe mitral

regurgitation caused by annular dilatation resulting in inadequate leaflet coaptation.

The recommended threshold for mitral valve repair in ischaemic regurgitation is a calculated effective regurgitant orifice area >20 mm^2 and/or a regurgitant volume >30 ml/beat [65]. Patients with mild to moderate mitral regurgitation, target vessels at adequate condition and evidence of reversible ischaemia posterolaterally, can be treated by revascularisation alone. Ischaemic mitral regurgitation should not be considered solely as simple failure of a single papillary muscle, but as a functional problem of unsuccessful coordination of the entire mitral apparatus. Surgical treatment is based on mitral annuloplasty with proper undersizing of the valve ring, in an attempt to restore leaflet coaptation depth [76]. Occurrence of systolic anterior motion (SAM) producing LV outflow tract obstruction should be avoided. The undersized valve ring remodels the base of the dilated heart, aiming to re-establish an ellipsoid shape to the LV. Results from the RIME study showed that mitral annuloplasty combined with CABG in patients with moderate ischemic mitral regurgitation is associated with improvement in functional capacity, LV reverse remodeling, regurgitation severity and B-type natriuretic peptide levels [77]. These results have been challenged by other studies which failed to show a clinically meaningful advantage of adding mitral valve repair to CABG at 1-year follow-up [78]. While mitral annuloplasty was advocated by the majority of surgeons in patients with moderate to severe mitral regurgitation undergoing CABG, results from Acker *et al.* revealed that chordal-sparing mitral valve replacement produced similar results to mitral valve repair in patients with severe ischemic mitral regurgitation, in terms of reducing LV reverse remodeling and the rate of major adverse cardiac or cerebrovascular events at 12 months [79]. Preservation of subvalvar apparatus in patients undergoing mitral valve replacement is crucial for maintaining LV geometry and function. Undoubtedly, mitral valve replacement provides a more durable correction of mitral regurgitation, which may significantly impact long-term outcomes. This benefit should be weighed against any potential disadvantage of implanting a prosthetic valve. Further studies are required to identify not only the optimal technique for the management of ischaemic mitral regurgitation, but also the risk factors associated with recurrence of mitral regurgitation.

MECHANICAL CIRCULATORY SUPPORT

Mechanical Circulatory Support (MCS) in Acute Heart Failure (HF)

In profound acute cardiogenic shock, immediate restoration of blood flow and perfusion pressure to end-organs (brain, liver, kidneys, gut) is of utmost importance in order to avoid permanent damage. Adequate RV function contributes significantly to prevention of central venous hypertension and end-organ venous congestion [80]. Modern circulatory support technology was developed on the principle that a failing pump could be repaired or replaced provided that the other organs show no signs of irreversible dysfunction. The landmark Randomized Evaluation of Mechanical Assistance for the Treatment of Congestive Heart Failure (REMATCH) study established the long-term benefit of LV assist devices (LVADs) regarding not only symptomatic relief, but also survival benefit in end-stage HF patients not eligible for heart transplantation [81]. Considering that survival in patients with refractory acute post-infarction cardiogenic shock cannot be achieved without mechanical circulatory support, adequtely-powered randomized trials are unlikely to be conducted and the role of blood pumps has yet to be defined. Data for the use of these devices in cardiogenic shock are derived from clinical experience in which a substantial number of survivors signify a positive outcome.

The pathophysiology behind mechanical off-loading of the LV is straightforward. The failing heart beats more than 100,000 times per day and pumps a total of 7,000 l of blood against increased afterload. A dilated heart is characterized by impaired subendocardial blood flow caused by elevated wall tension, thereby increasing myocardial oxygen consumption. Medical treatment with administration of inotropic agents results in a further increase in heart rate, afterload, wall tension and, thus oxygen consumption. On the other hand, an LVAD off-loads the heart, thereby reducing LV wall tension and improving coronary and systemic blood flow. Improved perfusion enhances myocardial and end-organ recovery. Short-term support devices are used as a first step in order to sustain the reperfused patient during a period of days or weeks after a myocardial infarction until ischaemic stunning resolves. In patients with an irreversible injury, these devices can be used as bridge to heart transplantation or implantation of a long-term LVAD [82]. Over the last decade, the safety and effectiveness of LVADs has improved significantly. However, still very few patients with potentially recoverable post-ischemic cardiogenic shock are offered the option of mechanical circulatory support even after early and effective revascularization, thus maintaining the persistent excessive mortality related to this condition [83].

Intra-aortic Balloon Pump (IABP)

Intra-aortic balloon pump (IABP) represents the first applicable and more convenient form of mechanical assistance that is available in most cardiac and coronary care units. It is easily implanted percutaneously through the femoral artery in the descending thoracic aorta. It assists the LV in patients with post-cardiotomy cardiogenic shock by decreasing end-diastolic pressure and LV afterload (Fig. **6**) [84]. For an average heart, coronary perfusion would be 2.75ml per beat without IABP support and 3.25 ml per beat after IABP support implementation. IABP also decreases end-diastolic and peak systolic aortic pressure, LV systolic work, and myocardial oxygen consumption.

Use of IABP can improve LV output by 20% [85, 86]. Class I indications for IABP use in acute myocardial infarction include: a) as a stabilizing measure for angiography and prompt revascularization, b) for mechanical complications of acute myocardial infarction; acute mitral regurgitation or ventricular septal rupture, c) for recurrent intractable ventricular arrhythmias with haemodynamic instability and d) for refractory postinfarction angina [87]. The influence of the IABP on ischaemic RV function is widely questioned. RV dysfunction presents after inferior wall infarctions and in 20-30% of patients post LVAD implantation. According to the porcine model of acute ischaemic right HF with cardiogenic shock constructed by Nordhaug and colleagues, use of an IABP did not affect LV and RV contractility; however, it was related to significantly improved cardiac output, lower PVR and increased RV efficiency [88]. Thus, IABP exerts an indirect beneficial effect on RV function by decreasing pulmonary arterial resistance.

Although IABP increases coronary blood flow, it does not significantly increase systemic blood flow, and, thus, becomes progressively less effective as hypotension develops [89]. IABP function is also influenced by balloon volume, inflation rate, positioning in the aorta, and presence of cardiac arrhythmias. IABP efficiency is limited in patients with highly compliant aortas. Lower limb ischemia due to mechanical obstruction, thrombosis, or embolism is the predominant complication occurring in 9-36% of patients. Risk factors for this serious complication include peripheral vascular disease, diabetes mellitus and female sex [90]. Other less frequent complications include mesenteric ischaemia or pancreatitis through atheroemboli in the celiac trunk.

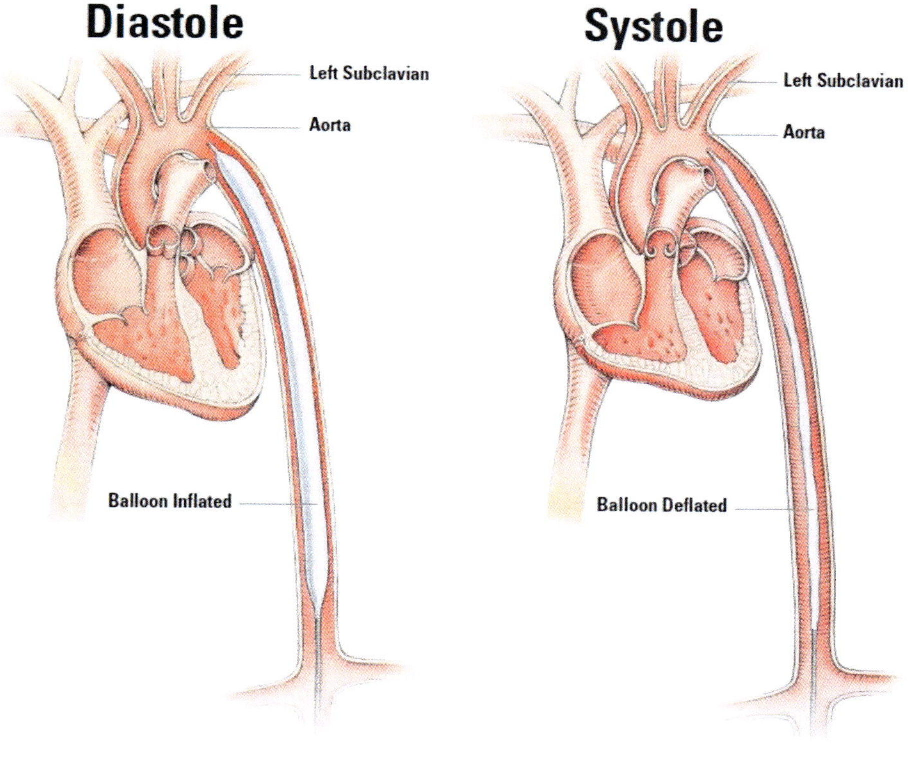

Fig. (6). Schematic representation of intra-aortic balloon pump. It is inserted in the descending aorta just distal to the left subclavian artery. It inflates in diastole just after the aortic valve closure, and deflates at the beginning of systole (Courtesy of Arrow International, http://www.arrowintl.com).

According to the SHOCK trial registry, patients who received IABP in addition to thrombolysis showed lower in-hospital mortality than those receiving thrombolysis alone. On the contrary, patients who were treated with primary PCI, according to NRMI-2 study, received no benefit from use of IABP [91, 92]. Recently, IABP-SHOCK II trial, in which 600 patients with cardiogenic shock were randomized, showed that IABP support did not reduce 12-month mortality in shock – complicated myocardial infarction cases, after early revascularization [93]. The lack of survival benefit could be explained by the fact that, despite experimental and clinical haemodynamic improvement with IABP, increase in cardiac output is only modest (estimated at approximately 0.5 l/min); thus, only partial mechanical circulatory support seems to be achieved [85].

Percutaneously Implanted Blood Pumps

Potentially reversible cardiogenic shock, such as after an extensive acute myocardial infarction, highlights the need for easily deployable, minimally-invasive LVADs that could be inserted percutaneously in the catheterization laboratory and provide effective off-loading of the acutely failing LV. Available percutaneous devices designed specifically to offer temporary circulatory support in the clinical practice are mainly Impella (Abiomed Inc, Danvers, MA, USA) and TandemHeart (CardiacAssist, Inc., Pittsburgh, PA, USA). When first introduced, these innovative LVADs were expected to be more effective in sustaining patients with cardiogenic shock compared to the IABP [94]. These devices have the ability to increase cardiac output and, thus, improve systemic blood flow and pressure, decrease LV wall stress, and improve coronary flow promoting functional recovery of the failing myocardium [95]. Experimental and clinical evidence showed that they could also limit infarct size [96, 97].

The catheter-based Impella models (Impella 2.5 and Impella CP) are percutaneously inserted *via* the femoral artery. These devices have a pump motor, which is positioned across the aortic valve in the cath lab, under fluoroscopic or echocardiographic guidance (Fig. **7**). The pump is connected to a 3 kg portable external pump console. It provides forward flow by sucking blood from the LV cavity and ejecting into the aorta. Impella 2.5 provides up to 2.5 l/min through a 12 Fr pump motor, while the more recent Impella CP provides up to 3.3 l/min of flow through a 14 Fr pump motor. They are indicated for short-term support (from 6 hours to 1 week). Although easily deployable and functionally effective, the Impella percutaneous VAD has a number of drawbacks including limited duration of support, insufficient cardiac output in larger patients (>100 kg body weight), and risk for displacement of the inflow pump out of the LV cavity. Lower limb ischemia can occur in patients with atherosclerotic aortas [98]. Finally, a diseased aortic valve, stenotic or regurgitant, or presence of a mechanical aortic prosthesis, preclude its use.

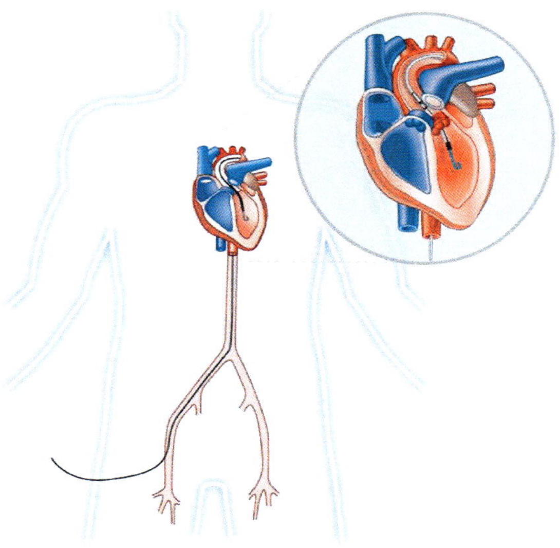

Fig. (7). The Impella microaxial blood pump (Courtesy of Abiomed Inc, http://www.abiomed.com/products).

TandemHeart is a short-term (<14 days) external percutaneously inserted centrifugal blood pump [99]. A long 21 Fr inflow cannula is inserted percutaneously through the right femoral vein and advanced towards the right atrium under fluoroscopic and echocardiographic guidance. After transatrial septal perforation, the tip of the inflow cannula is introduced into the left atrium. A 17 Fr cannula inserted in the femoral artery provides left heart bypass at a flow rate of approximately 4 l/min with a rotational speed between 2,500 and 4,500 rpm (Fig. **8**). RV support is also possible after performing transjugular cannulation of the right atrium with pulmonary artery cannulation *via* a femoral vein. Cohort studies in patients with cardiogenic shock verified the haemodynamic efficacy of the TandemHeart. Potential disadvantages include the risk of lower limb ischemia distal to the implantation site and limited device deployment in patients <70 kg body weight [95].

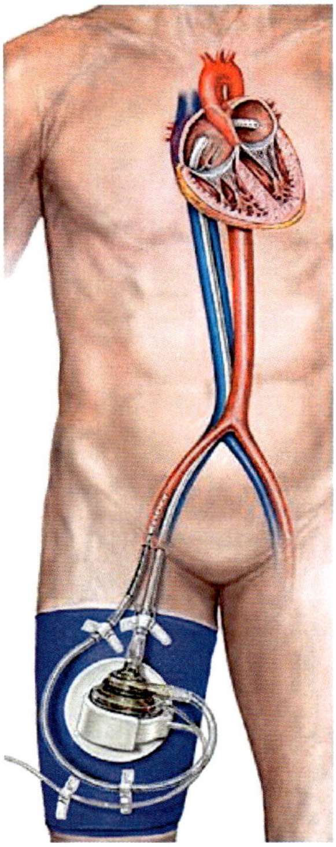

Fig. (8). The TandemHeart System.
(Courtesy of CardiacAssist Inc, http://www.cardiacassist.com/tandemheart-system/).

Irrespectively of numerous optimistic clinical reports, the haemodynamic effects of percutaneous LVADs in terms of improving clinical outcome in patients with cardiogenic shock remain debatable. Cheng *et al.* conducted a meta-analysis including three randomized clinical studies in patients with post-infarction shock; IABP was directly compared to TandemHeart in two studies, while the Impella 2.5 was compared to IABP in one study [100]. Percutaneous VADs improved cardiac index, mean arterial pressure and pulmonary capillary wedge pressure, in comparison to IABP; however, with no survival benefit. Moreover IABP showed a lower risk of complications, whereas the LVADs were linked to ten-times higher cost. These findings were surprising for those who expected pump flow to improve survival; however, there are several possible explanations; a) inadequate duration of support (<7 days) for sufficient recovery from myocardial stunning, b) inadequate off-loading of the failing LV, c) limited flow through peripherally inserted conduits insufficient to reverse multi-organ failure and d) a high incidence of limb ischaemia, which in some cases resulted in early removal of the device. Despite their limited use in specialized centres, percutaneous LVADs still have an important role in heamodynamically unstable patients undergoing high-risk primary PCI [101,102].

Extracorporeal Life Support (ECLS)

Extracorporeal Life Support (ECLS), commonly referred to as Extracorporeal Membrane Oxygenation (ECMO), is used to sustain physiological levels of blood flow in patients with cardiogenic shock, and more recently as a rescue system during cardiopulmonary resuscitation [103, 104]. The main characteristic of ECLS, over other forms of MCS, is that it offers both cardiac and pulmonary support for patients with cardiac and respiratory failure, who are often in profound hypoxia. An ECLS circuit includes a centrifugal blood pump, a membrane oxygenator and a heparin-coated circuit (Fig. **9**). It represents the simplest and most-rapid method of restoring systemic blood flow and, with modern peripheral percutaneous arterio-venous cannulation techniques, can be used in the catheterization laboratory or emergency room [105]. The circuit takes around 10-15 min to be assembled. Cannulation of the femoral artery and vein could be performed rapidly with a Seldinger technique, even during cardiac resuscitation. The tip of the venous drainage cannula is advanced into the lower right atrium. In post-cardiotomy setting, open surgical cannulation of the ascending aorta and the right atrium can be used. Central cannulation provides higher flows, but requires surgical decannulation and is associated with infectious and bleeding complications.

After the establishment of the circuit, the flow rate can be progressively increased to 3.5-4.0 l/min, which provides almost complete off-loading/decompression of the RV and restoration of a normal cardiac index. The mean arterial pressure is maintained at 75-85 mmHg. A narrow pulsatile arterial pressure tracing is indicative of residual myocardial contractility and, thus, decreased risk of intracardiac clot formation. When pulsatility disappears, volume expansion or inotropic support is indicated. ECLS enables rapid stabilization of haemodynamic status and correction of biochemical derangement, while it allows time to determine recovery, cardiac transplantation or a long-term LVAD (bridge to recovery, bridge to transplantation or bridge to LVAD). Drainage of blood from the circulation into the ECLS circuit leads to decreased right atrial and central venous pressure (CVP). This results in reduced RV ejection into the lungs and decreased pulmonary venous return to the left atrium, thus reducing LV end-diastolic volume and pressure. Decrease in end-diastolic volume and pressure limits wall stress, improves coronary perfusion and reduces work load posed to the ventricle, thereby promoting myocardial performance and contractility. The highly oxygenated blood that returns retrograde into the descending aorta can result in improved end-organ and coronary perfusion. Recovery of contractile function and arterial pulsation is a positive sign of myocardial recovery and the time required for the recovery has been related to survival [106]. Failure of ventricular recovery after 72 hours of ECLS support is an ominous sign associated with increased mortality [107].

It should be noted that veno-arterial ECLS offers optimal RV unloading and respiratory support. However, LV afterload and wall stress is elevated due to retrograde blood flow into the aorta. In cases when the failing LV is incapable of opening the aortic valve, loss of native ejection occurs, arterial pulsatility reduces and LVEDV and wall tension increase. Moreover, blood volume return from bronchial circulation and thebesian vessels directly into the left atrium further dilates the LV. Subsequent left atrial hypertension (left atrial pressure >20 mmHg) can lead to pulmonary oedema and impair gas exchange to the lungs related to a dismal prognosis. This condition mandates prompt institution of some type of LV decompression. The LV can be vented either by mini-thoracotomy and direct cannulation of the left atrium or LV, or percutaneously in the catheterization laboratory creating a small atrial septal defect (atrial septostomy) [108]. A minimally invasive technique has also been suggested using the pulsatile paracorporeal assist device iVAC 3L (PulseCath, Groningen, The Netherlands) through the right axillary artery [109]. In conclusion, ECLS provides effective RV offloading and respiratory support and can be implemented either in the catheterization laboratory or in the operating room as a bridge to recovery (such as post-acute myocardial infarction, pulmonary embolism or myocarditis), bridge to decision or bridge to long-term MCS.

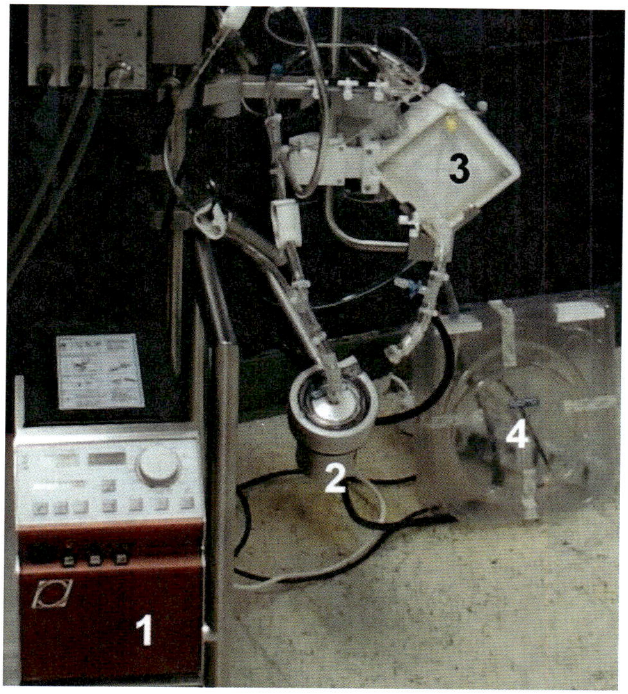

Fig. (9). The Extracorporeal Life Support (ECLS) circuit. Note the simplicity of the system which comprises of a controller (1); centrifugal pump (2); oxygenator (3); heparinized tubing (4).

Surgically Implanted Temporary Blood Pumps

Surgically implanted continuous-flow and pulsatile blood pumps are designed to provide full off-loading (up to 10 l/min) of either or both ventricles (LVAD, RVAD or BiVAD). The main characteristic of these devices is that they require surgical central cannulation of atria, ventricles and great arteries (aorta and main pulmonary artery) in order to bypass and off-load the failing ventricle. In contrast to percutaneously inserted systems that can be used from 6 hours to 14 days, all centrally implanted pumps can be used for periods ranging from weeks to several months. In cases showing no native heart recovery, temporary pumps can be replaced by long-term implanted LVADs (bridge to long-term LVAD).

The CentriMag ventricular assist system (Thoratec Corporation, Pleasanton, CA, USA) employs a magnetically levitated rotor spinning at 500–5,500 rpm to generate up to 10 l/min of blood flow. The device has no mechanical bearings and no contact between the rotor and pump housing, resulting in reduced haemolysis or thrombus formation [110]. Patients are heparinized to achieve an activated clotting time of >200 s. The system is suitable for both left and right heart support (Fig. **10**). The pump can be used effectively for at least 30 days. However, support durations of up to 3 months have been reported in patients awaiting heart transplantation [111, 112].

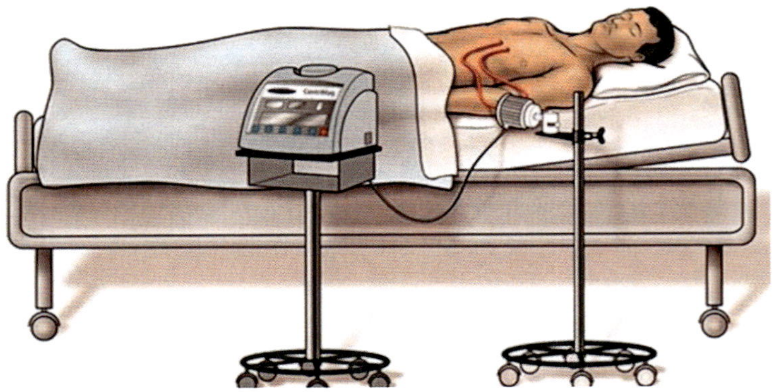

Fig. (10). The CentriMag ventricular assist device extracorporeal system (Courtesy of Thoratec Corporation, http://www.thoratec.com).

CentriMag provides effective ventricular off-loading with a relatively low cost. For these reasons this system gained wide acceptance throughout Europe and the USA. A recent meta-analysis published by Borisenko *et al.* included 53 observational studies of patients supported with CentriMag for temporary treatment of refractory cardiogenic shock. LV support was used in 93 patients, RV support in 198 patients and biventricular support in 179 patients [113]. Thirty-day survival was 66% in non-cardiotomy cardiogenic shock, 41% in post-cardiotomy cardiogenic shock, 54% in post-transplant graft rejection or failure, and 61% in post-LVAD implantation RV failure. In a retrospective review of 29 patients in whom the CentriMag system was used for RV support, Bhama *et al.* reported 48% 30-day mortality [114]. Overall, evidence suggests that immediate introduction of CentriMag support results in recovery of heart function and weaning from device in a significant proportion of patients [115]. By salvaging with CentriMag support, physicians gain time to evaluate the clinical condition dynamics and make informed decisions about referring the patient for heart transplantation or permanent VAD implantation.

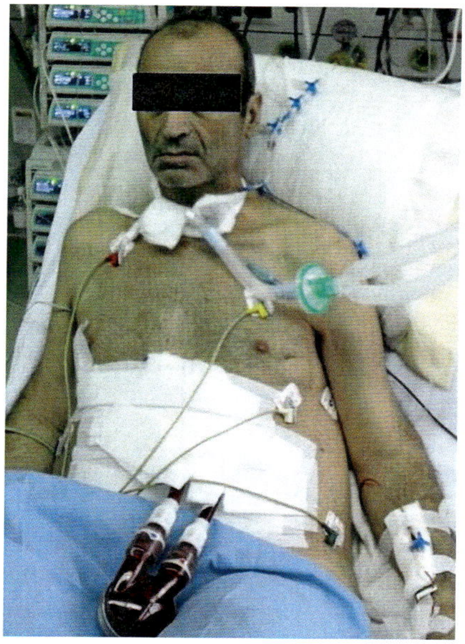

Fig. (11). Patient supported with ABIOMED AB5000 paracorporeal LVAD. Note the two cannulae (inflow and outflow) and the pneumatic pump chamber.
LVAD: left ventricular assist device.

Need for medium-term support in acute HF (one month to one year) mandates the use of portable pneumatic VADs. The AB5000 (Abiomed Inc.) paracorporeal ventricle is driven by a pneumatic console that delivers up to 6 l/min of blood flow and allows for patient ambulation. This system can support LV, RV or both ventricles. Left heart cannulation is achieved through the ventricular apex or the left atrium delivering blood to the ascending aorta (Fig. **11**), while right heart support is performed *via* the right atrium and main pulmonary artery. Other pneumatically-driven pumps with similar indications include Thoratec paracorporeal VAD (Thoratec PVADTM Thoratec Corporation, Pleasanton, CA, USA) and Excor VAD (BerlinHeart, Berlin, Germany). The latter is also indicated for pediatric patients offering pumps of variable volume. They are mainly implanted as medium-term LV or biventricular support (implantable LVAD or BiVAD) and represent an ideal solution for bridging patients to recovery, heart transplantation or implantation of a long-term LVAD for destination therapy.

Decision Making Regarding Temporary Mechanical Circulatory Support

The main characteristics of available systems that provide temporary MCS are summarized in Table **6**. The decision for system selection depends on the aetiology of acute HF, expected duration of support, intention to treat, cost, centre's availability and experience of the team. Taking all these parameters under account, IABP is implanted easily percutaneously and is associated with acceptable cost and low complications rate; although not associated with survival benefit as it could not provide off-loading of the failing LV. ECLS represents an easy-to-assemble off-the-shelf solution to conditions affecting primarily the RV, such as massive pulmonary embolism or acute myocardial infarction of the RV, as well as conditions in which myocardial recovery after days to weeks of support is anticipated, such as in acute fulminant myocarditis. ECLS provides effective unloading of the RV as well as respiratory support with a relatively low cost. Main use of percutaneously implantable pumps includes emergency cases in the catheterization laboratory, as they are easily deployable and provide immediate, though partial, LV support for a few hours.

Table 6. List of devices, used for temporary mechanical circulatory support. The rightward columns represent more invasive devices which offer improved support, though, with higher cost. It is of note that a stepwise strategy can be followed utilizing one or more devices (sequentially bridging one to the other) from left to right, as listed in the Table.

	IABP	**ECLS**	**Impella**	**Tandem Heart**	**CentriMag**	**Para-corporeal VADs**
Support	LV	RV, LV, lungs	LV	LV	RV, LV or BiVAD	RV, LV or BiVAD
max Flow (l/min)	0.5-1	4-6	2.5-3.3 (CP)	4	Up to 10	6
Mechanism	Pneumatic	Centrifugal	Axial flow	Centrifugal	Centrifugal	Pneumatic
Outflow	NR	17-19 Fr	NR	15-17 Fr	24 Fr	32 Fr
Inflow	NR	21-23 Fr	13 Fr	21 Fr	33 Fr	42 Fr
Insertion	PC	PC ±Surgical	PC	PC	Surgical	Surgical

(Table 6) contd.....

	IABP	ECLS	Impella	Tandem Heart	CentriMag	Para-corporeal VADs
Oxygenator	NR	YES	NR	NR	±	
Duration of use	<7 d	<28 d	6 h - 7 d	<14 d	<30 d	<12 m
Estimated cost (€)	1,500	1,500	8,000-15,000	5,000-8,000	3,000-5,000	20,000-30,000
Access complications (%)	0-5	5-10		20-30	5-10	30-35

ECLS: extracorporeal life support; IABP: intra-aortic balloon pump; LV: left ventricle; NR: not required; PC: percutaneous; RV: right ventricle; VAD: ventricular assist device.

Regarding post-cardiotomy acute HF, surgically implantable VADs (extracorporeal or paracorporeal) offer full offloading of both ventricles and have been used extensively with encouraging clinical results and lower rates of bleeding and infectious complications compared to ECLS. Extracorporeal and paracorporeal VADs are equally effective in unloading the LV, though the cost of paracorporeal devices is significantly higher compared to ECLS or extracorporeal VADs, which restricts their use as a first solution in a limited number of high-volume specialized centres. They are mainly used as a second step to recovery after the implantation of a temporary VAD that has supported circulation for a period of 1-4 weeks. Their main advantage is the medium-term duration of support (from one month to one year) and their portability that permits the patient to recover from critical state and mobilize.

Mechanical Circulatory Support in Chronic Heart Failure (HF)

Fully implantable, long-term rotary blood pumps have been used in chronic HF patients, after initial stabilization and reversal of multiorgan failure with a temporary VAD or ECMO. These pumps are designed to be mechanically durable for at least 5 years, with correspondingly low levels of haemolysis or risk of thromboembolism. They consist of a single moving part, the impeller, which provides 5–10 l/min of continuous axial or centrifugal blood flow without pulse pressure. Continuous flow is well tolerated in the long term, and the control and power systems are easily portable (Fig. **12**) [80]. The majority of the patients progressively regain pulse pressure as the native LV contractility improves. Second-generation continuous-flow LVADs are smaller in size, showing improved mechanical reliability and reduced complication rates compared to first-generation pneumatically-driven volume displacement LVADs.

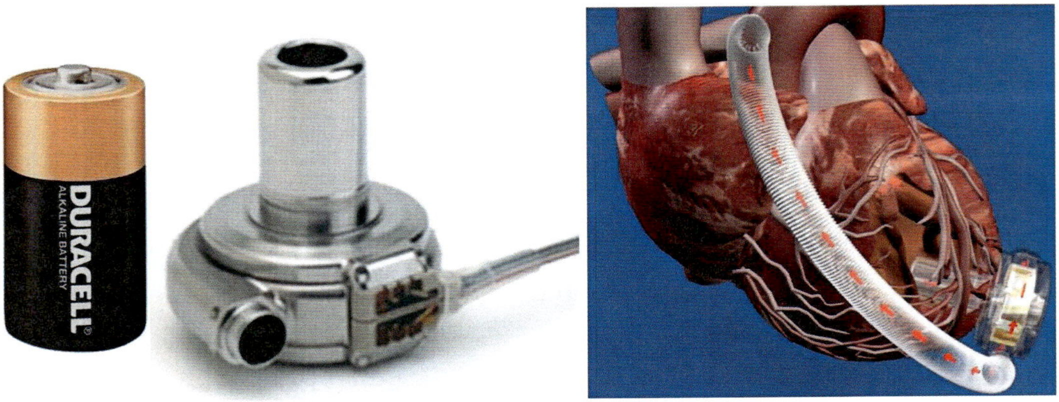

Fig. (12). Continuous flow left ventricular assist device (HeartWare HVAD) having the size of type C battery. The inflow part is inserted into the cavity of the LV. A centrifugal pump directs blood flow to the ascending aorta (Courtesy of HeartWare Inc, http://www.heartware.com).

Up to date, the longest duration of event-free survival (7.5 years) has been reported for a patient with a Jarvik 2000 'Flowmaker' (Jarvik, New York, NY, USA). Post-mortem examination of the device, following noncardiac-related death, showed no evidence of mechanical wear or thrombus formation (Fig. **13**). Other devices, including the HeartMate II, HeartWare (Miami Lakes, FL, USA), Incor (Berlin Heart, Berlin, Germany), and DuraHeart (Terumo Corporation, Shibuya-ku, Japan) LVADs are in widespread use and show excellent mechanical reliability [116 - 118]. Bleeding and thromboembolism are the main complications associated with these devices. Improvement in pump design and anticoagulants administration led to a significant reduction in the incidence of serious complications. Survival exceeding 5 years is now reported for a series of patients worldwide with rotary blood pumps and perhaps justifies their cost.

With the progressive decline in the number of available donor hearts and a gradual improvement in implantable blood-pump technology, the strategies for management of patients with end-stage (stage IV) HF are changing. Life-long implantation of an LVAD represents a more realistic option than transplantation for most patients with end-stage heart failure. A major issue becomes the appropriate management of other cardiac conditions, such as coronary artery or valvular disease, in this setting. Understandable concerns in terms of complicating LVAD implantation in the high-risk patient exist. Uncorrected aortic or tricuspid regurgitation are problematic. Functional tricuspid regurgitation can be dynamic and responsive to medical therapy. Dilatation of the mural annulus is the dominant mechanism. In the failing RV, there is septal shift due to increased diastolic pressure resulting in compression of the LV, which subsequently impairs LVAD filling. The LVAD itself decreases LV volume and may exacerbate tricuspid regurgitation acutely because of leftward shift of the interventricular septum and increased venous return. Liberal indications for tricuspid valve repair at the time of LVAD implantation exist [119]. Concomitant tricuspid annuloplasty during LVAD implantation does not seem to increase mortality, in contrast to concomitant aortic valve replacement or more extensive interventions.

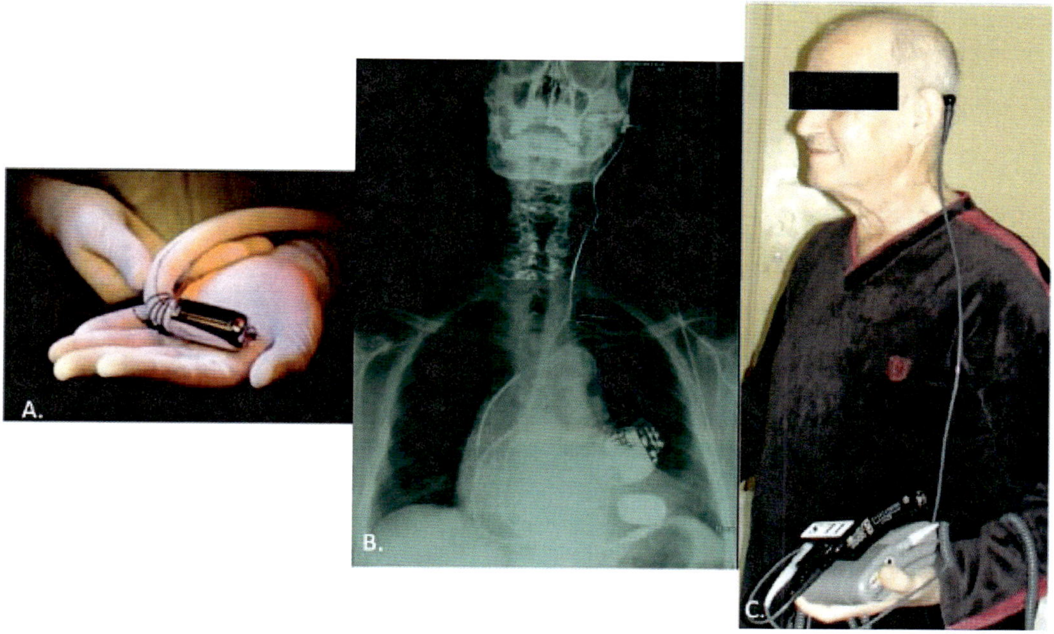

Fig. (13). A. The Jarvik Flowmaker device. **B.** Plain radiograph of a patient suffered from ischaemic cardiomyopathy. After cardiac resynchronization and placement of an implantable defibrillator, the patient was inotrope dependent in the hospital for 3 months. He received a Jarvik FlowMaker device with a skull pedestal power delivery. **C.** Twelve months later he was in New York Heart Association class I with objective evidence of improved myocardial perfusion and contractility.

Total Artificial Heart (TAH)

For decades, replacement of the failing heart with an artificial heart has been the "Holy Grail" for cardiac surgeons. Despite many efforts, the only available TAH in the market is Syncardia TAH (SynCardia, Tucson, Arizona, USA). The AbioCor TAH received FDA approval in 2006 for destination therapy and it was used to a limited number of patients; however, its clinical use has been discontinued. Syncardia TAH delivers pulsatile flow by filling two artificial ventricles lined with polyurethane, which eject blood *via* a four-layer, pneumatically driven, moving diaphragm [120]. Four mechanical valves (Medtronic Hall tilting disc) permit unidirectional flow. The device is connected to patient's circulatory system by cuffs sutured to the atria and vascular grafts sutured to the aorta and pulmonary artery. The maximal stroke volume is 70 ml. The device can deliver a cardiac output of more than 9 l/min (Fig. **14**). A smaller version (50 ml) has been designed, particularly for women and adolescents, and will soon enter into clinical trials.

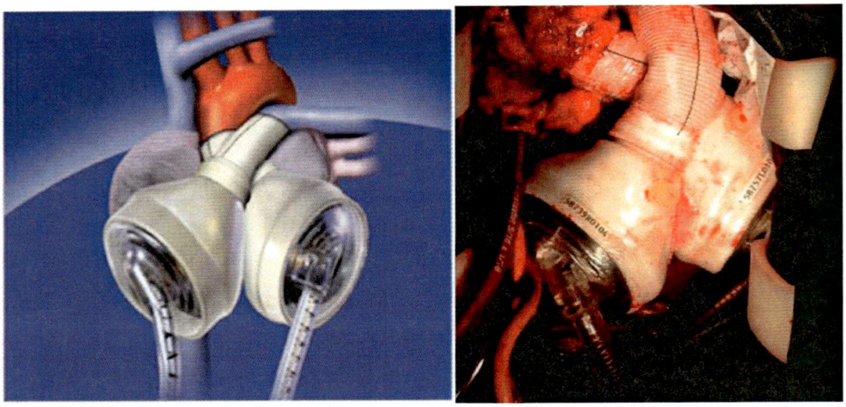

Fig. (14). Syncardia total artificial heart is implanted by removing both ventricles leaving atria cuffs and arterial ends for anastomosis.

There are several limitations including large peripherals, noisy function, high risk of infection due to wide drivelines tunnellized under the skin, as well as risk of thromboembolic events. Syncardia TAH is currently approved as a bridge to transplantation. Results from published clinical trials indicated a bridge to transplant rate 50-80% with a mean support time of 50-110 days [121, 122]. Early in 2015, it received FDA approval for conducting a clinical study of the effectiveness of TAH as destination therapy.

TAH that are under development include ReinHeart from Aahen University, which is in clinical testing in animals and the Carmat TAH (Carmat, Velizy, France) which is in clinical use in humans. The very promising electrically-driven biosynthetic Carmat TAH was first implanted into human in December 2013. The device contains two ventricles, each with a blood compartment and a driving fluid compartment, separated by a flexible hybrid membrane. The hybrid membrane has a polyurethane layer at the fluid-contacting surface and bovine pericardial tissue on the blood-contacting surface [123]. Electro-hydraulic pumps create a systolic and a diastolic phase by moving the silicone fluid and deploying the hybrid membrane. Pressure sensors located in the device detect preload alterations, resulting in automatic adaptation of stroke volume and beat rate. The generated pulsatile blood flow ranges from 2 to 9 l/min with a flow correction on the right side to adjust for the bronchial shunt. Bioprosthetic valves at the inlet and outlet of each blood compartment permit the forward flow. A percutaneous driveline delivers power to the prosthesis and permits exchange of data and inputs. The device is currently undergoing clinical investigation in humans.

HEART TRANSPLANTATION

It has been almost 5 decades since the first human heart transplantation performed in December 1967 in South Africa by Christiaan Barnard [124]. This great achievement was the result of many years of early pioneering experimental work by Alexis Carrel, Frank Mann, Richard Lower and Norman Shumway [125]. Over the next decades, survival in heart transplant recipients significantly improved with refinement of donor and recipient selection methods, better donor heart preservation as well as with the advances in immunosuppression. In the current era, 1-year survival approaches 90%, while 5-year survival reaches up to 70%, with a median overall survival exceeding 10 years (Fig. **15**) [126]. The field of heart transplantation is constantly evolving. With the improving results of cardiac transplantation, more patients with comorbidities are referred for transplantation evaluation, despite reasons for being characterized as non-suitable for transplantation candidates according to previous contraindications.

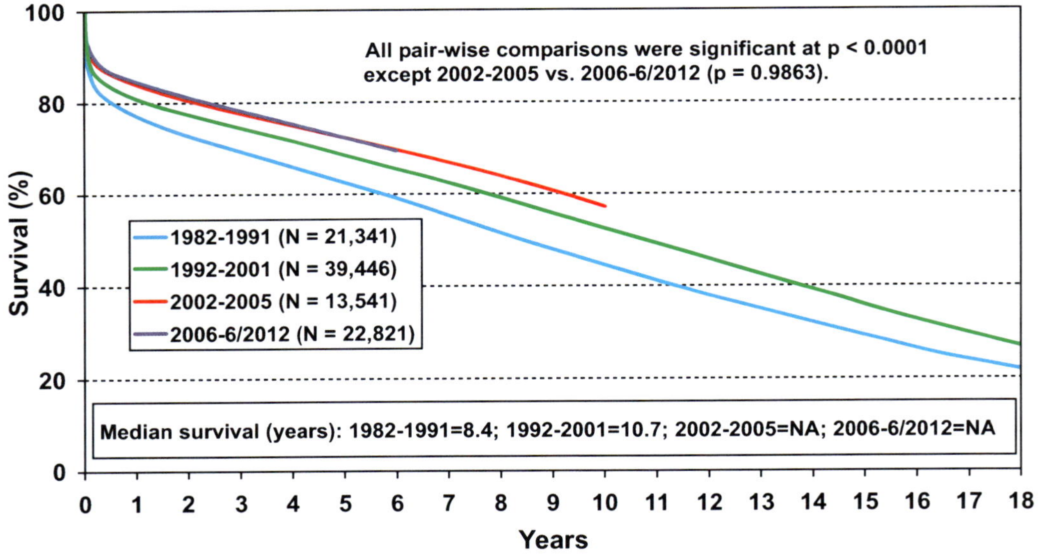

Fig. (15). Long-term survival curve of adult heart transplant recipients by era (Adapted from the 2014 Annual Report of the International Society of Heart and Lung Transplantation Registry, http://www.ishlt.org/registries).

Recipient Selection

The assesment of patients with end-stage HF to become potential candidates for cardiac transplantation is undertaken by a multidisciplinary team in order to ensure an equitable, objective and medically justified allocation of the limited donor organs to patients with the greatest chance of postoperative survival and rehabilitation. Accepted indications for heart transplantation are outlined in Table 7, while recipient selection criteria are outlined in Table **8**. The main objective is to identify those patients with end-stage HF (stage IV) refractory to optimal medical and surgical therapy, in a relatively good condition, who possess the potential to resume a normal active life and comply with a demanding medical regimen after heart transplantation [127].

When a patient with end-stage HF is referred to a transplant center, the initial evaluation requires assessment of the severity of HF, identification of any potentially reversible factors and evaluation of the adequacy of current medical therapy. In a patient with ICM this involves assessment of myocardial viability, whether in patients with valvular heart disease, the degree of severity of valvular disease needs to be evaluated, so as determine whether there are percutaneous or surgical options. Arrhythmias should be addressed and treated. Toxic agents such as persistent alcohol intake, illicit drug use, or salt-retaining drugs (such as non-steroidal agents), should be discontinued. Medical therapy should be optimized with upregulation of vasodilators, diuretics, and use of biventricular pacing as indicated. In most patients, a few months of optimal medical therapy is administered to assess therapeutic response. If no reversible causes are identified and therapy is thought to be at an optimal level with the presence of NYHA class IIIB/IV symptoms, then the transplant evaluation process begins. However, if on referral the patient is in cardiogenic shock or on parenteral inotropic agents and cannot be tapered because of hypotension, end-organ dysfunction, or symptoms, then the options for this patient are limited to urgent cardiac transplantation, mechanical device support or palliative care. Screening for transplantation involves an extensive evaluation to exclude significant comorbidities that can increase either the short-term perioperative risk or long-term survival [128].

Table 7. Indications for heart transplantation.

• Cardiogenic shock requiring continuous intravenous inotropic support or mechanical circulatory support with an IABP or VAD
• Persistent NYHA class IV congestive HF symptoms refractory to optimal medical therapy (LVEF <20%, peak VO_2 <12 ml/kg/min)
• Intractable or severe angina symptoms in patients with coronary artery disease not amenable to percutaneous or surgical revascularization
• Intractable life-threatening arrhythmias unresponsive to medical therapy, catheter ablation and/or ICD

IABP: intra-aortic balloon pump; ICD: implantable cardioverter defibrillator; LVEF: left ventricular ejection fraction; NYHA: New York Heart Association; VAD: ventricular assist device.

Table 8. Recipient selection for heart transplantation.

I. Systolic heart failure (ejection fraction < 35%)	**II. Ischaemic heart disease with intractable angina**
• Ischaemic	• Ineffective maximal medical therapy
• Dilated	• Not a candidate for myocardial revascularization
• Valvular	• Unsuccessful myocardial revascularization
• Hypertensive	
• Other	
• Excluded (amyloid, HIV infection, cardiac sarcoma)	

(Table 8) contd.....

III. Intractable arrhythmia • Uncontrolled with ICD • Not amenable to electrophysiology-guided or optimal medical therapy • Not a candidate for ablative therapy	**IV. Hypertrophic cardiomyopathy** • NYHA Class IV symptoms despite interventinal and medical therapies
V. Congenital heart disease without severe fixed pulmonary hypertension	**VI. Cardiac tumor** • No evidence of distant metastases

ICD: implantable cardioverter defibrillator; NYHA: New York Heart Association.

Contraindications to transplantation continue to evolve, with centers expanding criteria for acceptance. The traditional contraindications to transplantation are listed in Table **9**.

Table 9. Contraindications to heart transplantation.

Absolute contraindications	Relative contraindications
1. Systemic illness with a life expectancy <2 years 2. Fixed pulmonary hypertension - Pulmonary vascular resistence >5-6 Wood units - Pulmonary artery systolic pressure >60 mmHg - Transpulmonary gradient >15 mmHg 3. Significantly irreversible renal dysfunction (*e.g.* creatinine clearance <50 ml/min) 4. Significantly irreversible hepatic dysfunction (*e.g.* bilirubin > 3 mg/dl) 5. Active malignancy 6. Active infection	1. Age >65 years 2. Severe peripheral vascular or cerebrovascular disease 3. Active peptic ulcer disease 4. Diabetes mellitus with end-organ damage 5. Morbid obesity or cachexia 6. Chronic obstructive pulmonary disease 7. Active alcohol or drug abuse 8. Active mental illness or psychosocial instability 9. Noncompliance with medical care

The face of heart transplantation is continuously changing. Apart from older patients with acquired heart disease considered for heart transplantation, a significant proportion of younger patients being referred for evaluation have complex congenital heart disease, despite repair or palliation [129]. Congenital heart disease is identified as one of the strongest risk factors for one-year mortality after heart transplantation in adults according to the International Society for Heart and Lung Transplantation (ISHLT) database [130]. Moreover, there is also a steady rise in the number of patients on MCS that are being referred for heart transplantation as well as in the number of re-transplant candidates [126]. This changing patient population brings new challenges to the transplant centres [124]. The proportion of sensitized patients (having preformed antibodies directed against the donor heart) is crucial for preventing rejection and allograft vasculopathy [131]. Recipient age > 65 years, traditionally considered as absolute contraindication to transplantation, is now regarded as a relative contraindication. Older recipients show reduced risk of rejection, while the incidence of infection and allograft vasculopathy is increased [132].

During the last two decades, expansion in the clinical use of MCS has permited many severely ill adult and pediatric patients to survive until a suitable donor heart became available. Patients on MCS are at increased risk for rejection, infection, stroke and bleeding [124]. The mechanical devices and the history of blood transfusions are potential triggers of immunologic response [130]. The increasing number of patients transplanted at early ages, explains the increase in the rate of re-transplantation [126]. The likelihood of re-transplantation increases with the time passed after the surgical procedure, with the largest portion occurring 10 or more years after the primary transplant. Re-transplantation is more common in the group aged 18 to 39 years (5% *vs* 1-3% of all diagnoses in older age groups). Cardiac allograft vasculopathy and myopathy are the most common indications for re-transplantation. Primary graft failure and rejection make up approximately 25% of re-transplant indications in Europe and North America. Primary graft failure is the dominant cause for re-transplantation during the first month after the primary transplant, whereas allograft vasculopathy is the main indication at one year and thereafter. Overall survival rates after re-transplantation are significantly lower, probably due to the consequence of years of immunosuppression and allosensitization [133].

Donor Selection

The selection of donors for cardiac transplantation follows the guidelines outlined in Table **10**. A primary screen is performed by specialists from organ procurement organizations and information is collected regarding clinical course, cause of death, body size, ABO blood type, and serologies (including human immunodeficiency virus, hepatitis B virus, and hepatitis C virus). A secondary screen is then performed by a transplant physician, including review of relevant history, baseline electrocardiogram, chest radiograph, laboratory data, and echocardiogram. The final screen is performed by the procuring surgeon, who directly inspects the organ. Potential donors should meet requirements for brain death. Donors with a history of cardiac disease, including prior myocardial infarction and intractable ventricular arrhythmias, should be excluded [134]. Donor age of less than 55 years is preferable, although occasionally older donors are considered.

Table 10. Donor selection for heart transplantation.

Standard criteria	Extended donor criteria
1. Age < 55 years 2. No history of chest trauma or cardiac disease 3. No history of prolonged severe hypotension 4. Meets haemodynamic criteria 5. Mean arterial pressure >60 mm Hg 6. Central venous pressure 8-12 mm Hg 7. Inotropic support <10 μg/kg/min (dopamine or dobutamine) 8. Normal electrocardiogram 9. Normal echocardiogram 10. Negative hepatitis B and C antigens, HIV	1. Donor age >55 years 2. Cocaine use 3. Alcohol abuse 4. Significant inotrope requirement 5. Electrocardiography abnormalities (left ventricular hypertrophy, regional wall abnormality) 6. Long-standing diabetes mellitus 7. Prolonged ischaemic time (>4 h) 8. Malignant brain tumors 9. Single-vessel coronary artery disease 10. Undersized organ (mismatch >30%) in patients with pulmonary hypertension

Given the donor shortage and the increasing number of patients with end-stage HF that are potential candidates for heart transplantation, interest has focused on the use of marginal donors for marginal recipients. Expanded donor criteria include the use of donors substantially smaller than the recipients, donors with CAD that may require CABG, LV dysfunction or donors from older age groups [135, 136]. Limited information is available regarding the long-term durability of organs derived from this expanded pool, and there is some evidence that certain donor factors, such as older age and prolonged ischaemic time, may contribute to increased recipient mortality risk [137].

Current Trends in Immunosuppression

Prevention or management of allograft rejection through immunosuppression is very important. However, various immunosuppression – related health problems, such as drug toxicity, infections and malignancies, should be also addressed. Most immunosuppressive regimens include a combination of several agents used concurrently. Immunosuppressive regimens are classified as induction, maintenance or anti-rejection. Induction regimens provide intense early postoperative immune suppression while maintenance regimens are used throughout the patient's life to prevent both acute and chronic rejection. Three general principles should be followed regarding patients undergoing induction and maintenance immunosuppressive therapy regimens:

a. Considering that immune reactivity leading to graft rejection is more pronounced within the first three to six months after graft implantation, the highest intensity of immunosuppression is administered immediately after surgery and decreases gradually over the first year, eventually settling on the lowest maintenance levels of immunosuppression that offers prevention of graft rejection with minimal drug toxicity.
b. Use of a low-dose regime including multiple drugs with non-overlapping toxicities is preferable over higher (and more toxic) doses of fewer drugs.
c. Avoidance of over-immunosuppression, as it is associated to undesirable effects including susceptibility to infection and malignancy.

Induction therapy refers to the use of more intense immunosuppression in the initial days after transplantation, when the risk of allograft rejection is the highest. Agents administered for induction may be divided into 2 categories: a) depleting antibodies [*e.g.*, polyclonal antibodies (horse or rabbit antithymocyte globulin), anti-CD3 antibodies (OKT3), human monoclonal anti-CD52 (alentuzumab)] and b) non-depleting antibodies or fusion proteins [*e.g.* anti-CD25 antibodies (daclizumab, basiliximab) or fusion proteins with natural binding properties currently being studied, *e.g.* CTLA4-Ig (LEA29Y)] [124]. From a clinical perspective, induction therapy permits delayed initiation of nephrotoxic immunosuppressive drugs in patients with compromised renal function following surgery, while it allows some flexibility with respect to early glucocorticoid weaning or use of glucocorticoid-sparing baseline regimens after transplantation [137,138]. The overall utility of induction is uncertain and data comparing induction protocols are limited. Induction therapy decreases the possibility of early rejection; however, this beneficial effect may be negated by an increase in late rejection (after the completion of induction therapy), infection and malignancy [139]. Currently, evidence supports use of induction agents on a selective basis in highly sensitized patients or patients with severe renal failure at the time of transplantation.

The goal of maintenance immunosuppression is to achieve host-graft adaptation, while maintaining the risk of infection or cancer to the lowest possible level. The majority of cardiac transplant protocols include a triple maintenance therapy consisting of corticosteroids (usually prednisone), a calcineurin inhibitor (cyclosporine or tacrolimus) and an antiproliferative agent (usually mycophenolate mofetil). Prednisone is initiated early after heart transplantation and is usually tapered to low doses or withdrawn during the first year. Early withdrawal is performed within the first month after transplantation, while late withdrawal occurs between 6 to 12 months post-transplant. Late steroid withdrawal permits more intensive therapy in the first 6 months when the risk of rejection is still high [140]. International trends in the use of maintenance immunosuppressive agents at one year post-transplantation include a steady increase in tacrolimus, which is currently the most widely prescribed calcineurin inhibitor (89% of patients) in heart transplantation. Mycophenolate mofetil and mycophenolate sodium remain the predominant antimetabolite agents (91% of patients. Recently, rapamycin inhibitors or proliferation signal inhibitors (sirolimus and everolimus) have been associated with decreased progression of allograft vasculopathy and cancer as well as with resistance to rejection [141]. With respect to drug combinations, use of tacrolimus and mycophenolate mofetil with or without steroids was most common during the first year post-transplantation, followed by cyclosporine and mycophenolate mofetil with or without steroids [124]. In the future, individualization of immunosuppressive medication together with improved laboratory immune monitoring as well as the introduction of pharmacogenomics, will eventually play a greater role in optimization of therapy [142].

Is a lifetime Left Ventricular Assist Device (LVAD) a Realistic Alternative to Transplantation?

With expansion of the evidence base, patterns of care are emerging. Transplantation is the "restricted commodity" and is predominantly directed toward young patients with acute or chronic heart failure to prolong life. In contrast, the implantable rotary pumps are increasingly deployed electively for refractory symptoms in non-transplant eligible patients, those unlikely to receive a donor heart and the elderly [143]. Suggestions regarding the optimum candidate for transplant *versus* mechanical support are outlined in Table **11**. The differences indicate that the two approaches are complementary rather than competitive. Artificial differentiation between "bridge to transplant" or "destination therapy" groups is no longer useful in a sense that patients are switched from one strategy to the other depending on evolving patient preference and centers' experience. Even the so-called "fixed" pulmonary vascular resistance ($\geq$ 7.5 Wood units) has been shown to be reversible after LVAD support, allowing patients initially rejected for transplantation to receive a donor heart at a later time [144].

Table 11. Ideal candidates from a prognostic and economic standpoint [143].

Heart transplantation	Rotary LVAD
• Age <50 years • UNOS status I • No metabolic risk factors • No hepatic or renal dysfunction • Low pulmonary vascular resistance	• Age <70 years • UNOS status II • No right heart failure • No hepatic dysfunction • Not on renal replacement therapy • No contraindication to anticoagulation • Supportive family or equivalent

LVAD: left ventricular assist device; UNOS: United Network for Organ Sharing.

CONCLUDING REMARKS

We have reached the era when long-term LVAD therapy should be offered to literally all transplant candidates who face a prolonged waiting period for a donor heart (risking interim death) or be offered a marginal organ. Further refinements of the LVAD approach using adjuvant medical therapy or direct stem cell injection to improve myocardial contractility may eventually provide equivalence between transplant and LVAD [145, 146]. Lifetime circulatory support has the potential to supersede transplantation by a factor of 20:1 [143]. Many patients who are submitted for palliative care alone could gain symptomatic relief and several extra years of life with an appropriate blood pump. So far, this message has not reached the primary care physician. Given the potential demand as transplantation declines in some countries, lifetime LVAD therapy could reasonably be performed in tertiary centers that specialize in non-transplant heart failure surgery [126]. Devices are improving rapidly and can be made available in sufficient numbers to address heart failure epidemiology. Severe HF will then sit firmly in the surgical domain.

CONFLICT OF INTEREST

The authors confirm that they have no conflict of interest to declare for this publication.

ACKNOWLEDGEMENTS

Declared none.

REFERENCES

[1] Allender S, Scarborough P, Peto V, *et al.* European cardiovascular disease statistics. Available from: https://www.bhf.org.uk 2008.

[2] Nichols M, Townsend N, Scarborough P, Rayner M. Cardiovascular disease in Europe: epidemiological update. Eur Heart J 2013; 34(39): 3028-34. [http://dx.doi.org/10.1093/eurheartj/eht356] [PMID: 24014390]

[3] Tsuyuki RT, Shrive FM, Galbraith PD, Knudtson ML, Graham MM. Revascularization in patients with heart failure. CMAJ 2006; 175(4): 361-5. [http://dx.doi.org/10.1503/cmaj.060108] [PMID: 16908896]

[4] Gheorghiade M, Filippatos G. Reassessing treatment of acute heart failure syndromes: the ADHERE Registry. Eur Heart J Suppl 2005; 7 (Suppl. B): B13-9. [http://dx.doi.org/10.1093/eurheartj/sui008]

[5] Gheorghiade M, Bonow RO. Chronic heart failure in the United States: a manifestation of coronary artery disease. Circulation 1998; 97(3): 282-9. [http://dx.doi.org/10.1161/01.CIR.97.3.282] [PMID: 9462531]

[6] Guha K, McDonagh T. Heart failure epidemiology: European perspective. Curr Cardiol Rev 2013; 9(2): 123-7. [http://dx.doi.org/10.2174/1573403X11309020005] [PMID: 23597298]

[7] Zile MR, Brutsaert DL. New concepts in diastolic dysfunction and diastolic heart failure: Part I: diagnosis, prognosis, and measurements of diastolic function. Circulation 2002; 105(11): 1387-93. [http://dx.doi.org/10.1161/hc1102.105289] [PMID: 11901053]

[8] Morrow DA, Gersh BJ. Chronic Coronary Artery Disease. In: Libby P, Bonow RO, Mann DL, Zipes DP, Eds. Braunwald's Heart Disease. Philadelphia: Saunders Elsevier Editions 2007; pp. 1353-404.

[9] Gheorghiade M, Sopko G, De Luca L, *et al.* Navigating the crossroads of coronary artery disease and heart failure. Circulation 2006; 114(11): 1202-13. [http://dx.doi.org/10.1161/CIRCULATIONAHA.106.623199] [PMID: 16966596]

[10] Canty JM Jr. Coronary blood flow and myocardial ischemia. In: Libby P, Bonow RO, Mann DL, Zipes DP, Eds. Braunwald's Heart Disease. Philadelphia: Saunders Elsevier Editions 2007; pp. 1184-90.

[11] Phillips HR, O'Connor CM, Rogers J. Revascularization for heart failure. Am Heart J 2007; 153(4) (Suppl.): 65-73. [http://dx.doi.org/10.1016/j.ahj.2007.01.026] [PMID: 17394905]

[12] Shanmugam G, Légaré JF. Revascularization for ischaemic cardiomyopathy. Curr Opin Cardiol 2008; 23(2): 148-52.
[http://dx.doi.org/10.1097/HCO.0b013e3282f43011] [PMID: 18303528]

[13] Bax JJ, van der Wall EE, Harbinson M. Radionuclide techniques for the assessment of myocardial viability and hibernation. Heart 2004; 90 (Suppl. 5): v26-33.
[http://dx.doi.org/10.1136/hrt.2002.007575] [PMID: 15254006]

[14] Laude K, Thuillez C, Richard V. Coronary endothelial dysfunction after ischemia and reperfusion: a new therapeutic target? Braz J Med Biol Res 2001; 34(1): 1-7.
[http://dx.doi.org/10.1590/S0100-879X2001000100001] [PMID: 11151023]

[15] Kinlay S, Behrendt D, Wainstein M, *et al.* Role of endothelin-1 in the active constriction of human atherosclerotic coronary arteries. Circulation 2001; 104(10): 1114-8.
[http://dx.doi.org/10.1161/hc3501.095707] [PMID: 11535565]

[16] Piérard LA, Carabello BA. Ischaemic mitral regurgitation: pathophysiology, outcomes and the conundrum of treatment. Eur Heart J 2010; 31(24): 2996-3005.
[http://dx.doi.org/10.1093/eurheartj/ehq411] [PMID: 21123277]

[17] Mahrholdt H, Klem I, Sechtem U. Cardiovascular MRI for detection of myocardial viability and ischaemia. Heart 2007; 93(1): 122-9.
[http://dx.doi.org/10.1136/hrt.2005.071290] [PMID: 17170353]

[18] Ling LF, Marwick TH, Flores DR, *et al.* Identification of therapeutic benefit from revascularization in patients with left ventricular systolic dysfunction: inducible ischemia *versus* hibernating myocardium. Circ Cardiovasc Imaging 2013; 6(3): 363-72.
[http://dx.doi.org/10.1161/CIRCIMAGING.112.000138] [PMID: 23595888]

[19] Beller GA, Ragosta M. Extent of myocardial viability in regions of left ventricular dysfunction by rest-redistribution thallium-201 imaging: a powerful predictor of outcome. J Nucl Cardiol 1998; 5(4): 445-8.
[http://dx.doi.org/10.1016/S1071-3581(98)90152-0] [PMID: 9715991]

[20] Bhatia M. Evaluation of ischemic heart disease and viability by cardiac MRI. Indian Heart J 2014; 66(1): 143-4.
[http://dx.doi.org/10.1016/j.ihj.2013.10.006] [PMID: 24581114]

[21] McMurray JJ, Adamopoulos S, Anker SD, *et al.* ESC Guidelines for the diagnosis and treatment of acute and chronic heart failure 2012. Eur Heart J 2012; 33(14): 1787-847.
[http://dx.doi.org/10.1093/eurheartj/ehs104] [PMID: 22611136]

[22] Bonow RO, Maurer G, Lee KL, *et al.* Myocardial viability and survival in ischemic left ventricular dysfunction. N Engl J Med 2011; 364(17): 1617-25.
[http://dx.doi.org/10.1056/NEJMoa1100358] [PMID: 21463153]

[23] Chareonthaitawee P, Gersh BJ, Araoz PA, Gibbons RJ. Revascularization in severe left ventricular dysfunction: the role of viability testing. J Am Coll Cardiol 2005; 46(4): 567-74.
[http://dx.doi.org/10.1016/j.jacc.2005.03.072] [PMID: 16098417]

[24] Di Sciascio G, Patti G, D'Ambrosio A, Nusca A. Coronary stenting in patients with depressed left ventricular function: acute and long-term results in a selected population. Catheter Cardiovasc Interv

2003; 59(4): 429-33.
[http://dx.doi.org/10.1002/ccd.10533] [PMID: 12891600]

[25] Vlaar PJ, de Smet BJ. Impact of heart failure on outcome after percutaneous coronary intervention: is it the patient or the intervention? Eur J Heart Fail 2011; 13(4): 364-5.
[http://dx.doi.org/10.1093/eurjhf/hfr027] [PMID: 21436362]

[26] Steg PG, Dabbous OH, Feldman LJ, *et al.* Determinants and prognostic impact of heart failure complicating acute coronary syndromes: observations from the Global Registry of Acute Coronary Events (GRACE). Circulation 2004; 109(4): 494-9.
[http://dx.doi.org/10.1161/01.CIR.0000109691.16944.DA] [PMID: 14744970]

[27] Stenestrand U, Wallentin L. Early revascularisation and 1-year survival in 14-day survivors of acute myocardial infarction: a prospective cohort study. Lancet 2002; 359(9320): 1805-11.
[http://dx.doi.org/10.1016/S0140-6736(02)08710-X] [PMID: 12044375]

[28] Hochman JS, Sleeper LA, Webb JG, *et al.* Early revascularization and long-term survival in cardiogenic shock complicating acute myocardial infarction. JAMA 2006; 295(21): 2511-5.
[http://dx.doi.org/10.1001/jama.295.21.2511] [PMID: 16757723]

[29] Carluccio E, Biagioli P, Alunni G, *et al.* Effect of revascularizing viable myocardium on left ventricular diastolic function in patients with ischaemic cardiomyopathy. Eur Heart J 2009; 30(12): 1501-9.
[http://dx.doi.org/10.1093/eurheartj/ehp125] [PMID: 19389790]

[30] Brener SJ, Lytle BW, Casserly IP, Schneider JP, Topol EJ, Lauer MS. Propensity analysis of long-term survival after surgical or percutaneous revascularization in patients with multivessel coronary artery disease and high-risk features. Circulation 2004; 109(19): 2290-5.
[http://dx.doi.org/10.1161/01.CIR.0000126826.58526.14] [PMID: 15117846]

[31] Comparison of coronary bypass surgery with angioplasty in patients with multivessel disease. N Engl J Med 1996; 335(4): 217-25.
[http://dx.doi.org/10.1056/NEJM199607253350401] [PMID: 8657237]

[32] Berger PB, Velianou JL, Aslanidou Vlachos H, *et al.* Survival following coronary angioplasty *versus* coronary artery bypass surgery in anatomic subsets in which coronary artery bypass surgery improves survival compared with medical therapy. Results from the Bypass Angioplasty Revascularization Investigation (BARI). J Am Coll Cardiol 2001; 38(5): 1440-9.
[http://dx.doi.org/10.1016/S0735-1097(01)01571-6] [PMID: 11691521]

[33] Kappetein AP, van Mieghem NM, Head SJ. Revascularization Options: Coronary Artery Bypass Surgery and Percutaneous Coronary Intervention. Heart Fail Clin 2016; 12(1): 135-9.
[http://dx.doi.org/10.1016/j.hfc.2015.08.011] [PMID: 26567980]

[34] Gioia G, Matthai W, Gillin K, *et al.* Revascularization in severe left ventricular dysfunction: outcome comparison of drug-eluting stent implantation *versus* coronary artery by-pass grafting. Catheter Cardiovasc Interv 2007; 70(1): 26-33.
[http://dx.doi.org/10.1002/ccd.21072] [PMID: 17585381]

[35] Windecker S, Kolh P, Alfonso F, *et al.* 2014 ESC/EACTS Guidelines on myocardial revascularization. Eur Heart J 2014; 35(37): 2541-619.
[http://dx.doi.org/10.1093/eurheartj/ehu278] [PMID: 25173339]

[36] Levine GN, Bates ER, Blankenship JC, *et al.* 2011 ACCF/AHA/SCAI Guideline for Percutaneous Coronary Intervention: a report of the American College of Cardiology Foundation/American Heart Association Task Force on Practice Guidelines and the Society for Cardiovascular Angiography and Interventions. Circulation 2011; 124(23): e574-651. [http://dx.doi.org/10.1161/CIR.0b013e31823ba622] [PMID: 22064601]

[37] Yancy CW, Jessup M, Bozkurt B, *et al.* 2013 ACCF/AHA guideline for the management of heart failure: a report of the American College of Cardiology Foundation/American Heart Association Task Force on practice guidelines. Circulation 2013; 128(16): e240-327. [http://dx.doi.org/10.1161/CIR.0b013e31829e8807] [PMID: 23741058]

[38] Abraham WT, Hayes DL. Cardiac resynchronization therapy for heart failure. Circulation 2003; 108(21): 2596-603. [http://dx.doi.org/10.1161/01.CIR.0000096580.26969.9A] [PMID: 14638522]

[39] Brignole M, Auricchio A, Baron-Esquivias G, *et al.* 2013 ESC Guidelines on cardiac pacing and cardiac resynchronization therapy: the Task Force on cardiac pacing and resynchronization therapy of the European Society of Cardiology (ESC). Developed in collaboration with the European Heart Rhythm Association (EHRA). Eur Heart J 2013; 34(29): 2281-329. [http://dx.doi.org/10.1093/eurheartj/eht150] [PMID: 23801822]

[40] Baldasseroni S, Opasich C, Gorini M, *et al.* Left bundle-branch block is associated with increased 1-year sudden and total mortality rate in 5517 outpatients with congestive heart failure: a report from the Italian network on congestive heart failure. Am Heart J 2002; 143(3): 398-405. [http://dx.doi.org/10.1067/mhj.2002.121264] [PMID: 11868043]

[41] Zareba W, Klein H, Cygankiewicz I, *et al.* Effectiveness of Cardiac Resynchronization Therapy by QRS Morphology in the Multicenter Automatic Defibrillator Implantation Trial-Cardiac Resynchronization Therapy (MADIT-CRT). Circulation 2011; 123(10): 1061-72. [http://dx.doi.org/10.1161/CIRCULATIONAHA.110.960898] [PMID: 21357819]

[42] Grines CL, Bashore TM, Boudoulas H, Olson S, Shafer P, Wooley CF. Functional abnormalities in isolated left bundle branch block. The effect of interventricular asynchrony. Circulation 1989; 79(4): 845-53. [http://dx.doi.org/10.1161/01.CIR.79.4.845] [PMID: 2924415]

[43] Owen JS, Khatib S, Morin DP. Cardiac resynchronization therapy. Ochsner J 2009; 9(4): 248-56. [PMID: 21603451]

[44] Hayes DL, Zipes DP. Cardiac Pacemakers and Cardioverter-Defibrillators. In: Libby P, Bonow RO, Mann DL, Zipes DP, Eds. Braunwald's Heart Disease. Philadelphia: Saunders Elsevier Editions 2007; pp. 847-51.

[45] Mann DL. Management of Heart Failure Patients with Reduced Ejection Fraction. In: Libby P, Bonow RO, Mann DL, Zipes DP, Eds. Braunwald's Heart Disease. Philadelphia: Saunders Elsevier Editions 2007; p. 636.

[46] McMurray JJ. Clinical practice. Systolic heart failure. N Engl J Med 2010; 362(3): 228-38. [http://dx.doi.org/10.1056/NEJMcp0909392] [PMID: 20089973]

[47] McAlister FA, Ezekowitz J, Hooton N, *et al.* Cardiac resynchronization therapy for patients with left

ventricular systolic dysfunction: a systematic review. JAMA 2007; 297(22): 2502-14. [http://dx.doi.org/10.1001/jama.297.22.2502] [PMID: 17565085]

[48] António N, Teixeira R, Coelho L, *et al.* Identification of 'super-responders' to cardiac resynchronization therapy: the importance of symptom duration and left ventricular geometry. Europace 2009; 11(3): 343-9. [http://dx.doi.org/10.1093/europace/eup038] [PMID: 19240109]

[49] Goldenberg I, Kutyifa V, Klein HU, *et al.* Survival with cardiac-resynchronization therapy in mild heart failure. N Engl J Med 2014; 370(18): 1694-701. [http://dx.doi.org/10.1056/NEJMoa1401426] [PMID: 24678999]

[50] Kaszala K, Ellenbogen KA. When right may not be right: right bundle-branch block and response to cardiac resynchronization therapy. Circulation 2010; 122(20): 1999-2001. [http://dx.doi.org/10.1161/CIRCULATIONAHA.110.986943] [PMID: 21041687]

[51] Ruschitzka F, Abraham WT, Singh JP, *et al.* Cardiac-resynchronization therapy in heart failure with a narrow QRS complex. N Engl J Med 2013; 369(15): 1395-405. [http://dx.doi.org/10.1056/NEJMoa1306687] [PMID: 23998714]

[52] Steinberg JS. Desperately seeking a randomized clinical trial of resynchronization therapy for patients with heart failure and atrial fibrillation. J Am Coll Cardiol 2006; 48(4): 744-6. [http://dx.doi.org/10.1016/j.jacc.2006.05.031] [PMID: 16904543]

[53] Wilton SB, Leung AA, Ghali WA, Faris P, Exner DV. Outcomes of cardiac resynchronization therapy in patients with *versus* those without atrial fibrillation: a systematic review and meta-analysis. Heart Rhythm 2011; 8(7): 1088-94. [http://dx.doi.org/10.1016/j.hrthm.2011.02.014] [PMID: 21338711]

[54] Linde C, Leclercq C, Rex S, *et al.* Long-term benefits of biventricular pacing in congestive heart failure: results from the MUltisite STimulation in cardiomyopathy (MUSTIC) study. J Am Coll Cardiol 2002; 40(1): 111-8. [http://dx.doi.org/10.1016/S0735-1097(02)01932-0] [PMID: 12103264]

[55] Gasparini M, Auricchio A, Regoli F, *et al.* Four-year efficacy of cardiac resynchronization therapy on exercise tolerance and disease progression: the importance of performing atrioventricular junction ablation in patients with atrial fibrillation. J Am Coll Cardiol 2006; 48(4): 734-43. [http://dx.doi.org/10.1016/j.jacc.2006.03.056] [PMID: 16904542]

[56] Ganesan AN, Brooks AG, Roberts-Thomson KC, Lau DH, Kalman JM, Sanders P. Role of AV nodal ablation in cardiac resynchronization in patients with coexistent atrial fibrillation and heart failure a systematic review. J Am Coll Cardiol 2012; 59(8): 719-26. [http://dx.doi.org/10.1016/j.jacc.2011.10.891] [PMID: 22340263]

[57] Tracy CM, Epstein AE, Darbar D, *et al.* 2012 ACCF/AHA/HRS focused update of the 2008 guidelines for device-based therapy of cardiac rhythm abnormalities: a report of the American College of Cardiology Foundation/American Heart Association Task Force on Practice Guidelines. J Am Coll Cardiol 2012; 60(14): 1297-313. [http://dx.doi.org/10.1016/j.jacc.2012.07.009] [PMID: 22975230]

[58] Thompson KA, Philip KJ, Barbagelata A, Schwarz ER. Review article: the new concept of interventional heart failure therapy-part 1: electrical therapy, treatment of CAD, fluid removal, and

ventricular support. J Cardiovasc Pharmacol Ther 2010; 15(2): 102-11.
[http://dx.doi.org/10.1177/1074248410366447] [PMID: 20435990]

[59] Bernard ML, Gold MR. Economic implications and cost-effectiveness of implantable cardioverter defibrillator and cardiac resynchronization therapy. Heart Fail Clin 2011; 7(2): 241-250, ix.
[http://dx.doi.org/10.1016/j.hfc.2010.12.007] [PMID: 21439502]

[60] Glikson M, Friedman PA. The implantable cardioverter defibrillator. Lancet 2001; 357(9262): 1107-17.
[http://dx.doi.org/10.1016/S0140-6736(00)04263-X] [PMID: 11297981]

[61] Epstein AE, DiMarco JP, Ellenbogen KA, *et al.* ACC/AHA/HRS 2008 Guidelines for Device-Based Therapy of Cardiac Rhythm Abnormalities: a report of the American College of Cardiology/American Heart Association Task Force on Practice Guidelines (Writing Committee to Revise the ACC/AHA/NASPE 2002 Guideline Update for Implantation of Cardiac Pacemakers and Antiarrhythmia Devices): developed in collaboration with the American Association for Thoracic Surgery and Society of Thoracic Surgeons. Circulation 2008; 117(21): e350-408.
[http://dx.doi.org/10.1161/CIRCUALTIONAHA.108.189742] [PMID: 18483207]

[62] Bardy GH, Lee KL, Mark DB, *et al.* Amiodarone or an implantable cardioverter-defibrillator for congestive heart failure. N Engl J Med 2005; 352(3): 225-37.
[http://dx.doi.org/10.1056/NEJMoa043399] [PMID: 15659722]

[63] A comparison of antiarrhythmic-drug therapy with implantable defibrillators in patients resuscitated from near-fatal ventricular arrhythmias. N Engl J Med 1997; 337(22): 1576-83.
[http://dx.doi.org/10.1056/NEJM199711273372202] [PMID: 9411221]

[64] Moss AJ, Zareba W, Hall WJ, *et al.* Prophylactic implantation of a defibrillator in patients with myocardial infarction and reduced ejection fraction. N Engl J Med 2002; 346(12): 877-83.
[http://dx.doi.org/10.1056/NEJMoa013474] [PMID: 11907286]

[65] Westaby S. Non-transplant surgery for heart failure. Heart 2000; 83(5): 603-10.
[http://dx.doi.org/10.1136/heart.83.5.603] [PMID: 10768919]

[66] Velazquez EJ, Lee KL, Jones RH. Coronary-artery bypass surgery in patients with ischemic cardiomyopathy. N Engl J Med 2016; 374: 1511-20.
[http://dx.doi.org/10.1161/01.CIR.90.6.2645] [PMID: 7994804]

[67] Castelvecchio S, Menicanti L, Donato MD. Surgical ventricular restoration to reverse left ventricular remodeling. Curr Cardiol Rev 2010; 6(1): 15-23.
[http://dx.doi.org/10.2174/157340310790231626] [PMID: 21286274]

[68] Jones RH, Velazquez EJ, Michler RE, *et al.* Coronary bypass surgery with or without surgical ventricular reconstruction. N Engl J Med 2009; 360(17): 1705-17.
[http://dx.doi.org/10.1056/NEJMoa0900559] [PMID: 19329820]

[69] White HD, Norris RM, Brown MA, Brandt PW, Whitlock RM, Wild CJ. Left ventricular end-systolic volume as the major determinant of survival after recovery from myocardial infarction. Circulation 1987; 76(1): 44-51.
[http://dx.doi.org/10.1161/01.CIR.76.1.44] [PMID: 3594774]

[70] Migrino RQ, Young JB, Ellis SG, *et al.* End-systolic volume index at 90 to 180 minutes into

reperfusion therapy for acute myocardial infarction is a strong predictor of early and late mortality. The Global Utilization of Streptokinase and t-PA for Occluded Coronary Arteries (GUSTO)-I Angiographic Investigators. Circulation 1997; 96(1): 116-21.
[http://dx.doi.org/10.1161/01.CIR.96.1.116] [PMID: 9236425]

[71] Di Donato M, Castelvecchio S, Menicanti L. End-systolic volume following surgical ventricular reconstruction impacts survival in patients with ischaemic dilated cardiomyopathy. Eur J Heart Fail 2010; 12(4): 375-81.
[http://dx.doi.org/10.1093/eurjhf/hfq020] [PMID: 20185429]

[72] Witkowski TG, ten Brinke EA, Delgado V, *et al.* Surgical ventricular restoration for patients with ischemic heart failure: determinants of two-year survival. Ann Thorac Surg 2011; 91(2): 491-8.
[http://dx.doi.org/10.1016/j.athoracsur.2010.09.074] [PMID: 21256300]

[73] Michler RE, Rouleau JL, Al-Khalidi HR, *et al.* Insights from the STICH trial: change in left ventricular size after coronary artery bypass grafting with and without surgical ventricular reconstruction. J Thorac Cardiovasc Surg 2013; 146(5): 1139-1145.e6.
[http://dx.doi.org/10.1016/j.jtcvs.2012.09.007] [PMID: 23111018]

[74] Kolh P, Windecker S, Alfonso F, *et al.* 2014 ESC/EACTS Guidelines on myocardial revascularization: the Task Force on Myocardial Revascularization of the European Society of Cardiology (ESC) and the European Association for Cardio-Thoracic Surgery (EACTS). Developed with the special contribution of the European Association of Percutaneous Cardiovascular Interventions (EAPCI). Eur J Cardiothorac Surg 2014; 46(4): 517-92.
[http://dx.doi.org/10.1093/ejcts/ezu366] [PMID: 25173601]

[75] David TE. Techniques and results of mitral valve repair for ischemic mitral regurgitation. J Card Surg 1994; 9(2) (Suppl.): 274-7.
[http://dx.doi.org/10.1111/j.1540-8191.1994.tb00940.x] [PMID: 8186580]

[76] Bach DS, Bolling SF. Early improvement in congestive heart failure after correction of secondary mitral regurgitation in end-stage cardiomyopathy. Am Heart J 1995; 129(6): 1165-70.
[http://dx.doi.org/10.1016/0002-8703(95)90399-2] [PMID: 7754949]

[77] Chan KM, Punjabi PP, Flather M, *et al.* Coronary artery bypass surgery with or without mitral valve annuloplasty in moderate functional ischemic mitral regurgitation: final results of the Randomized Ischemic Mitral Evaluation (RIME) trial. Circulation 2012; 126(21): 2502-10.
[http://dx.doi.org/10.1161/CIRCULATIONAHA.112.143818] [PMID: 23136163]

[78] Smith PK, Puskas JD, Ascheim DD, *et al.* Surgical treatment of moderate ischemic mitral regurgitation. N Engl J Med 2014; 371(23): 2178-88.
[http://dx.doi.org/10.1056/NEJMoa1410490] [PMID: 25405390]

[79] Acker MA, Parides MK, Perrault LP, *et al.* Mitral-valve repair versus replacement for severe ischemic mitral regurgitation. N Engl J Med 2014; 370(1): 23-32.
[http://dx.doi.org/10.1056/NEJMoa1312808] [PMID: 24245543]

[80] Westaby S, Anastasiadis K, Wieselthaler GM. Cardiogenic shock in ACS. Part 2: Role of mechanical circulatory support. Nat Rev Cardiol 2012; 9(4): 195-208.
[http://dx.doi.org/10.1038/nrcardio.2011.205] [PMID: 22231716]

[81] Rose EA, Gelijns AC, Moskowitz AJ, *et al.* Long-term use of a left ventricular assist device for end-

stage heart failure. N Engl J Med 2001; 345(20): 1435-43.
[http://dx.doi.org/10.1056/NEJMoa012175] [PMID: 11794191]

[82] Arzamendi D, Garcia-Alvarez A, Roig E, *et al.* New insights in the management of cardiogenic shock complicating myocardial infarction: role of urgent heart transplantation. J Heart Lung Transplant 2008; 27(9): 984-9.
[http://dx.doi.org/10.1016/j.healun.2008.06.011] [PMID: 18765190]

[83] Reynolds HR, Hochman JS. Cardiogenic shock: current concepts and improving outcomes. Circulation 2008; 117(5): 686-97.
[http://dx.doi.org/10.1161/CIRCULATIONAHA.106.613596] [PMID: 18250279]

[84] Kolyva C, Pantalos GM, Pepper JR, Khir AW. How much of the intraaortic balloon volume is displaced toward the coronary circulation? J Thorac Cardiovasc Surg 2010; 140(1): 110-6.
[http://dx.doi.org/10.1016/j.jtcvs.2009.10.015] [PMID: 20080266]

[85] Scheidt S, Wilner G, Mueller H, *et al.* Intra-aortic balloon counterpulsation in cardiogenic shock. Report of a co-operative clinical trial. N Engl J Med 1973; 288(19): 979-84.
[http://dx.doi.org/10.1056/NEJM197305102881901] [PMID: 4696253]

[86] Malliaras K, Charitos E, Diakos N, *et al.* Effects of intra-aortic balloon pump counterpulsation on left ventricular mechanoenergetics in a porcine model of acute ischemic heart failure. J Cardiovasc Transl Res 2014; 7(9): 810-20.
[http://dx.doi.org/10.1007/s12265-014-9600-6] [PMID: 25376149]

[87] Ryan TJ, Antman EM, Brooks NH, *et al.* 1999 update: ACC/AHA guidelines for the management of patients with acute myocardial infarction. A report of the American College of Cardiology/American Heart Association Task Force on Practice Guidelines (Committee on Management of Acute Myocardial Infarction). J Am Coll Cardiol 1999; 34(3): 890-911.
[http://dx.doi.org/10.1016/S0735-1097(99)00351-4] [PMID: 10483976]

[88] Nordhaug D, Steensrud T, Muller S, Husnes KV, Myrmel T. Intraaortic balloon pumping improves hemodynamics and right ventricular efficiency in acute ischemic right ventricular failure. Ann Thorac Surg 2004; 78(4): 1426-32.
[http://dx.doi.org/10.1016/j.athoracsur.2003.12.077] [PMID: 15464508]

[89] Westaby S, Balacumaraswami L, Sayeed R. Maximizing survival potential in very high risk cardiac surgery. Heart Fail Clin 2007; 3(2): 159-80.
[http://dx.doi.org/10.1016/j.hfc.2007.05.001] [PMID: 17643920]

[90] Christenson JT, Cohen M, Ferguson JJ III, *et al.* Trends in intraaortic balloon counterpulsation complications and outcomes in cardiac surgery. Ann Thorac Surg 2002; 74(4): 1086-90.
[http://dx.doi.org/10.1016/S0003-4975(02)03854-7] [PMID: 12400750]

[91] Hochman JS, Buller CE, Sleeper LA, *et al.* Cardiogenic shock complicating acute myocardial infarction-etiologies, management and outcome: a report from the SHOCK Trial Registry. SHould we emergently revascularize Occluded Coronaries for cardiogenic shocK? J Am Coll Cardiol 2000; 36(3) (Suppl. A): 1063-70.
[http://dx.doi.org/10.1016/S0735-1097(00)00879-2] [PMID: 10985706]

[92] Barron HV, Every NR, Parsons LS, *et al.* The use of intra-aortic balloon counterpulsation in patients with cardiogenic shock complicating acute myocardial infarction: data from the National Registry of

Myocardial Infarction 2. Am Heart J 2001; 141(6): 933-9.
[http://dx.doi.org/10.1067/mhj.2001.115295] [PMID: 11376306]

[93] Thiele H, Zeymer U, Neumann FJ, *et al.* Intra-aortic balloon counterpulsation in acute myocardial infarction complicated by cardiogenic shock (IABP-SHOCK II): final 12 month results of a randomised, open-label trial. Lancet 2013; 382(9905): 1638-45.
[http://dx.doi.org/10.1016/S0140-6736(13)61783-3] [PMID: 24011548]

[94] Henriques JP, de Mol BA. New percutaneous mechanical left ventricular support for acute MI: the AMC MACH program. Nat Clin Pract Cardiovasc Med 2008; 5(2): 62-3.
[http://dx.doi.org/10.1038/ncpcardio1060] [PMID: 18043597]

[95] Thiele H, Sick P, Boudriot E, *et al.* Randomized comparison of intra-aortic balloon support with a percutaneous left ventricular assist device in patients with revascularized acute myocardial infarction complicated by cardiogenic shock. Eur Heart J 2005; 26(13): 1276-83.
[http://dx.doi.org/10.1093/eurheartj/ehi161] [PMID: 15734771]

[96] Meyns B, Stolinski J, Leunens V, Verbeken E, Flameng W. Left ventricular support by catheter-mounted axial flow pump reduces infarct size. J Am Coll Cardiol 2003; 41(7): 1087-95.
[http://dx.doi.org/10.1016/S0735-1097(03)00084-6] [PMID: 12679206]

[97] Sjauw KD, Remmelink M, Baan J Jr, *et al.* Left ventricular unloading in acute ST-segment elevation myocardial infarction patients is safe and feasible and provides acute and sustained left ventricular recovery. J Am Coll Cardiol 2008; 51(10): 1044-6.
[http://dx.doi.org/10.1016/j.jacc.2007.10.050] [PMID: 18325447]

[98] Sjauw KD, Konorza T, Erbel R, *et al.* Supported high-risk percutaneous coronary intervention with the Impella 2.5 device the Europella registry. J Am Coll Cardiol 2009; 54(25): 2430-4.
[http://dx.doi.org/10.1016/j.jacc.2009.09.018] [PMID: 20082934]

[99] Burkhoff D, Cohen H, Brunckhorst C, O'Neill WW. A randomized multicenter clinical study to evaluate the safety and efficacy of the TandemHeart percutaneous ventricular assist device *versus* conventional therapy with intraaortic balloon pumping for treatment of cardiogenic shock. Am Heart J 2006; 152(3): 469.e1-8.
[http://dx.doi.org/10.1016/j.ahj.2006.05.031] [PMID: 16923414]

[100] Cheng JM, den Uil CA, Hoeks SE, *et al.* Percutaneous left ventricular assist devices *vs.* intra-aortic balloon pump counterpulsation for treatment of cardiogenic shock: a meta-analysis of controlled trials. Eur Heart J 2009; 30(17): 2102-8.
[http://dx.doi.org/10.1093/eurheartj/ehp292] [PMID: 19617601]

[101] Vranckx P, Meliga E, De Jaegere PP, Van den Ent M, Regar ES, Serruys PW. The TandemHeart, percutaneous transseptal left ventricular assist device: a safeguard in high-risk percutaneous coronary interventions. The six-year Rotterdam experience. EuroIntervention 2008; 4(3): 331-7.
[http://dx.doi.org/10.4244/EIJV4I3A60] [PMID: 19110806]

[102] Mahmoudi M, Syed AI, Waksman R. The role of percutaneous circulatory assist devices in acute myocardial infarction and high-risk percutaneous coronary intervention in the 21st century. Cardiovasc Revasc Med 2011; 12(4): 237-42.
[http://dx.doi.org/10.1016/j.carrev.2010.10.003] [PMID: 21130711]

[103] Sheu JJ, Tsai TH, Lee FY, *et al.* Early extracorporeal membrane oxygenator-assisted primary

percutaneous coronary intervention improved 30-day clinical outcomes in patients with ST-segment elevation myocardial infarction complicated with profound cardiogenic shock. Crit Care Med 2010; 38(9): 1810-7.
[http://dx.doi.org/10.1097/CCM.0b013e3181e8acf7] [PMID: 20543669]

[104] Fujimoto K, Kawahito K, Yamaguchi A, *et al.* Percutaneous extracorporeal life support for treatment of fatal mechanical complications associated with acute myocardial infarction. Artif Organs 2001; 25(12): 1000-3.
[http://dx.doi.org/10.1046/j.1525-1594.2001.06792.x] [PMID: 11843768]

[105] Yamauchi T, Masai T, Takeda K, Kainuma S, Sawa Y. Percutaneous cardiopulmonary support after acute myocardial infarction at the left main trunk. Ann Thorac Cardiovasc Surg 2009; 15(2): 93-7. [PMID: 19471222]

[106] Duncan BW, Hraska V, Jonas RA, *et al.* Mechanical circulatory support in children with cardiac disease. J Thorac Cardiovasc Surg 1999; 117(3): 529-42.
[http://dx.doi.org/10.1016/S0022-5223(99)70333-8] [PMID: 10047657]

[107] Thiagarajan RR, Yarlagadda V, Bratton SL. Cardiac failure: Principles and physiology. In: Annich G, Lynch W, MacLaren G, Wilson J, Bartlett R, Eds. ECMO Extracorporeal cardiopulmonary support in critical care. 4th ed. Extracorporeal Life Support Organization 2012; pp. 33-9.

[108] Avalli L, Maggioni E, Sangalli F, Favini G, Formica F, Fumagalli R. Percutaneous left-heart decompression during extracorporeal membrane oxygenation: an alternative to surgical and transeptal venting in adult patients. ASAIO J 2011; 57(1): 38-40.
[http://dx.doi.org/10.1097/MAT.0b013e3181fe5d0b] [PMID: 21048495]

[109] Anastasiadis K, Chalvatzoulis O, Antonitsis P, Tossios P, Papakonstantinou C. Left ventricular decompression during peripheral extracorporeal membrane oxygenation support with the use of the novel iVAC pulsatile paracorporeal assist device. Ann Thorac Surg 2011; 92(6): 2257-9.
[http://dx.doi.org/10.1016/j.athoracsur.2011.05.063] [PMID: 22115242]

[110] John R, Liao K, Lietz K, *et al.* Experience with the Levitronix CentriMag circulatory support system as a bridge to decision in patients with refractory acute cardiogenic shock and multisystem organ failure. J Thorac Cardiovasc Surg 2007; 134(2): 351-8.
[http://dx.doi.org/10.1016/j.jtcvs.2007.01.085] [PMID: 17662772]

[111] Slaughter MS, Tsui SS, El-Banayosy A, *et al.* Results of a multicenter clinical trial with the Thoratec Implantable Ventricular Assist Device. J Thorac Cardiovasc Surg 2007; 133(6): 1573-80.
[http://dx.doi.org/10.1016/j.jtcvs.2006.11.050] [PMID: 17532959]

[112] Kaczorowski DJ, Datta J, Kamoun M, Dries DL, Woo YJ. Profound hyperacute cardiac allograft rejection rescue with biventricular mechanical circulatory support and plasmapheresis, intravenous immunoglobulin, and rituximab therapy. J Cardiothorac Surg 2013; 8: 48.
[http://dx.doi.org/10.1186/1749-8090-8-48] [PMID: 23497431]

[113] Borisenko O, Wylie G, Payne J, *et al.* Thoratec CentriMag for temporary treatment of refractory cardiogenic shock or severe cardiopulmonary insufficiency: a systematic literature review and meta-analysis of observational studies. ASAIO J 2014; 60(5): 487-97.
[http://dx.doi.org/10.1097/MAT.0000000000000117] [PMID: 25010916]

[114] Bhama JK, Kormos RL, Toyoda Y, *et al.* Clinical experience using the Levitronix CentriMag system

for temporary right ventricular for temporary right ventricular mechanical circulatory support. J Heart Lung Transplant 2009; 28: 971-6.
[http://dx.doi.org/10.1016/j.healun.2009.04.015] [PMID: 19716053]

[115] Shuhaiber JH, Jenkins D, Berman M, *et al.* The Papworth experience with the Levitronix CentriMag ventricular assist device. J Heart Lung Transplant 2008; 27(2): 158-64.
[http://dx.doi.org/10.1016/j.healun.2007.10.015] [PMID: 18267221]

[116] Slaughter MS, Rogers JG, Milano CA, *et al.* Advanced heart failure treated with continuous-flow left ventricular assist device. N Engl J Med 2009; 361(23): 2241-51.
[http://dx.doi.org/10.1056/NEJMoa0909938] [PMID: 19920051]

[117] Strueber M, O'Driscoll G, Jansz P, Khaghani A, Levy WC, Wieselthaler GM. Multicenter evaluation of an intrapericardial left ventricular assist system. J Am Coll Cardiol 2011; 57(12): 1375-82.
[http://dx.doi.org/10.1016/j.jacc.2010.10.040] [PMID: 21414534]

[118] Morshuis M, El-Banayosy A, Arusoglu L, *et al.* European experience of DuraHeart magnetically levitated centrifugal left ventricular assist system. Eur J Cardiothorac Surg 2009; 35(6): 1020-7.
[http://dx.doi.org/10.1016/j.ejcts.2008.12.033] [PMID: 19233673]

[119] Westaby S. Tricuspid regurgitation in left ventricular assist device patients. Eur J Cardiothorac Surg 2012; 41(1): 217-8.
[http://dx.doi.org/10.1016/j.ejcts.2011.06.019] [PMID: 21820908]

[120] Morris RJ. Total artificial heart-concepts and clinical use. Semin Thorac Cardiovasc Surg 2008; 20(3): 247-54.
[http://dx.doi.org/10.1053/j.semtcvs.2008.08.006] [PMID: 19038735]

[121] Gerosa G, Scuri S, Iop L, Torregrossa G. Present and future perspectives on total artificial hearts. Ann Cardiothorac Surg 2014; 3(6): 595-602.
[PMID: 25512901]

[122] Copeland JG, Smith RG, Arabia FA, *et al.* Cardiac replacement with a total artificial heart as a bridge to transplantation. N Engl J Med 2004; 351(9): 859-67.
[http://dx.doi.org/10.1056/NEJMoa040186] [PMID: 15329423]

[123] Mohacsi P, Leprince P. The CARMAT total artificial heart. Eur J Cardiothorac Surg 2014; 46(6): 933-4.
[http://dx.doi.org/10.1093/ejcts/ezu333] [PMID: 25228743]

[124] Hunt SA. Taking heart-cardiac transplantation past, present, and future. N Engl J Med 2006; 355(3): 231-5.
[http://dx.doi.org/10.1056/NEJMp068048] [PMID: 16855261]

[125] Ventura HO, Muhammed K. Historical perspectives on cardiac transplantation: the past as prologue to challenges for the 21st century. Curr Opin Cardiol 2001; 16(2): 118-23.
[http://dx.doi.org/10.1097/00001573-200103000-00007] [PMID: 11224643]

[126] Lund LH, Edwards LB, Kucheryavaya AY, *et al.* The registry of the International Society for Heart and Lung Transplantation: thirty-first official adult heart transplant report-2014; focus theme: retransplantation. J Heart Lung Transplant 2014; 33(10): 996-1008.
[http://dx.doi.org/10.1016/j.healun.2014.08.003] [PMID: 25242124]

[127] Nwakanma LU. Shah AS, Conte JV, Baumgartner WA. Heart transplantation. In: Cohn LH, Ed. Cardiac Surgery in the Adult. New York: McGraw-Hill 2008; pp. 1539-77.

[128] Mancini D, Lietz K. Selection of cardiac transplantation candidates in 2010. Circulation 2010; 122(2): 173-83.
[http://dx.doi.org/10.1161/CIRCULATIONAHA.109.858076] [PMID: 20625142]

[129] Taylor DO, Edwards LB, Boucek MM, *et al.* Registry of the International Society for Heart and Lung Transplantation: twenty-fourth official adult heart transplant report-2007. J Heart Lung Transplant 2007; 26(8): 769-81.
[http://dx.doi.org/10.1016/j.healun.2007.06.004] [PMID: 17692781]

[130] Kerman RH. Understanding the sensitized patient. Heart Fail Clin 2007; 3(1): 1-9.
[http://dx.doi.org/10.1016/j.hfc.2007.03.003] [PMID: 17545004]

[131] Aliabadi AZ, Zuckermann AO, Grimm M. Immunosuppressive therapy in older cardiac transplant patients. Drugs Aging 2007; 24(11): 913-32.
[http://dx.doi.org/10.2165/00002512-200724110-00004] [PMID: 17953459]

[132] Hosseinpour AR, Cullen S, Tsang VT. Transplantation for adults with congenital heart disease. Eur J Cardiothorac Surg 2006; 30(3): 508-14.
[http://dx.doi.org/10.1016/j.ejcts.2006.06.007] [PMID: 16857376]

[133] Johnson MR, Aaronson KD, Canter CE, *et al.* Heart retransplantation. Am J Transplant 2007; 7(9): 2075-81.
[http://dx.doi.org/10.1111/j.1600-6143.2007.01902.x] [PMID: 17640316]

[134] Harringer W, Haverich A. Heart and heart-lung transplantation: standards and improvements. World J Surg 2002; 26(2): 218-25.
[http://dx.doi.org/10.1007/s00268-001-0209-y] [PMID: 11865352]

[135] Laks H, Marelli D, Fonarow GC, *et al.* Use of two recipient lists for adults requiring heart transplantation. J Thorac Cardiovasc Surg 2003; 125(1): 49-59.
[http://dx.doi.org/10.1067/mtc.2003.62] [PMID: 12538985]

[136] Chen JM, Russo MJ, Hammond KM, *et al.* Alternate waiting list strategies for heart transplantation maximize donor organ utilization. Ann Thorac Surg 2005; 80(1): 224-8.
[http://dx.doi.org/10.1016/j.athoracsur.2005.01.022] [PMID: 15975371]

[137] Del Rizzo DF, Menkis AH, Pflugfelder PW, *et al.* The role of donor age and ischemic time on survival following orthotopic heart transplantation. J Heart Lung Transplant 1999; 18(4): 310-9.
[http://dx.doi.org/10.1016/S1053-2498(98)00059-X] [PMID: 10226895]

[138] Rosenberg PB, Vriesendorp AE, Drazner MH, *et al.* Induction therapy with basiliximab allows delayed initiation of cyclosporine and preserves renal function after cardiac transplantation. J Heart Lung Transplant 2005; 24(9): 1327-31.
[http://dx.doi.org/10.1016/j.healun.2004.08.003] [PMID: 16143252]

[139] Yamani MH, Taylor DO, Czerr J, *et al.* Thymoglobulin induction and steroid avoidance in cardiac transplantation: results of a prospective, randomized, controlled study. Clin Transplant 2008; 22(1): 76-81.
[PMID: 18251036]

[140] Beniaminovitz A, Itescu S, Lietz K, *et al.* Prevention of rejection in cardiac transplantation by blockade of the interleukin-2 receptor with a monoclonal antibody. N Engl J Med 2000; 342(9): 613-9. [http://dx.doi.org/10.1056/NEJM200003023420902] [PMID: 10699160]

[141] Miller LW, Wolford T, McBride LR, Peigh P, Pennington DG. Successful withdrawal of corticosteroids in heart transplantation. J Heart Lung Transplant 1992; 11(2 Pt 2): 431-4. [PMID: 1571342]

[142] Eisen HJ. Immunosuppression on the horizon. Heart Fail Clin 2007; 3(1): 43-9. [http://dx.doi.org/10.1016/j.hfc.2007.03.002] [PMID: 17545008]

[143] Macphee IA, Fredericks S, Tai T, *et al.* Tacrolimus pharmacogenetics: polymorphisms associated with expression of cytochrome p4503A5 and P-glycoprotein correlate with dose requirement. Transplantation 2002; 74(11): 1486-9. [http://dx.doi.org/10.1097/00007890-200212150-00002] [PMID: 12490779]

[144] Westaby S. Cardiac transplant or rotary blood pump: contemporary evidence. J Thorac Cardiovasc Surg 2013; 145(1): 24-31. [http://dx.doi.org/10.1016/j.jtcvs.2012.08.048] [PMID: 23244251]

[145] Mikus E, Stepanenko A, Krabatsch T, *et al.* Reversibility of fixed pulmonary hypertension in left ventricular assist device support recipients. Eur J Cardiothorac Surg 2011; 40(4): 971-7. [PMID: 21354812]

[146] Anastasiadis K, Antonitsis P, Doumas A, *et al.* Stem cells transplantation combined with long-term mechanical circulatory support enhances myocardial viability in end-stage ischemic cardiomyopathy. Int J Cardiol 2012; 155(3): e51-3. [http://dx.doi.org/10.1016/j.ijcard.2011.07.062] [PMID: 21852003]

CHAPTER 10

Novel Therapies for Heart Failure: The Gene and Cell Methods

Eleni Papanikolaou and **Nicholas P. Anagnou***

Laboratory of Cell and Gene Therapy, Biomedical Research Foundation of the Academy of Athens, Athens, Greece

Laboratory of Biology, National & Kapodistrian University of Athens, Medical School, Athens, Greece

Abstract: Heart disease still remains one of the leading causes of mortality in the developed world. Therefore, finding the right cure for cardiovascular disease remains a current umnet medical need. However, the recent advances in understanding the molecular basis of myocardial dysfunction, the characterization of novel properties of cardiac progenitors, the identification of the plasticity of several subpopulations of cardiac cells and the development of more efficient gene transfer technologies, has made heart failure another excellent candidate for cell and gene-based therapies.

Keywords: Acute myocardial infarction, β-adrenergic system, Calcium cycling proteins, Cardiac stem cells, Gene therapy, Heart failure, Hematopoietic stem cells, Insertional mutagenesis, Lentiviral vector, Retroviral integration.

INTRODUCTION

By definition, gene therapy is a strategy aiming to manipulate an individual's abnormal genes expression or to correct mutated genes by employing administration of a specific DNA or RNA sequence. These therapeutic sequences, termed transgenes, are delivered to the patient's cells enclosed inside specific vectors. In most types of viral vectors, the transgene is integrated into the host

* **Corresponding author Nicholas P Anagnou:** Laboratory of Cell and Gene Therapy, Biomedical Research Foundation of the Academy of Athens, Athens, Greece; Tel: +30 210 746 2356; Fax: +30 210 746 2412; E-mail: anagnou@med.uoa.gr

Panagiotis Georgoulias (Ed.)

genome and is expected to be expressed throughout the entire life of the patient, thus leading to the successful treatment of the given disease [1]. It should be emphasized, however, that gene transfer in general, is not applicable to diseases with complex phenotypes linked to networks of affected genes. Thus, excluding cancer, gene therapy is mostly suited to treat monogenic disorders, such as certain hereditary diseases caused by specific mutations and is especially applicable for treatment of certain blood diseases such as hemoglobinopathies or immunodeficiencies [2].

The definition of cell therapy though, differs in the sense that cell therapy refers to the administration of modified over unmodified cell populations to the patient, or the induction of maturation of a specific cell population [1].

Therefore, while in cell therapy the aim is to restore or regenerate the damaged tissue, in gene therapy the aim is to correct the damaged cells through genetic manipulations. These two notions are complementary, *i.e.* it is conceivable to characterize gene therapy as cell therapy of genetically corrected cells.

Although in the original concept gene therapy was specifically designed for treatment of monogenic diseases, the latest advances towards the understanding of the molecular basis of myocardial dysfunction, the characterization of novel properties of cardiac progenitors, the identification of the plasticity of several subpopulations of cardiac cells and the development of more efficient gene transfer strategies, has made heart failure another excellent candidate for cell and gene-based therapies.

GENE THERAPY

Gene therapy is considered successful when there is adequate correction of the phenotype of the disease. This implies that the therapeutic vector has to be efficient in terms of a) gene delivery, b) tissue specificity, c) stability and d) safety. Furthermore, the selection of the appropriate cell type for correction is of critical importance, and depends on the type of organ(s) and/or tissues in which the abnormal phenotype is manifested.

As a general principle, the cells under manipulation are the stem cells since they are the only cell type that confers life-long correction. However, when the disease phenotype affects a solid organ, then the challenging issue is to target each individual population of stem cells within the specified organ. Therefore, there are three main types of gene therapy/gene delivery approaches:

a. *In situ* gene therapy, which employs direct administration of the vector carrying the therapeutic genetic material to the affected tissue, such as by an injection into an organ or a tumor nodule [1]. This type of therapy is suitable for gene transfer to the heart.
b. *Ex vivo* gene therapy, which employs isolation of stem cells from the affected individual, correction of these cells at the laboratory by co-cultivation with the therapeutic vector and infusion of the corrected cell material back to the patient from whom they were originally derived [1]. In this sense, this type of gene therapy can be considered as autologous transplantation of genetically corrected cells and assumes that the cells can be easily removed from the patients. Ex-vivo gene therapy applies for diseases of the blood such as hemoglobinopathies and immunodeficiencies.
c. *In vivo* gene therapy which employs direct administration of the therapeutic vector to a live animal. The vector can be administered either by an intravenous injection or by other physical means such as hypodermic injection, aerosol, or employing other routes [1].

Gene Therapy Vectors

The most important part in a gene therapy setting is the construction of the appropriate vehicles to deliver the therapeutic gene to the patient or to the selected cell population. Specifically for the heart, the strategy must be designed considering both the tissue-specific and spatial patterns of the cardiovascular pathophysiological process and taking into account whether the aim is to treat heart failure which is a broader process *versus* a focal damage such as nodal dysfunction. Since the cardiac stem cells cannot be removed in order to be processed, it is mandatory that the optimal vector format must first demonstrate broad transduction efficiency to the majority of cardiomyocytes to ensure significant impact on ventricular function and second be able to effectively deliver and drive sustained transgene expression to guarantee long term therapy. For safety reasons, the designed vector should also pose the least possible cytotoxic effects.

Generally, vector delivery systems can be divided in two large categories: those that derive from genetically modified viruses and those deriving from non-viral formulations such as those manufactured by the use of nanotechnology [3]. Non-viral vectors include: a) naked plasmid DNA, b) oligonucleotides, c) liposomes and d) DNA polymer-carrying particles [4]. Recombinant viruses employed as vectors in cardiac gene therapy are:

a. Retroviruses: From the family of Retroviridae only two subfamilies are used, the subfamily of *Oncoretroviridae* (*e.g.* Murine Leukemia Virus- related) and *Lentiviridae* (*e.g.* Human Immunodeficience Virus- related). Oncoretroviruses are also called gamma retroviruses.
b. Adeno-Associated viruses.
c. Adenoviruses.

Basically, since each virus presents different tropism, it is anticipated that each individual vector delivery system will exhibit unique specificity and a separate molecular expression pattern. Therefore, it is critical to choose or design the appropriate delivery system to ensure the therapy's success, to properly implement the therapeutic strategy and to drive efficient expression of the therapeutic genes in the myocardium.

Specifically for gene therapy of the heart, the vectors can be delivered to the myocardium by the following ways: a) Coronary artery and venous infusion, b) direct intramyocardial injection and c) pericardial delivery [4]. Since for cardiovascular diseases, the *in situ* gene therapy scheme is employed and the patients are under general anaesthesia, it is absolutely critical to assess both the invasiveness of vector delivery method and the patient's safety prior to initiating gene therapy trials.

Retroviruses

Retroviruses constitute probably the largest viral family employed as efficient tools for stem cell gene therapy, because of their unique ability to integrate their genome into the host cell's genome. This is accomplished through reverse transcription, during which the viral single-stranded (ss) RNA is converted to double-stranded (ds) DNA. Once reverse transcription is finalized, integration of the retroviral DNA into the host cell genome occurs and thus the viral genomes become permanently fixed as proviruses into the DNA of the host.

Among retroviruses two specific families are mostly employed in clinical gene therapy: The oncoretroviruses (also called gamma-retroviruses) and the lentiviruses. A basic difference between these two families is their ability to integrate depending, or not, on the disassociation of the nuclear envelope. More specifically, for oncoretroviruses, integration fails to occur in quiescent cells and can only occur in cycling cells, because during mitosis the nuclear membrane disassembles, rendering the chromosomes accessible to the virus. This fact suggests that successful infection by oncoretroviruses, such as MLV, requires cell division [5].

Lentiviruses on the other hand, can efficiently infect both dividing and non-dividing cells as they do not require dissociation of the nuclear envelope in order to integrate their genome into the host's genome, as it has been previously documented [6]. This is a crucial characteristic for genetically modifying tissues, such as the liver, muscle, brain and the hematopoietic system, as they are able to correct even non-dividing cells that reside in the G_o phase of the cell cycle.

Both families consist of a phospholipid envelope layer around a protein capsid that contains a plus (+) strand RNA genome ranging from 7 to 10 kb. Their genome is flanked by the Long Terminal Repeats (LTRs) which are approximately 600 bp in size. Within the LTR there is a powerful enhancer and promoter that drives the expression of the viral genes, namely the *gag*, *pol* and *env* genes. The *gag* gene encodes for the capsid proteins, *pol* encodes the reverse transcriptase enzyme and also an integrase activity, while *env* expresses the envelope glycoproteins. Retroviruses have a natural tropism for hematopoietic cells, including hemopoietic stem cells. More specifically, the advantages of oncoretroviral vectors include: a) their ability to promote efficient and stable gene transfer, b) high fidelity gene transfer because they integrate intact and do not cause chromosomal rearrangements and c) they can transduce up to 40% of hematopoietic stem cells in non-human primates. Unfortunately, a serious drawback in their clinical setting occurred when several patients during the gene therapy clinical trial for X-linked severe combined immunodeficiency (X-SCID) conducted in France, developed T-cell acute lymphoblastic leukemia, due to integration of the viral genome in the second intron of the LMO-2 proto-oncogene [7]. Furthermore, additional safety issues were raised after utilization of a gamma-retroviral vector for chronic granulomatous disease [8] that led to genomic instability and myelodysplasia following EVI1 activation after gene therapy. Therefore, it is anticipated that lentiviral vectors will progressively displace oncoretroviral vectors at least in the field of hemopoietic gene therapy [9]. However in the context of cardiac stem cells and cardiomyocytes regeneration, there are only few studies that have been conducted to date. Thus, this field represents an additional challenge, since there are still basic issues that remain to be fully addressed regarding the level of myocyte regeneration [10].

Wild-type HIV naturally infects $CD4^+$ T-cells of the hemopoietic system. However, in the gene therapy context, HIV-based vectors bear a different glycoprotein on their envelope, derived from vesicular stomatitis virus (VSV), namely the VSV-G envelope glycoprotein. This process, *i.e.* the replacement of the wild type HIV envelope glycoprotein with the VSV-G glycoprotein, is called pseudotyping. VSV-G confers significant advances in terms of tropism for many cells, including stem cells of the hematopoietic and the cardiac system. VSV-G pseudotyped lentiviral vectors can also be easily purified and concentrated by ultracentrifugation leading to increased vector titers. Titer is defined as the number of virions/ml. Lentiviral vectors present the same advantages as oncoretroviral vectors, but exhibit higher titers than oncoretroviral vectors. Lentiviral vectors are currently utilized in several promising human clinical trials for various disorders including ADA-deficient SCID [11], β-thalassemia [12], Wiskott-Aldrich syndrome [13] and metachromatic leukodystrophy [14]. Clearly, lentiviral vectors have outperformed oncoretroviral vectors in terms of safety and efficiency and thus, represent a potent future agent that can be employed effectively in the cardiac gene therapy field. Moreover, successful lentiviral transduction has been documented in cardiomyocytes, cardiac micro-vascular endothelial cells, cardiac stem cells and progenitors [15 - 18]. However, it seems that utilization of lentiviral vectors in the cardiac gene therapy field is still far from reaching the clinical practice, mainly due to the fact that lentiviruses naturally do not exhibit tropism for the heart.

Although retroviruses are potent tools in gene therapy, they still present one major drawback which is the risk for insertional mutagenesis. Insertional mutagenesis is defined as the activation of proto-oncogenes or down-regulation of tumour suppressor genes upon viral integration. While this possibility had been originally estimated to be extremely low based on the assumption that pro-viral integration into the genome was random, clinical trials in gene therapy were halted due to this specific adverse effect [7, 12, 19 - 21]. Mapping studies of retroviral integration sites in cell lines documented that retroviral integration is actually not a random process and that each virus exhibits a unique pattern of integration. Thus, MLV-based vectors mainly integrate around transcriptional start sites, while lentiviral vectors strongly prefer to integrate inside transcription units and gene-dense regions of the genome. Still, the basis for these preferences is unknown [22 - 26].

Gene therapy based on retroviral vectors can be made safer by utilization of specific DNA elements called insulators. Insulators can block enhancer activity and simultaneously maintain the chromatin status of distinct chromosomal regions. Moreover, when insulators were introduced in gene therapy retroviral vectors, they diminished variable expression and silencing of the transgene and most importantly, reduced the risk of insertional mutagenesis [27, 28]. Therefore, gene therapy by utilization of lentiviral vectors was made safer by deletion of the U3 region of the LTR in the self-inactivating (SIN) configuration and the simultaneous incorporation of insulators. These modifications have paved the way in the broad utilization of lentiviral vectors in the fields of stem cell biology, haematology, neuroscience, developmental biology and transgenesis.

Adeno-associated Viruses (AAV)

Adeno-associated viruses (AAV) belong to the family of Parvoviridae. These are viruses with no known pathogenicity and contain a non-enveloped capsid that comprises a 4.7 kb single-stranded DNA genome. Their genome has two genes, the *cap* gene encoding the structural proteins of the viral capsid, and the *rep* gene that encodes the non-structural proteins necessary for viral replication and assembly. Their genome is also flanked by short inverted terminal repeats (ITR) that are smaller in size compared to the retroviral LTR. Their life cycle is divided in two phases, the replicative and the latent phase. In the productive phase, the AAV is able to co-infect the host cell only with the presence of a helper virus [29]. In most cases the helper virus belongs to the family of Adenoviridae. In the absence of a helper virus, AAV often enters the latent phase, integrating into the human genome, commonly within a specific region of chromosome 19, although this has been reported only in cell lines. This specific site is considered one of the few "safe harbors" within the human genome in the sense that integration of any genetic element in this specific site does not cause serious adverse effects associated with cancer.

In contrast to adenoviruses that are especially immunogenic, the main advantage of AAVs is the minor inflammatory response they cause to the host and this is the principle reason that AAVs are employed in the gene therapy setting. AAVs are engineered to become gene therapy vectors by the complete deletion of the viral *cap* and *rev* genes, while the inverted terminal repeats which are necessary for packaging and integration remain intact. Thus, AAV vectors are rendered replication-deficient because the viral coding sequences are entirely removed and can serve as efficient and safe transgene vehicles to mediate long-term gene expression in dividing and non-dividing cells of various tissues. However, naturally occurring AAV variants are typically inefficient in infecting human embryonic stem cells [29].

Thirteen different serotypes of AAV based on the structure of the capsid protein have been described who also display distinct tissue tropism. However, the most cardiotropic serotypes AAV-1, 6, 8 and 9 also confer significant transduction in non-target tissues such as the lung, the skeletal muscles and the liver [4]. Several methods have been introduced in order to enhance AAV cardiotropism and novel viral capsid AAV libraries were constructed through DNA shuffling and chimeric strain production. Chimeric strain production was employed as a strategy to simultaneously enhance tissue tropism and help AAV-based vectors to avoid naturally occurring neutralizing antibodies [30 - 34]. These strategies were imperative because a large percentage of the human population (20-80% approximately) already had neutralizing antibodies to various AAV serotypes, severely limiting the efficient use of AAV and compromising its therapeutic potency. Also, the presence of such antibodies constitutes a major exclusion criterion in many AAV-based clinical trials [35]. Nevertheless, there are many studies reporting the efficient transduction of cardiac cells by AAV vectors and it seems that AAVs constitute the most effective way for gene transfer in cardiac cells to date [36, 37]. Finally, there are several on-going gene therapy clinical trials for HF employing AAV vectors.

Adenoviruses

Human adenoviruses constitute another viral family used in gene therapy approaches. Adenoviruses are non-enveloped, double-stranded (ds) DNA viruses with large protein complexes on their capsid that bind to CD46 or to Coxsackie-adenovirus receptor (CAR). Their genome size ranges between 30 and 35 kb, and contains five segments that encode early gene products (E1a, E1b, E2a, E2b, E3, and E4), and five segments that encode late gene products (L1–L5). The E1, E2, and E4 gene products regulate transcription and translation of the late genes and therefore, are necessary for viral replication [38]. Depending on the serotype for viral binding and cellular entry, adenoviruses are classified into 51 immunologically distinct serotypes divided into 6 subgroups, namely subgroups A–F. Upon cellular entry, the dsDNA is transported to the nucleus across nuclear pores. Thus, Adenoviruses efficiently transduce both mitotic and non-mitotic cells. This, combined with their broad tropism of several different cell types, has rendered adenoviral vectors one of the most promising vehicles for *in vivo* treatment of several human diseases such as cystic fibrosis and hemophilia. Adenoviral vectors present the following advantages: a) they exhibit particularly high titers (over 10^{11} vector particles/ml), b) they are credible in terms of gene transfer because the vector genomes are genetically stable, c) they can achieve particularly high transgene expression due to their ability to deliver many genome copies per target cell, and d) they can efficiently carry large therapeutic genes of approximately 25-30 kb in size.

However, despite the fact that adenoviral replication-deficient vectors can be easily produced and at high titers, there are two important drawbacks: a) Due to their inability to integrate into the host's genome, they confer only transient expression of the therapeutic gene that typically lasts 1-2 months in non-dividing cells and significantly less in dividing cells and b) they are able to induce significant cellular and humoral immune response of the host. Thus, adenoviral vectors, especially of the first generation are preferable where short-term expression and single dosing is desirable, such as cancer vaccine therapies. However, initial enthusiasm for first-generation adenoviral vectors in gene therapy has decreased, because not only they did fail to confer long-term transgene expression, but also caused significant toxicity and resulted in the death of an individual [38]. Another critical parameter is the pre-existing immunity against adenoviruses in patients that hamper gene delivery and expression. Although, third-generation gutless or helper-dependent adenoviral vectors are attenuated in terms of immunogenic potential, there is still a significant risk. Finally, there is presence of CAR receptors in the liver that limit adenoviral tissue specificity. Therefore, due to the aforementioned limiting factors, adenoviral mediated strategies are limited in cardiovascular gene therapy trials [39].

Non-viral Vectors

Non-viral vectors are most frequently plasmids and typically include a well-characterized and constitutive promoter sequence such as the cytomegalovirus (CMV) or Rous sarcoma virus (RSV) promoters, combined with enhancer sequences to confer tissue specificity of the transgene. Plasmids are double-stranded circular DNA molecules of about 2-12 kb in size, bearing several characteristics such as an origin of replication, to ensure replication in bacteria and in certain cases eukaryotic cells, and an antibiotic resistance gene. Non-viral, *i.e.* plasmid-based DNA vector systems have several advantages: a) They are low cost constructs, b) they are extremely easy to manufacture, and c) do not provoke systemic responses of the patient's immune system. In any molecular biology setting, plasmids are readily delivered in *in vitro* cultured cells by a technique called transfection that includes lipofection, electroporation and calcium phosphate precipitation. The idea is to introduce the plasmid DNA within the cells of a stable cell line. This type of plasmid transfection is being globally employed in cell lines during the production of adenoviral, AAV and lentiviral based vectors. However, it is a different issue to transfect stable cell lines in the laboratory and a different issue to deliver naked plasmids to tissues in a gene therapy setting. The latter has been shown to be both inefficient and challenging because plasmids are rapidly and systematically degraded inside the cell due to their intracellular compartmentalization to the endosomes leading to short-term expression. Moreover, transient expression is related with histone modification and heterochromatin formation and *de novo* methylation. All these implications hamper the use of plasmids as potent transgene vectors.

Several approaches have been developed to overcome these issues such as incorporation of the recently identified matrix attachment region (MAR) elements that have exhibited inhibition of DNA methylation and therefore, have shown to prevent transgene silencing [40]. Moreover, these elements effectively insulate the transgene, creating independent euchromatin domains. Plasmids can be also made more stable inside the cells when combined with liposomal and polymer systems that serve as carrier molecules. This strategy shields the DNA within these complexes and thus, protects plasmids from systemic degradation. These polymers are made of polyethylenimines (PEI) and polyamidoamine complexes (PAA) and have conferred enhanced plasmid uptake from the cells combined with protection from endosomal degradation and reduced cytotoxicity. However, even by this method, the DNA is rapidly cleared from the circulation and concentrated mainly in the lungs [41].

Molecular Targets

Before reaching any clinical trial, the appropriate gene target must be determined. During the last decade, extensive knowledge towards the understanding of the pathophysiology of heart failure at the molecular and cellular level has been provided. This knowledge has paved the way towards developing new therapeutic approaches based on gene-transfer technology. Currently, the main targets in the field of cardiac gene therapy can be divided into two main categories: a) molecular targets of the β-adrenergic system and b) molecular targets of calcium cycling proteins. Any of these targets is validated first in well characterized animal models of heart failure where they are considered successful if they provide rescue of cardiac function, do not cause arrhythmogenesis and can establish a gene-dose effect.

The β-Adrenergic System

A common denominator in HF is the down-regulation and desensitization of the β-adrenergic receptor (β-AR). Therefore, a rationale based on gene transfer for overexpression of β-AR is a simple way to overcome β-AR down-regulation in a relevant gene therapy setting. Overexpression of the human β_1-ARs has been shown to cause severe cardiomyopathy in transgenic mice [42]. On the contrary, cardiac overexpression of β_2-AR demonstrated increased basal myocardial adenylate cyclase activity with increased LV function [43] in other mouse models. Hence, direct and intracoronary myocardial delivery of adenovirus containing the human β_2-AR transgene led to enhanced cardiac function in rodents and mammalian models [44].

A second potent molecular target for heart gene therapy is the G protein-coupled receptor kinase 2 (GRK2). GRK2 is the most abundantly expressed GRK in the heart and has been associated with the pathogenesis of dysfunctional cardiac β-AR signalling. GRKs phosphorylate the agonist-occupied receptors, resulting in functional uncoupling. In mice, selective GRK2 ablation after HF induced by MI, resulted in better survival, halted ventricular remodelling, and improved cardiac contractile performance [45]. Finally, βARKct, a peptide that inhibits GRK2-mediated β-AR desensitization, has been evaluated *in vivo* in animals. Intra-coronary administration of adenovirus-mediated βARKct transgene to rabbits three weeks after induced MI, was linked to a marked reversal of ventricular dysfunction [46]. However, the latest findings of Schumacher *et al.* suggest that the selective serotonin reuptake inhibitor (SSRI) paroxetine inhibits GRK2 with selectivity over other GRKs and thus, confers beneficial effects markedly greater than those of β-blocker therapy [47]. These results severely challenge the use of gene therapy methods for this specific molecular target, if this novel therapeutic approach proves to be equally successful in heart failure.

The last target of the β-adrenergic system is adenylate cyclase 6 (ADCY6) which catalyses the formation of cAMP by ATP. Up-regulation of ADCY6 had a neutral effect on basal cardiac function and was not related to structural heart abnormalities [48]. Overexpression of ADCY6 in transgenic mice improved cardiac function in response to adrenergic stimulation and increased cAMP production in isolated cardiomyocytes. Moreover, intra-coronary administration of adenovirus encoding ADCY6 in a pacing model of HF in pigs, resulted in improved LV function and remodelling which was linked to increased cAMP-generating capacity [49]. These promising effects of up-regulation of ADCY6 in preclinical studies are currently under investigation for the initiation of clinical trials in HF patients [43].

Calcium Cycling Proteins

An important discovery revealed that calcium cycling is disordered in human HF regardless of the etiology, partially due to decreased sarcoplasmic reticulum Ca^{2+} ATPase 2a (SERCA2a) activity [4, 50]. Consequently, a wide range of reports concerning gene transfer of SERCA2a has shown enhancement in cardiac contractility in a large number of experimental models of HF, restoration of the normal cardiac metabolism, decrease in ventricular arrhythmias, and improvement of coronary flow through activation of endothelial nitric oxide synthase (eNOS) in endothelial cells [51 - 55].]. Therefore, it was a logical step to utilize SERCA2a as the first molecular target for gene transfer in the context of heart failure gene therapy. This strategy was further advanced by the identification of several miRNAs that suppress intracellular calcium levels in myocardium, by interacting with mRNA encoding SERCA2a [56]. Specifically, the expression of *miR-25* was increased in HF, both in mice and humans. Further corroboration of this finding was provided *via* adeno-associated virus 9 (AAV9)-mediated overexpression of *miR-25 in vivo*, which led to a significant loss of contractile function. Consequently, injection of an antisense oligonucleotide against *miR-25*, significantly halted HF in a mouse model, improving cardiac function and survival compared to controls. These data reveal that endogenous *miR-25* contributes to declining cardiac function during HF and suggest that it might be targeted therapeutically to restore function.

Other Targets

Recently, the ability of the stromal derived factor 1 (SDF1) to activate the homing of endogenous stem cells *via* the chemokine receptor type 4 (CCR4) to the infracted myocardium, has prompted their use as therapeutic targets in ischemic

HF [57]. To this end, there is currently one clinical trial with the aim to investigate the therapeutic benefit of SDF1 overexpression in ischemic cardiomyopathy by gene transfer of SDF1 incorporated in a naked plasmid (see next Section).

Finally, other molecules have emerged as candidates for gene therapy for heart failure such as phospholamban (PLN), protein phosphatase 1 (PP1) and S100. Several different strategies were employed. For example, in the case of PLN there was inhibition through RNAi technology [58]. On the other hand, inhibition of PP1 was mediated by direct gene addition of the protein phosphatase-1 inhibitor-1 [59]. The gene strategy concerning S100 was up-regulation of the protein by gene addition. S100 belongs to a family of Ca^{2+}-modulated proteins involved in intracellular regulatory activities. S100 enhances the activity of both ryanodine receptors (RYRs) and SERCA2a and thus, promotes cardiac contractile and relaxation function. Therefore, gene transfer of S100A1 by an AAV9-based vector in a preclinical model of ischemic cardiomyopathy induced dramatic improvements in contractile function, suggesting that a gene therapy clinical trial for human heart failure might be possible in the future [4] by gene addition of S100A1.

Gene Therapy Clinical Trials

Heart failure (HF) is one of the leading causes of mortality in the United States, with an estimated prevalence of >37.7 million individuals globally [60]. Device-based treatments and pharmacotherapies have improved patient survival, but HF eventually results in degeneration and death. The 5-year survival for individuals with HF is approximately 50%, and in end-stage the HF 1-year survival is as low as 22% regardless of therapy.

Therefore, the need to improve current therapeutic approaches to treat HF is mandatory. To this end, several clinical trials employing gene transfer have taken place. The so-called CUPID trial was the first clinical trial of gene therapy in the United States and was initiated in 2007 [61]. The trial's concept was entirely based on gene delivery of the SERCA2 cDNA *via* a recombinant AAV1 (AAV1.SERCA2a) for calcium up-regulation in patients with advanced heart failure. The study was a two-part, phase 1/2 multi-center trial designed to evaluate the safety and the biological effects of gene transfer of the SERCA2a cDNA *via* the recombinant AAV1. During the first part of the study, participants were administered a single intracoronary infusion of AAV1.SERCA2a in an open-label approach. Follow-up of these patients after twelve months, documented an acceptable safety pattern and moreover, improvement was detected in several patients suggesting that gene transfer of AAV1.SERCA2a conferred a quantitative biological benefit. During the second part of the trial, 39 patients with advanced HF as defined by New York Heart Association (NYHA) class III/IV, exhibiting ejection fraction (EF) ≤30% and maximal oxygen uptake <16 mL/kg per minute, received the AAV1-mediated SERCA2a transgene in one or three doses of DNase resistant particles (DRPs), *i.e.* low dose (6×10^{11} DRPs), middle dose (3×10^{12} DRPs), and high dose (1×10^{13} DRPs), or placebo [39, 60]]. The results during the first year, showed that the cumulative recurrent cardiovascular events such as death, heart failure admission, left ventricular assist device (LVAD) insertion, cardiac transplantation, and myocardial infarction, increased in the placebo group but not in the low and middle-dose AAV1.SERCA2a groups, which demonstrated diminished recurrent cardiovascular events for the first six months. It should be emphasized however, that these groups demonstrated events that were similar to placebo from months 6 to 12. On the other hand, the high-dose AAV1.SERCA2a group, continued to do significantly better than the rest of the groups at 12 months without any increase in adverse events, laboratory abnormalities, or arrhythmias [62]. Unfortunately, these promising results were not reproduced in the follow-up CUPID 2 Phase 2b trial (NCT01643330) that was designed to evaluate whether increasing SERCA2a activity *via* gene therapy, improves clinical outcome. CUPID 2 is a randomized, double-blind, placebo-controlled, phase 2b trial that included 250 symptomatic heart failure patients with left ventricular ejection fractions of <35%. Patients were randomized to receive a single intracoronary infusion of 1×10^{13} DNase-resistant particles of AAV1/SERCA2a ($n = 123$) or placebo ($n = 127$). The primary endpoint was the time to recurrent events (hospital admission because of heart failure or ambulatory treatment for worsening heart failure) with a median follow-up of 17.5 months. Sadly, treatment with AAV1/SERCA2a did not improve time to recurrent events compared to placebo (104 *vs.* 128 events; hazard ratio, $p = 0.81$) since 16% of patients died in the placebo group and 21% of patients died in the AAV1/SERCA2a group [63]. Thus, the authors concluded that AAV1/SERCA2a at the dose tested did not improve the clinical course of patients with heart failure and reduced ejection fraction. The authors also elaborate the reasons for this inconsistency. First, no obvious important differences in study population characteristics were recorded between the trials. Second, a review of the vector's manufacturing processes identified variations in the proportion of empty viral capsids (containing only the protein capsid and not the single-stranded DNA) between CUPID 1 (85%) and CUPID 2 (25%), which could have affected transduction efficiency. Thus, one of the main possible reasons for the discrepancies between the two CUPID trials, may be due to the reduced transduction efficiency. Accordingly, the authors suggested that the use of a higher dose or a higher percentage of empty capsids serving as decoys for neutralising antibodies, or both, might have beneficial effects.

Furthermore, the authors assessed the presence of AAV1/SERCA2a DNA in cardiac tissues from patients, whose condition deteriorated, requiring either transplantation or mechanical circulatory support device implantation, and cardiac tissue obtained from deceased patients. The amount of vector DNA in these tissues (approximate median 43 copies per μg DNA) were at the lower end of the threshold for dose–response curves in pharmacology studies (<500 copies per μg DNA). Although the number of cells that were transduced is difficult to determine because of the variable ploidy of cardiomyocytes, these levels are most consistent with the likelihood that only a very small proportion of cardiomyocytes were expressing AAV1-delivered SERCA2a in the myocardium of these patients. Finally, it is also possible that SERCA2a is not the right target in human heart failure, despite the success in mouse models. Nevertheless, and despite this trial's failure to improve the clinical outcome of the recruited patients, several important conclusions were drawn: a) gene therapy with AAV1 may be feasible using different transgenes and b) no safety issues emerged under these conditions. The latter is a critical fact for a gene therapy trial.

Still, the results of the CUPID clinical trial, have prompted researchers to conduct two other clinical trials targeting SERCA2a. The first trial, which is conducted in the United Kingdom, enrolles patients with advanced HF who received LVAD at least one month prior to treatment. These patients will be treated either with

AAV1.SERCA2a or saline as the placebo. Simultaneously, a Phase 2, single-center, double-blind, randomized, placebo-controlled, parallel-group study will be conducted at the Institute de Cardiologie Pitié-Salpêtrière in Paris, France, with the primary objective of investigating the impact of AAV1.SERCA2a on cardiac remodelling parameters in patients who suffer from severe heart failure [4].

In a different approach, a Phase 1 clinical trial was recently completed showing that SDF-1 gene therapy improved HF symptoms in patients suffered from ischemic cardiomyopathy [64]. As previously described, the study was based on preclinical results indicating that adult stem cells induce tissue repair by activating endogenous stem cells through the SDF1/CCR4 axis. In the respective clinical trial JVS-100, a DNA plasmid encoding SDF-1, was injected in the endomyocardial tissue of 17 patients with ischemic cardiomyopathy. The primary objective of this Phase 1, open-label, dose-escalation study with 12 months of follow-up, was to document if JVS-100 improves clinical parameters. Efficacy end points were change in quality of life, NYHA class criteria, 6-minute walk distance, single photon emission computed tomography, N-terminal pro-brain natriuretic peptide (NT-proBNP), and echocardiography at 4 and 12 months. The primary safety end point was met. At 4 months, all of the cohorts exibited improvements in 6-minute walk distance, quality of life, and NYHA class criteria. Subjects in the 15 and 30-mg dose groups demonstrated improvements in 6-minute walk distance (15 mg: median 41 minutes [range 3-61 minutes]; 30 mg: median 31 minutes [range 22-74 minutes]) and quality of life (15 mg: median -16 points [range +1 to -32 points]; 30 mg: median -24 points [range +17 to -38 points]) over baseline. At 12 months, improvements in symptoms were sustained. The data clearly demonstrate the importance of defining the molecular mechanisms of stem cell-based tissue repair and suggest that overexpression of SDF-1 *via* gene therapy can be proposed as a strategy for improving HF symptoms in patients with ischemic cardiomyopathy.

CELL THERAPY

In theory, cells that were lost after a heart attack or during a chronic cardiovascular disease should be replaced and/or repaired in order for the patient to recover. However, the adult mammalian heart has been generally considered to be a terminally differentiated organ and cardiomyocytes were assumed to be fully post-mitotic cells based on their specific characteristics that include: a) a complex and well-developed cytoskeleton that physically impedes the formation of the mitotic spindle and b) their multinucleated and polyploeidic state. Despite these features, Beltrami *et al.* in 2001 altered this dogma and demonstrated that the human adult heart possesses a population of cardiomyocytes with proliferative potential [65]. Since this discovery, a fair number of publications, which were very well reviewed by Aguirre *et al.*, showed that adult human cardiomyocytes renew very slowly, in decreasing numbers with advancing age, and therefore this cell pool is insufficient to heal the heart after MI [66]. Consequently it is an established principle that post-natal cardiomyocyte renewal occurs in humans at a rate of 1.5% per year at the age of 25 years [67]. Although this rate has been controversial in the literature, it is a rather accepted fact that regeneration in the adult human heart occurs in slow rates and aims to preserve long-term homeostatic maintenance of the heart's function rather than leading to a rapid renewal after a heart attack.

Over the past decade two theories emerged trying to explain the source of adult cardiac regeneration in mammals: a) progenitor or stem cells give rise to new cardiomyocytes, and b) mature cardiomyocytes re-enter the mitotic cell cycle and generate new cardiomyocytes [68]. There are data to support both hypotheses and the major issue that remains to be elucidated is to define the source of regenerated cardiomyocytes during aging and injury.

However, the acquisition of this knowledge has paved the way to stem cell therapy and tissue engineering for the treatment of heart disease. To this end, several strategies have been developed some of which were also utilized in clinical trials. In a number of cell therapy trials, autologous stem cells were applied employing transplantation of bone marrow, which includes several numbers of stem cells, as a treatment for heart attacks. An alternative strategy involved the use of endogenous cardiac stem cells for the treatment of HF. Other groups are developing "off the shelf" non-autologous stem cell products to treat patients such as embryonic stem cells or induced pluripotent stem cells. One of the major challenges in the field of heart cell therapy involves the ability of the new cells to make sufficient connections with the existing heart cells. These connections are required in order to preserve the electrical currents that are needed for the heart to beat in an organized and efficient manner. Various cell therapies for the treatment of scar tissue due to a heart attack are being investigated in Phase I, II or III clinical trials [68, 69].

It is therefore clear that a number of cell populations combined with various delivery methods have been utilized in several clinical trials for cell therapy of heart disease. A brief description of the cell types administered, as well as the results obtained in the clinical setting are presented in the second part of this chapter.

Stem Cell Types Used for Cardiac Repair

Allogeneic Stem Cells

Allogeneic bone marrow transplantation is a routinely used medical intervention to treat a large number of hemopoietic diseases, such as leukemias and hemoglobinopathies. In that sense, allogeneic cells from human donors may have greater success after implantation. Allogeneic stem cells include umbilical cord-derived cells, fetal cardiomyocytes and embryonic mesenchymal stem cells (EMSCs). The use of fetal originating cells, such as the EMSCs and the fetal cardiomyocytes, has been hampered due to ethical and legal issues and shifted the existing attention to other alternative sources for stem cell therapy, such as the cord blood. To this end, human umbilical cord blood-derived cells have been exploited. Cord blood stem cells, namely $CD34^+$ hematopoietic progenitor/stem cells, are currently used for repopulating bone marrow in patients suffering from blood diseases such as acute leukemia. Human cord blood contains a fair number of non-hematopoietic stem cells that express decreased class II human leukocyte antigens and seem not to trigger an immune response, thus minimising the risk of rejection. This reduced immunological activity offers a striking option for regenerative therapy [70]. A significant reduction in infarct size has also been demonstrated after intra-myocardial injection of human cord blood-derived cells in animal models [70].

Autologous Stem Cells

To eliminate the potential for allogeneic rejection, autologous cells have become a central focus of heart cell therapy. This category of cells includes skeletal myoblasts, adipose-derived stem cells (AdSCs), resident cardiac stem cells (RCSCs), bone marrow-derived (BMD) stem cells, induced pluripotent stem cells (iPSCs), multipotent adult progenitor cells such as the circulating progenitor cells (CPCs), endothelial progenitor cells (EPCs) and endogenous cardiac progenitors in the form of cardiospheres. Of these types, AdSCs, RCSCs, BMD cells, CPCs and cardiospheres have been administered in the clinical setting.

Induced Pluripotent Stem Cells (iPSCs)

iPSCs derive from differentiated adult cells that have been induced to a state of pluripotency through a process of genetic reprogramming mediated by over-expression of certain master genes, such as the octamer-binding protein 3/4 (OCT3/4), the SRY-box 2 (SOX2), the Krüppel-like factor 4 (KLF4), and the *myc* proto-oncogene protein (c-MYC). Alternative methods to induce pluripotency have now been developed to promote reprogramming *via* SOX2 and OCT4, or by over-expression of NANOG, LIN28, OCT4, and SOX2 [70]. Interestingly, generation of iPSC without c-MYC has been demonstrated to favor generation of iPSCs with a greater tendency towards cardiac differentiation [71]. This experimental process mitigates the ethical concerns associated with the isolation and use of embryonic stem cells. iPSCs are capable of differentiating into the cardiac lineage by utilizing a variety of tissues, including fibroblasts, keratinocytes, human cord blood, human foreskin fibroblasts, and peripheral blood T-lymphocytes. However, developing procedures to efficiently and cost-effectively produce sufficient numbers of autologous cells for transplantation within a therapeutic time frame remains a major issue. It should be noted, however, that iPSCs have not yet been utilized in the clinical setting as there have been several reports of tumour formation in laboratory animals after iPSCs administration. Finally, another important issue with iPSCs is to achieve long-term stability and integration into the myocardium as there have been observations of incomplete differentiation of cardiomyocytes compared to mature cells [66].

Skeletal Myoblasts

Skeletal myoblasts are harvested by muscle biopsy from the individual and then grafted to the cardiac tissue. Although preclinical assays verified their ability to engraft, create myotubules, and improve cardiac function after transfer into infarcted myocardium, their eventual use in the MAGIC (Myoblast Autologous Grafting in Ischemic Cardiomyopathy) clinical trial yielded poor results [69]. A major limitation to their use is that they remain committed to the skeletal muscle lineage and have been associated with arrhythmias due to the separation of cardiomyocytes by islands of skeletal muscle cells, therefore interfering with the propagation of electrical potentials [69].

Adipose-derived Stem Cells (AdSCs)

AdSCs derive from the adipose tissue that includes a heterogeneous mixture of mesenchymal stem cells (MSCs), hematopoietic stem cells (HSCs), and endothelial progenitor cells (EPCs). AdSCs have been considered as a credible source of adult stem cells for cardiac repair because of their major clinical advantage of availability, easy harvesting, and relatively low cost. The amount of mesenchymal stem cells in freshly isolated adipose tissue is ~2.500-fold greater than that of freshly aspirated bone marrow, therefore cell culture is not necessary to generate therapeutically sufficient cells [72]. In average, 20 to 40 million cells can be isolated and prepared within 2 h after liposuction from as little as 200 g of lipoaspirate, enabling the treatment of acute myocardial infarction (AMI) patients within hours after the primary percutaneous coronary intervention (PPCI).

Preclinical studies have demonstrated that AdSCs are linked to improvement in ventricular function in animal models of AMI. The predominant working mechanism of AdSCs therapy in AMI seems to be through paracrine release of anti-apoptotic, immunomodulatory, and pro-angiogenic factors. These factors evoke cardiomyocyte salvage and stimulate neo-angiogenesis in the infarct border zone and eventually lead to decreased infarct scar formation and adverse cardiac remodelling. There have been two different clinical trials involving AdSCs, the PRECISE trial with poor results and the APOLLO study with positive results (see next section Cell Therapy Clinical Trials).

Resident Cardiac Stem Cells (RCSCs) or Cardiac Progenitor Cells

This cell population was originally described by Beltrami *et al.* in 2001 and contains a population of cardiomyocytes with proliferative potential [65]. Subsequent studies have further characterized and isolated RCSCs and demonstrated efficient differentiation into cardiomyocytes or vascular cells [67]. These cells are isolated from cardiac tissue obtained during heart surgery or endocardiac biopsy and then expanded in culture for use in autologous transplantation. Preclinical studies in rodents demonstrated reduction in the infarct size and improvement of left ventricular function after RCSC culture and injection [67]. The best-characterized and most well-studied RCSC population is c-kit^{+}/Lin^{-} cells, originally described in the rat heart. The c-kit^{+}/Lin^{-} RCSCs, isolated and expanded in culture, exhibit all the properties of stem cells. However, the use of a single marker to isolate cardiac progenitors is still an issue, as it is susceptible to contamination of non-progenitor cells and therefore, effective harvesting and expanding techniques need to be perfected.

Cardiospheres (CSs)

Cardiospheres (CSs) are self-assembling multicellular clusters derived by the cellular expansion of cardiac explants cultured in non-adhesive substrates [73]. They contain a core of primitive, proliferating cells, and an outer layer of mesenchymal/stromal cells and differentiating cells that express cardiomyocyte proteins and connexin 43 [73]. Cardiospheres exhibit the following phenotype: they are negative for CD34, CD45, positive for c-kit (core), CD31 (periphery), CD90, CD105 (periphery), αMHC (periphery), cTnI (periphery), CD133 (periphery), MDR-1 (periphery), connexin 43, Nkx2.5 (core) and desmin (core) [69]. They represent an attractive cell source for cardiac regeneration because they contain both primitive cells and committed progenitors for the three major cell types present in the heart, *i.e.* cardiomyocytes, endothelial cells, and smooth muscle cells, and also because they can derive from percutaneous endomyocardial biopsies. Cardiospheres have been successfully used in preclinical studies and resulted in improved cardiac function after MI [73].

Bone Marrow-derived (BMD) Stem Cells and Circulating Progenitor Cells (CPCs)

Bone marrow is rich in several stem cell and progenitor cell populations as it contains, among others, hematopoietic stem cells, namely $CD34^+$ cells and mesenchymal stem cells. BMD stem cells can differentiate *in vitro* to a variety of cells including cardiomyocytes and vascular endothelial cells. Their major advantage is the fact that they can be harvested easily, safely and in large numbers and that there is also an extended clinical experience. Some of these stem cells are also released in the circulation and represent the circulating progenitor cells that can be isolated from the blood's mononuclear fraction. Encouraging results have been reported in animal models of ischemic HF [69]. BMD stem cells have been also utilized in the majority of clinical trials with controversial results.

Cell Therapy Clinical Trials

Stem cell biology holds significant promise for treating diseases of the heart. In the preclinical setting, autologous cardiac cell therapy appeared to be safe, and therefore, investigators have aggressively advanced into clinical cell therapy. In this section some of the clinical studies are mentioned in respect to the timeframe of the intervention (early *vs.* late) and the disease's type (chronic *vs.* acute, ischemic *vs.* non-ischemic). These data are summarized in Tables **1 - 4**.

Table 1. Clinical trials of cell therapy for acute ischemic heart failure, early intervention (<7 d).

Name	Cell source	Delivery mode	Result
TOPCARE-AMI	BMD and CPC	Intracoronary	Positive
BOOST	BMD	Intracoronary	Positive but transient
ASTAMI	BMD	Intracoronary	No change
REPAIR-AMI	BMD	Intracoronary	Positive
REGENT	BMD and $CD34^+$	Intracoronary	No significant change
APOLLO	AdSC	Intracoronary	Positive but not significant

AdSC: adipocyte-derived stem cells; BMD: bone marrow-derived cells; CPC: circulating progenitor cells. For further information regarding the trials refer to the text.

Table 2. Clinical trials of cell therapy for acute ischemic heart failure, late intervention (>7 d).

Name	Cell source	Delivery mode	Result
MYSTAR	BMD	Intracoronary / intramyocardial	Positive
SWISS-AMI	BMD	Intracoronary	No change
LateTIME	BMD	Intracoronary	No change
CADUCEUS	Cardiospheres	Intracoronary	No change

BMD: bone marrow-derived cells.
For further information regarding the trials refer to the text.

Table 3. Clinical trials of cell therapy for chronic ischemic heart failure.

Name	Cell source	Delivery mode	Result
PRECISE	AdSC	Transendocardial	No change
TOPCARE-CHD	BMD or CPC	Intracoronary	No change
POSEIDON	MSC	Transendocardial	No change
StarHEART	BMD	Intracoronary	Positive
SCIPIO	RCSC	Intracoronary	Positive
PROMETHEUS	MSC	Intramyocardial	Positive

AdSC: adipocyte-derived stem cells; BMD: bone marrow-derived cells; CPC: circulating progenitor cells; MSC: mesenchymal stem cells; RCSC: resident cardiac stem cells.
For further information regarding the trials refer to the text.

Table 4. Clinical trial of cell therapy for chronic non-ischemic heart failure.

Name	Cell source	Delivery mode	Result
TOPCARE-DCM	BMD	Intracoronary	Positive

BMD: bone marrow-derived cells.
For further information regarding the trial refer to the text.

For acute ischemic heart disease, the discrimination is based on the time of intervention and is divided in clinical trials in which intervention took place within the first 7 days after the cardiac event and late in which intervention took place later, *i.e.* after 7 days. Therefore, all the included studies are characterized in terms of the increase in left ventricular ejection fraction (LVEF), the improved exercise time, and the improved functional class (as per the NYHA Functional

Classification) compared with placebo and the overall incidents of adverse effects (https://clinicaltrials.gov/ct2/home).

Early Intervention

TOPCARE-AMI Study: Transplantation Of Progenitor Cells And Regeneration Enhancement in Acute Myocardial Infarction

The TOPCARE-AMI trial was the first randomized study investigating the effects of intracoronary infusion of circulating (CPC) or bone BMD in 59 patients with AMI 4 days after the infarction. In the five-year follow-up, data of 55 patients confirmed no signs of intra-myocardial calcification or tumors. One patient died during the initial hospitalization, no patient was re-hospitalized for HF and 16 patients underwent target vessel revascularization (TVR). Serum levels of NT-proBNP (see also TOPCARE-CHD study) remained significantly reduced indicating the absence of HF. Magnetic Resonance Imaging (MRI) subgroup analysis in 31 patients demonstrated a persistent improvement of LVEF (from 46 ± 10% at baseline to 57 ± 10% at 5 years, $p < 0.001$). Simultaneously, there was a reduction ($p<0.001$) in functional infarct size assessed as late enhancement volume normalized to LV mass. However, despite stability of LV end-systolic volume, LV end-diastolic volume increased significantly.

BOOST Study: BOne marrOw transfer to enhance ST-elevation infarct regeneration

This study was conducted after percutaneous coronary intervention with stent implantation of the infarct-related artery in 60 patients that were randomized 1:1 to a control group with optimal post-infarction therapy and a BMD transfer group that also underwent an intracoronary BMD infusion 4.8 ± 1.3 days after PCI. Cardiac MRI was performed 3.5 ± 1.5 days, 6 ± 1 months and 18 ± 6 months after PCI. Although there were no adverse effects related to BMD cells transfer, in the control group, the mean global LVEF increased by 0.7 and 3.1 percentage points after 6 and 18 months, respectively, while the LVEF in the BMD group increased by 6.7 and 5.9 percentage points. The difference in LVEF improvement between groups was significant after 6 months but not after 18 months ($p = 0.27$). However, the speed of LVEF recovery over the course of 18 months was significantly higher in the BMC transfer group (p = 0.001). Therefore, in this study, a single dose of intracoronary BMDs did not offer long-term benefit regarding LV systolic function after AMI compared with a randomized control group.

ASTAMI Study: Autologous Stem-cell Transplantation in Acute Myocardial Infarction

This study was a randomized, controlled, prospective trial that included 49 patients with acute anterior wall ST-elevation myocardial infarction (STEMI), treated with acute PCI. The patients were randomized in a 1:1 way to receive either intracoronary transplantation of autologous mononuclear bone marrow cells (*i.e.* circulating progenitor cells) 5-8 days after PCI, or conventional therapy. LV function, exercise capacity, biochemical status, functional class, quality of life and complications were validated at baseline and during a 12-month follow-up. Twenty-four patients have been randomized to intracoronary BMD stem cell transplantation. Twenty patients showed chest pain and 16 patients had ischemic electrocardiographic (ECG) changes during the BMD stem cell transplantation procedure. One patient had ventricular fibrillation 24 h after transplantation. Intracoronary transplantation of autologous BMC in the acute phase after AMI was feasible and appears safe in the short term. However, there was no significant advantage compared to the control group.

REPAIR-AMI: Reinfusion of Enriched Progenitor cells And Infarct Remodeling in Acute Myocardial Infarction

This study was conducted in a total of 58 patients and aimed to investigate the effects of intracoronary infusion of BMD cells on coronary blood flow regulation in patients with re-perfused AMI. The patients were divided in the BMD group (n = 30) and the placebo group (n = 28). Coronary flow reserve (CFR) in the infarct artery and a reference vessel was evaluated by intracoronary Doppler at the time of study therapy (4.2 ± 0.1 days after AMI and at the 4-month follow-up). Initial CFR was decreased in the infarct artery compared with the reference vessel in both groups (p = 0.05). At the 4-month follow-up, CFR in the infarct artery had slightly improved in the placebo group (0.88 ± 0.18; p = 0.001 *versus* initial) but it was significantly increased by 90% (1.80 ± 0.25; p = 0.005 *versus* placebo) in BMD-treated patients, resulting in a normalization of CFR *versus* initial measurements and placebo at 4 months.

Therefore, this study showed that intracoronary BMD cell therapy after AMI restores microvascular function of the infarct-related artery, which is linked to a significant improvement in maximal vascular conductance capacity. These data provide clinical evidence of concept that progenitor cell transplantation promotes vascular repair.

REGENT: Myocardial REGENeraTion by intracoronary infusion of selected population of stem cells in acute myocardial infarction

This study aimed to compare intracoronary infusion of BMD unselected mononuclear cells (UNSEL) and selected $CD34^+$ $CXCR4^+$ cells (SEL) in patients with AMI that showed a <40% reduction in LVEF. For that purpose, two hundred patients were randomized to intracoronary infusion of UNSEL (n = 80) or SEL (n = 80) BMD cells or to the control group without BMD cell treatment. The primary end point was defined as change of LVEF and volumes, measured by MRI before and 6 months after the procedure. After 6 months, LVEF increased by 3% (p = 0.01) in patients treated with UNSEL, 3% in patients receiving SEL (p = 0.04) and remained unchanged in control group (p = 0.73). However, there were no significant differences in absolute changes of LVEF between the groups, while absolute changes of LV end-systolic volume and LV end-diastolic volume were also not significantly different in all groups. Finally, there were no differences in major cardiovascular events (death, re-infarction, stroke, target vessel revascularization) between groups. The study therefore concluded that in patients with AMI and impaired LVEF, treatment with BMD cells does not result in a significant improvement of LVEF or volumes.

APOLLO study: AdiPOse-derived Stem ceLLs in the treatment of patients with ST-elevation myOcardial infarction

As previously mentioned, administration of freshly isolated AdSCs in pre-clinical animal models of AMI, immediately after the AMI, improved function and myocardial perfusion.

The APOLLO trial was a randomized, double-blind, placebo-controlled, phase I/IIa study designed to evaluate the safety and feasibility of intracoronary infusion of AdSCs in the treatment of patients in the acute phase of a large ST-segment elevation acute myocardial infarction (STEMI). Patients were eligible for enrolment if interventional treatment for the AMI was successful and the area of LV hypokinesia or akinesia corresponded to the culprit lesion. The residual LVEF needed to be between 30% and 50%, as assessed by transthoracic echocardiography after the PPCI. After informed consent, the patients underwent a liposuction procedure of the periumbilical region, AdSCs were isolated and within 24 h after the PPCI were infused intra-coronarily, under careful monitoring for coronary flow–related side effects.

A total of 14 patients presenting with an anterior wall AMI were included in the trial and randomized 3:1 to receive an intracoronary infusion of either 20 million AdSC (n = 10) or placebo solution (n = 4) in the culprit artery. Sestamibi – single photon emission computed tomography (MIBI-SPECT) analysis depicted a +4% improvement in global LVEF in AdSC-treated patients from 52.1% to 56.1%, whereas the placebo group deteriorated by −1.7% (52.0% to 50.3%), rendering an absolute difference between the treatment groups of +5.7% (p = 0.114). A similar positive trend of improved cardiac function was reported by cardiac magnetic resonance (CMR) analysis, which demonstrated a +4.6% improvement of global LVEF in the AdSCs-treated group from baseline to 6-month follow-up (p = 0.091). The percentage of the LV infarct was decreased by −52% (31.6 ± 5.3% to 15.3 ± 2.6% at 6-month follow-up; p = 0.002) in the AdSC-treated patients, as opposed to no change in the placebo-treated AMI patients. These results overall suggest that AdSCs infusion led to a trend toward improved cardiac function, accompanied by a significant improvement of the perfusion defect and a 50% reduction of myocardial scar formation.

Late Intervention

This type of intervention is defined as the process during which the infusion took place later than the first 7 days after the cardiac event.

MYSTAR Study: MYocardial STem cell Administration after acute myocardial infarction

MYSTAR study is a multi-center, prospective, randomized, single-blind clinical trial designed to compare the early and late intracoronary or combined (percutaneous intra-myocardial and intra-coronary) administration of BMD stem-cells to patients after AMI with re-perfused infarct-related artery.

The hypothesis relied on the differential homing of the stem cells within the first 21 days after the incident of MI but no later than 42 days. Patients were divided into four groups: early intra-coronary non-selected BMD stem cells (between 21 and 42 days), early combined intra-coronary with intra-myocardial BMD stem cells, late (3 months) intra-coronary injection, and late combined injections.

The results indicated that the early and late delivery of cells induced mild, but not clinically relevant, improvements. There was a reduction in infarct size and an improvement in LVEF at both 3 months and 9 to 12 months after acute myocardial ischemia. The main improvements in the early and late groups were an estimated 3.5% and 3.9% improvement in LVEF, respectively, as well as a 3.5% and 3.4% improvement in infarct size, respectively. MYSTAR was the first randomized trial to investigate the effects of the combined (intra-myocardial and intra-coronary) and the intra-coronary mode of delivery of BMD cell therapy in the early and late periods after AMI.

SWISS-AMI Study: SWiss multicenter Intracoronary Stem cells Study in AMI

In this multi-center trial performed entirely in Switzerland, 192 patients with AMI successfully treated by PCI of the infarct-related artery, were randomized in a 1:1:1 ratio to one control and two BMD stem cell therapy treatment groups. The control group was treated with state-of-the-art medical therapy. The treatment groups received intra-coronary administration of autologous BMD cells at 5 to 7 days or 3 to 4 weeks after the initial event, respectively. LV function as well as scar size, transmural extension, and regional wall motion score were evaluated by CMR studies at baseline and after 4 and 12 months.

The primary end point was the change in global LVEF by CMR at 4 months as compared to baseline. The results showed no substantial improvement in LVEF measured after 6 months.

LateTIME Study: Use of Adult Autologous Stem Cells in Treating Patients two to three Weeks after the Heart Attack

This was a randomized, double-blind, placebo-controlled trial of the National Heart, Lung, and Blood Institute-sponsored Cardiovascular Cell Therapy Research Network of 87 patients with significant LV dysfunction (LVEF ≤45%) following successful PPCI of a major coronary artery after a moderate-to-large infarction, between July 2008 and February 2011. Patients received intra-coronary infusion of 150 × 10^6 autologous BMD cells (total nucleated cells) or placebo (BMD:placebo, 2:1). The primary end points were changes in global LVEF and regional (wall motion) LV function, in the infarct and border zone between baseline and 6 months, measured by CMR. The results showed no significant difference between the treated and the placebo groups.

CADUCEUS Study: CArdiosphere-Derived aUtologous stem CElls to reverse ventricUlar dySfunction

In the CADUCEUS study, 12.5 to 25 × 10^6 autologous cardiosphere derived cells grown from endomyocardial biopsy specimens, were infused *via* the intra-coronary route in 17 patients with LV dysfunction 1.5 to 3 months after MI. Eight patients were followed as routine-care control patients. There was a significant decrease in the scar size and increase in viable myocardium at 6 and 12 months in the treatment group compared to control group, but there was no significant difference between the two groups at 6 months regarding EF improvement.

Chronic Ischemic Heart Disease

PRECISE Study: adiPose-deRived stEm and regenerative Cells In the treatment of patients with non-revaScularizable ischEmic myocardium

This was the first-in-man study to assess the safety and feasibility of AdSCs after trans-endocardial delivery, in patients with non-revascularizable ischemic myocardium. For that purpose, 27 patients with no option for revascularization were randomized (3:1) to receive 44 ± 17 × 10^6 of AdSCs isolated from subcutaneous adipose tissue from the abdomen or placebo. Feasibility endpoints (infarct size measured by MRI as percent of LV infracted and peak VO2) were evaluated at baseline and 6 months. The results showed that there were no adverse events related to AdSCs harvesting or delivery. In the AdSCs group, infarct size remained stable from baseline to 6 months while significant worsening was observed in controls (–3.0 ± 3.8% and 5.2 ± 3.4%, respectively; $p = 0.04$) but there were no significant differences in LVEFs and LV volumes between the two groups.

TOPCARE-CHD Study: Transplantation Of Progenitor Cells And REcovery of left ventricular function in patients with Chronic ischemic Heart Disease

This study targeted MI patients with an attack of more than 3 months who were stable on medical therapy since MI. Autologous BMD stem cells in the form of mononuclear cells (mean number 214 ± 98 × 10^6) were injected through the intra-coronary route. A major goal of this study was the assessment of natriuretic peptide serum levels as objective markers of HF and the occurrence of cardiac death in relation to the functional capacity of the infused cells in a consecutive series of 121 patients. The results showed that both NT-proBNP and N-terminal pro-atrial natriuretic peptide (NT-proANP) serum levels were significantly decreased in patients with established post infarction HF 3 months after trans-coronary progenitor cell administration. Moreover, patients receiving a higher number of colony-forming cells were significantly less likely to die than those patients receiving low numbers of colony-forming cells ($p = 0.01$). Taken together, the results confirmed that patients with objective evidence of post-infarction HF demonstrate a significant reduction of both NT-proBNP and NT-proANP serum levels within 3 months following intra-coronary infusion of BMD and that infusion of progenitor cells with a high clonogenic capacity is related to a significantly lower mortality during further follow-up.

POSEIDON Study: PercutaneOus StEm cell Injection Delivery effects On Neomyogenesis: Comparison of allogeneic versus autologous bone marrow-derived mesenchymal stem cells delivered by trans-endocardial injection in patients with ischemic cardiomyopathy

In the initial study (POSEIDON pilot) the researchers attempted to assess the effects of neo-myogenesis after autologous or allogeneic transfer of mesenchymal stem cells derived from the bone marrow. MSCs have been reported to be immunoprivileged and immunosuppressive, because they do not express major histocompatibility class II antigens and they secrete T-helper type 2 cytokines [74]. Therefore, the potential benefits of allogeneic cell transfer include use as an "off-the-shelf" therapeutic, thus avoiding the necessity for additional procedures for patients and delays in therapy. In the pilot study, the patients were divided into three groups according to the number of infused cells: 20×10^6 for the first group, 100×10^6 for the second group, and 200×10^6 for the third group. No placebo group was employed. Treatment was linked to lower rates of treatment-emergent serious adverse effects, including immunologic reactions. MSC injection favourably affected patient quality of life, functional capacity, and ventricular remodelling. A continuation of this study, the so-called POSEIDON-DCM study is underway, but results have not been reported yet [75].

STAR-heart Study: The acute and long-term effects of intracoronary Stem cell Transplantation in patients with chronic heARt failure

The aim of this study was to quantitatively investigate ventricular hemodynamics, geometry, and contractility as well as the long-term clinical outcome of BMD cell therapy-treated patients with reduced LVEF due to chronic ischemic cardiomyopathy (n = 391; LVEF ≤ 35%). The control group (mean NYHA class 3.06) consisted of 200 patients with comparable LVEF. The study employed assessments of hemodynamics at rest and exercise, quantitative ventriculography, spiroergometry, 24 h Holter ECG, late potentials, and heart rate for a period of over 3 months to 5 years after intra-coronary BMD therapy. The results showed that there was a significant improvement in hemodynamics (*e.g.* LVEF, cardiac index), exercise capacity, oxygen uptake, and LV contractility in the treated group and a significant decrease in long-term mortality compared with the control group.

No side effects were observed.

SCIPIO Study: Stem Cell Infusion in Patients with Ischemic cardiOmyopathy

The SCIPIO study is one of the few trials in which purified stem cells are injected to the patients. Preclinical studies had shown that c-kit^{+} lineage- resident cardiac stem cells (RCSCs) improve post- LV dysfunction in animals; therefore, the SCIPIO trial aimed to assess their therapeutic potential in humans. The SCIPIO trial is a Phase I, randomized, open-label study of RCSCs in patients with post-infarction LV dysfunction (EF $\leq$40%) who underwent coronary bypass surgery. Autologous RCSCs were isolated from the right atrial appendage and re-infused intra-coronarily 4 ± 1 months after surgery, while patients in the control group received no treatment. In Stage A, 9 treated and 4 control patients were consecutively enrolled to evaluate the feasibility and short-term safety of RCSCs while in Stage B, patients were randomized to the treated or control arm in a 2:3 ratio. The results showed that autologous RCSCs were successfully isolated and expanded in 80 out of 81 patients. In 16 treated patients, no RCSC-related adverse effects have been reported. LVEF increased from 30.3 ± 1.9% before RCSC infusion to 38.5 ± 2.8% at 4 months after infusion, ($p = 0.001$). This was linked to an improvement in regional wall motion score index ($p = 0.005$), NYHA functional class ($p = 0.003$), and quality of life ($p < 0.0001$). In contrast, in 7 control patients, none of these variables changed appreciably during the corresponding time-interval. Importantly, the therapeutic effects of RCSCs were more pronounced at 1 year (increased LVEF, $p = 0.0007$, $n = 8$), suggesting that RCSCs continue to improve LV function beyond the first 4 months. Overall, the study presented initial results in humans that are very encouraging, and suggest that infusion of autologous RCSCs is effective in improving LV systolic function and decreasing infarct size.

PROMETHEUS Study: Prospective Randomized assessment Of MEsenchymal stem cell THErapy in patients Undergoing Surgery

This study was funded through the National Heart, Lung, and Blood Institute's Specialized Center for Cell Therapeutics and enrolled patients who required coronary artery bypass surgery and had EF between 0.20 and 0.50 due to a previous MI that caused segmental LV akinesis or dyskinesis. The patients entered the study if a) they met enrolment criteria, b) consented to participate, and c) if the patient's cardio-surgeons and independent clinicians estimated that it is safe to wait 4 to 5 weeks between bone-marrow harvest and treatment. The period of 4 to 5 weeks was necessary in order to amplify the autologous MSCs with which patients were treated at the time of surgery. No placebo control group was employed. Results have been presented for six patients who were injected with autologous MSCs into akinetic/hypokinetic myocardial territories. MRI was used to measure scar tissue, perfusion, wall thickness, and contractility at baseline and at 3, 6, and 18 months, and to compare structural and functional recovery in regions that received either MSC injections alone, or revascularization alone, or none of these modalities. A composite score of MRI variables was used to assess concordance of anti-fibrotic effects, perfusion, and contraction at different regions. After 18 months, subjects receiving MSCs demonstrated increased LVEF ($p = 0.0002$) and decreased scar mass ($p < 0.0001$) compared with baseline. MSC-injected segments had concordant reduction in scar size, perfusion, and contractile improvement, whereas revascularized and non-treated segments demonstrated non-concordant changes ($p < 0.0001$) *versus* injected segments. Therefore, this study overall demonstrated that intra-myocardial injection of autologous MSCs into akinetic yet non-revascularized segments produces comprehensive regional functional restitution and improvement in global LV function. These findings, although inconclusive because of lack of the placebo group, may lead to important therapeutic and mechanistic hypothesis-generating conclusions. Notably, no adverse effects have been reported.

Chronic Non-ischemic Heart Failure (HF)

There have been attempts to effectively treat chronic non ischemic HF. The TOPCARE-DCM study, *i.e.* transplantation of progenitor cells and recovery of LV function in patients with non-ischemic dilative cardiomyopathy (DCM), has utilized intra-coronary infusion of $259 \pm 135 \times 10^6$ BMD cells in 33 patients with dilated cardiomyopathy. The results showed that the treated group was linked to an improvement in regional contractile and microvascular function and a decrease in NT-proBNP serum levels, suggesting a beneficial effect on LV remodelling. Interestingly, the increase of regional contractile function was directly proportional to the functionality of the infused cells, as measured by their colony-forming capacity.

CONCLUDING REMARKS

Novel insights about the molecular mechanisms related to HF combined with the identification and development of vectors with the best cardiotropic properties, have made both gene therapy and cell therapy promising alternatives treatments to mechanical and pharmacological therapies for HF. However, many important issues such as the mechanism(s) of action of stem cells, their long-term engraftment potential, their mechanisms of aging as related to cardiovascular disease, the optimal cell type(s) to be infused or genetically corrected, the ideal dose of both cells and vectors to be administered and the route and frequency of cell administration, still remain to be resolved and elucidated. Moreover, we are still lacking definite knowledge about the basic physiology of heart in terms of regeneration and most importantly it should be emphasized that the pre-clinical studies have been performed in mouse models of heart failure without taking into account the heart's regeneration potential and physiological differences between species. Although the results from the clinical trials of gene therapy have been definite, still no cell therapy has been conclusively shown to be effective. The negative results of the CUPID 2 trial can be interpreted in many different ways: First it is true, that in terms of actual therapy, the trial failed to prove that a gene therapy approach is superior to the current pharmacological approaches for heart failure. However, this is a common issue when comparing novel molecular therapies with conventional therapies. During the initial gene therapy trials, there were several adverse effects reported including the death of an individual due to systemic inflammation from use of an adenoviral vector [76] and the development of leukemia in several pediatric patients as a result of insertional mutagenesis from an oncoretroviral vector [76]. However, despite these adverse effects, significant knowledge was acquired. First, the field utilized different strains of adenoviruses that are less immunogenic, second there was a gradual replacement of oncoretroviral vectors by lentiviral vectors, and third, important insights were gained about the minimum vector copy number/cell in order to reach a therapeutic result. From a gene therapist's point of view, the fact that specifically for the heart, "decoy" virions from AAV are necessary, represents an extremely important step forward and provides further guidance towards the generation of efficient vectors. Another extremely important issue is safety. The patients enrolled in the CUPID 2 trial received a fair amount of vector particles within a relatively short period of time, without raising safety issues in terms of immunogenicity and most importantly insertional mutagenesis. Thus, although the trial did not succeed in efficient therapy, still it provides valuable information of major importance regarding the feasibility, the efficiency and the safety of the whole approach. Furthermore, the ongoing parallel approaches world-wide to validate the therapeutic effects of cell-based regenerative medicine in heart failure, will immensely contribute to the advancement of rational therapies targeting cardiovascular disease. It is unclear whether any gene or cell therapy strategy will become medical routine within the next 5-10 years, but in the future, extensive research for the identification of novel targets, further improvement of vector systems and the ideal type of cell with cardioregenerative potential, will undoubtedly lead to even safer and more effective clinical trials. Specifically, the improvement of the technology of the iPSCs, is anticipated to provide unlimited supply of unique patient-specific cell types, which will enable the accurate modelling of cardiovascular disorders. This can lead to important mechanistic insights and in turn to the development of novel drugs tailored on patient-specific needs at the cellular level [77]. Finally, it should be emphasized that any single administration therapy, such as gene therapy, is far more superior to any current conventional pharmacological approach, since it maximizes the effect of the therapeutic agent but also because it dramatically improves the quality of life of the patients.

CONFLICT OF INTEREST

This study was supported by a Grant No. 11E-RARE-09-155 by the European Research Projects on Rare Diseases (ERA-Net) of the EU to N.P. A.

ACKNOWLEDGEMENTS

Declared none.

REFERENCES

[1] Dassanayaka S, Jones SP. Recent Developments in Heart Failure. Circ Res 2015; 117(7): e58-63.

[http://dx.doi.org/10.1161/CIRCRESAHA.115.305765] [PMID: 26358111]

[2] O'Connor TP, Crystal RG. Genetic medicines: treatment strategies for hereditary disorders. Nat Rev Genet 2006; 7(4): 261-76.
[http://dx.doi.org/10.1038/nrg1829] [PMID: 16543931]

[3] Yang F, Green JJ, Dinio T, *et al.* Gene delivery to human adult and embryonic cell-derived stem cells using biodegradable nanoparticulate polymeric vectors. Gene Ther 2009; 16(4): 533-46.
[http://dx.doi.org/10.1038/gt.2008.182] [PMID: 19129861]

[4] Hajjar RJ. Potential of gene therapy as a treatment for heart failure. J Clin Invest 2013; 123(1): 53-61.
[http://dx.doi.org/10.1172/JCI62837] [PMID: 23281410]

[5] Miller DG, Adam MA, Miller AD. Gene transfer by retrovirus vectors occurs only in cells that are actively replicating at the time of infection. Mol Cell Biol 1990; 10(8): 4239-42.
[http://dx.doi.org/10.1128/MCB.10.8.4239] [PMID: 2370865]

[6] Naldini L. Lentiviruses as gene transfer agents for delivery to non-dividing cells. Curr Opin Biotechnol 1998; 9(5): 457-63.
[http://dx.doi.org/10.1016/S0958-1669(98)80029-3] [PMID: 9821272]

[7] Hacein-Bey-Abina S, von Kalle C, Schmidt M, *et al.* A serious adverse event after successful gene therapy for X-linked severe combined immunodeficiency. N Engl J Med 2003; 348(3): 255-6.
[http://dx.doi.org/10.1056/NEJM200301163480314] [PMID: 12529469]

[8] Stein S, Ott MG, Schultze-Strasser S, *et al.* Genomic instability and myelodysplasia with monosomy 7 consequent to EVI1 activation after gene therapy for chronic granulomatous disease. Nat Med 2010; 16(2): 198-204.
[http://dx.doi.org/10.1038/nm.2088] [PMID: 20098431]

[9] Ariga T. A possible turning point in the hematopoietic stem cell gene therapy for primary immunodeficiency diseases? Lentiviral vectors could take the place of retroviral vectors. Expert Rev Clin Immunol 2013; 9(11): 1015-8.
[http://dx.doi.org/10.1586/1744666X.2013.850416] [PMID: 24168409]

[10] Wasala NB, Shin JH, Duan D. The evolution of heart gene delivery vectors. J Gene Med 2011; 13(10): 557-65.
[http://dx.doi.org/10.1002/jgm.1600] [PMID: 21837689]

[11] Hassan A, Booth C, Brightwell A, *et al.* Outcome of hematopoietic stem cell transplantation for adenosine deaminase-deficient severe combined immunodeficiency. Blood 2012; 120(17): 3615-24.
[http://dx.doi.org/10.1182/blood-2011-12-396879] [PMID: 22791287]

[12] Cavazzana-Calvo M, Payen E, Negre O, *et al.* Transfusion independence and HMGA2 activation after gene therapy of human β-thalassaemia. Nature 2010; 467(7313): 318-22.
[http://dx.doi.org/10.1038/nature09328] [PMID: 20844535]

[13] Aiuti A, Biasco L, Scaramuzza S, *et al.* Lentiviral hematopoietic stem cell gene therapy in patients with Wiskott-Aldrich syndrome. Science 2013; 341(6148): 1233151.
[http://dx.doi.org/10.1126/science.1233151] [PMID: 23845947]

[14] Biffi A, Montini E, Lorioli L, *et al.* Lentiviral hematopoietic stem cell gene therapy benefits metachromatic leukodystrophy. Science 2013; 341(6148): 1233158.

[http://dx.doi.org/10.1126/science.1233158] [PMID: 23845948]

[15] Kuang L, Feng J, He G, Jing T. Knockdown of Nrf2 inhibits the angiogenesis of rat cardiac microvascular endothelial cells under hypoxic conditions. Int J Biol Sci 2013; 9(7): 656-65. [http://dx.doi.org/10.7150/ijbs.5887] [PMID: 23904790]

[16] Du Y, Zhu H, Li D, *et al.* Lentiviral-mediated overexpression of Akt1 reduces anoxia-reoxygenation injury in cardiomyocytes. Cell Biol Int 2014; 38(4): 488-96. [http://dx.doi.org/10.1002/cbin.10234] [PMID: 24375547]

[17] Zanetti BF, Gomes WJ, Han SW. Identification, selection, and enrichment of cardiomyocyte precursors. Biomed Res Int 2013:390789. [http://dx.doi.org/10.1155/2013/390789]

[18] Barth AS, Kizana E, Smith RR, *et al.* Lentiviral vectors bearing the cardiac promoter of the Na+-Ca2+ exchanger report cardiogenic differentiation in stem cells. Mol Ther 2008; 16(5): 957-64. [http://dx.doi.org/10.1038/mt.2008.30] [PMID: 18388932]

[19] Cornetta K, Morgan RA, Anderson WF. Safety issues related to retroviral-mediated gene transfer in humans. Hum Gene Ther 1991; 2(1): 5-14. [http://dx.doi.org/10.1089/hum.1991.2.1-5] [PMID: 1863639]

[20] Moolten FL, Cupples LA. A model for predicting the risk of cancer consequent to retroviral gene therapy. Hum Gene Ther 1992; 3(5): 479-86. [http://dx.doi.org/10.1089/hum.1992.3.5-479] [PMID: 1420447]

[21] Katz MG, Fargnoli AS, Williams RD, Bridges CR. Gene therapy delivery systems for enhancing viral and nonviral vectors for cardiac diseases: current concepts and future applications. Hum Gene Ther 2013; 24(11): 914-27. [http://dx.doi.org/10.1089/hum.2013.2517] [PMID: 24164239]

[22] Elleder D, Pavlícek A, Paces J, Hejnar J. Preferential integration of human immunodeficiency virus type 1 into genes, cytogenetic R bands and GC-rich DNA regions: insight from the human genome sequence. FEBS Lett 2002; 517(1-3): 285-6. [http://dx.doi.org/10.1016/S0014-5793(02)02612-1] [PMID: 12062454]

[23] Schröder AR, Shinn P, Chen H, Berry C, Ecker JR, Bushman F. HIV-1 integration in the human genome favors active genes and local hotspots. Cell 2002; 110(4): 521-9. [http://dx.doi.org/10.1016/S0092-8674(02)00864-4] [PMID: 12202041]

[24] Laufs S, Gentner B, Nagy KZ, *et al.* Retroviral vector integration occurs in preferred genomic targets of human bone marrow-repopulating cells. Blood 2003; 101(6): 2191-8. [http://dx.doi.org/10.1182/blood-2002-02-0627] [PMID: 12424203]

[25] Mitchell RS, Beitzel BF, Schroder AR, *et al.* Retroviral DNA integration: ASLV, HIV, and MLV show distinct target site preferences. PLoS Biol 2004; 2(8): E234. [http://dx.doi.org/10.1371/journal.pbio.0020234] [PMID: 15314653]

[26] Wu X, Li Y, Crise B, Burgess SM. Transcription start regions in the human genome are favored targets for MLV integration. Science 2003; 300(5626): 1749-51. [http://dx.doi.org/10.1126/science.1083413] [PMID: 12805549]

[27] Papanikolaou E, Georgomanoli M, Stamateris E, *et al.* The new self-inactivating lentiviral vector for

thalassemia gene therapy combining two HPFH activating elements corrects human thalassemic hematopoietic stem cells. Hum Gene Ther 2012; 23(1): 15-31.
[http://dx.doi.org/10.1089/hum.2011.048] [PMID: 21875313]

[28] Hanawa H, Yamamoto M, Zhao H, Shimada T, Persons DA. Optimized lentiviral vector design improves titer and transgene expression of vectors containing the chicken β-globin locus HS4 insulator element. Mol Ther 2009; 17(4): 667-74.
[http://dx.doi.org/10.1038/mt.2009.1] [PMID: 19223867]

[29] Mays LE, Wilson JM. The complex and evolving story of T cell activation to AAV vector-encoded transgene products. Mol Ther 2011; 19(1): 16-27.
[http://dx.doi.org/10.1038/mt.2010.250] [PMID: 21119617]

[30] Asokan A, Conway JC, Phillips JL, *et al.* Reengineering a receptor footprint of adeno-associated virus enables selective and systemic gene transfer to muscle. Nat Biotechnol 2010; 28(1): 79-82.
[http://dx.doi.org/10.1038/nbt.1599] [PMID: 20037580]

[31] Wang J, Faust SM, Rabinowitz JE. The next step in gene delivery: molecular engineering of adeno-associated virus serotypes. J Mol Cell Cardiol 2011; 50(5): 793-802.
[http://dx.doi.org/10.1016/j.yjmcc.2010.10.017] [PMID: 21029739]

[32] Mitchell AM, Nicolson SC, Warischalk JK, Samulski RJ. AAV's anatomy: roadmap for optimizing vectors for translational success. Curr Gene Ther 2010; 10(5): 319-40.
[http://dx.doi.org/10.2174/156652310793180706] [PMID: 20712583]

[33] Li W, Asokan A, Wu Z, *et al.* Engineering and selection of shuffled AAV genomes: a new strategy for producing targeted biological nanoparticles. Mol Ther 2008; 16(7): 1252-60.
[http://dx.doi.org/10.1038/mt.2008.100] [PMID: 18500254]

[34] Ying Y, Müller OJ, Goehringer C, *et al.* Heart-targeted adeno-associated viral vectors selected by *in vivo* biopanning of a random viral display peptide library. Gene Ther 2010; 17(8): 980-90.
[http://dx.doi.org/10.1038/gt.2010.44] [PMID: 20393510]

[35] Jaski BE, Jessup ML, Mancini DM, *et al.* Calcium upregulation by percutaneous administration of gene therapy in cardiac disease (CUPID Trial), a first-in-human phase 1/2 clinical trial. J Card Fail 2009; 15(3): 171-81.
[http://dx.doi.org/10.1016/j.cardfail.2009.01.013] [PMID: 19327618]

[36] Wang D, Zhong L, Nahid MA, Gao G. The potential of adeno-associated viral vectors for gene delivery to muscle tissue. Expert Opin Drug Deliv 2014; 11(3): 345-64.
[http://dx.doi.org/10.1517/17425247.2014.871258] [PMID: 24386892]

[37] Asokan A, Samulski RJ. An emerging adeno-associated viral vector pipeline for cardiac gene therapy. Hum Gene Ther 2013; 24(11): 906-13.
[http://dx.doi.org/10.1089/hum.2013.2515] [PMID: 24164238]

[38] Lasaro MO, Ertl HC. New insights on adenovirus as vaccine vectors. Mol Ther 2009; 17(8): 1333-9.
[http://dx.doi.org/10.1038/mt.2009.130] [PMID: 19513019]

[39] Naim C, Yerevanian A, Hajjar RJ. Gene therapy for heart failure: where do we stand? Curr Cardiol Rep 2013; 15(2): 333.
[http://dx.doi.org/10.1007/s11886-012-0333-3] [PMID: 23307169]

[40] Argyros O, Wong SP, Harbottle RP. Non-viral episomal modification of cells using S/MAR elements. Expert Opin Biol Ther 2011; 11(9): 1177-91.
[http://dx.doi.org/10.1517/14712598.2011.582035] [PMID: 21548848]

[41] Yockman JW, Kastenmeier A, Erickson HM, *et al.* Novel polymer carriers and gene constructs for treatment of myocardial ischemia and infarction. J Control Release 2008; 132(3): 260-6.
[http://dx.doi.org/10.1016/j.jconrel.2008.06.024] [PMID: 18662730]

[42] Milano CA, Allen LF, Rockman HA, *et al.* Enhanced myocardial function in transgenic mice overexpressing the beta 2-adrenergic receptor. Science 1994; 264(5158): 582-6.
[http://dx.doi.org/10.1126/science.8160017] [PMID: 8160017]

[43] Maurice JP, Hata JA, Shah AS, *et al.* Enhancement of cardiac function after adenoviral-mediated *in vivo* intracoronary beta2-adrenergic receptor gene delivery. J Clin Invest 1999; 104(1): 21-9.
[http://dx.doi.org/10.1172/JCI6026] [PMID: 10393695]

[44] Shah AS, Lilly RE, Kypson AP, *et al.* Intracoronary adenovirus-mediated delivery and overexpression of the beta(2)-adrenergic receptor in the heart : prospects for molecular ventricular assistance. Circulation 2000; 101(4): 408-14.
[http://dx.doi.org/10.1161/01.CIR.101.4.408] [PMID: 10653833]

[45] Raake PW, Vinge LE, Gao E, *et al.* G protein-coupled receptor kinase 2 ablation in cardiac myocytes before or after myocardial infarction prevents heart failure. Circ Res 2008; 103(4): 413-22.
[http://dx.doi.org/10.1161/CIRCRESAHA.107.168336] [PMID: 18635825]

[46] Shah AS, White DC, Emani S, *et al. In vivo* ventricular gene delivery of a beta-adrenergic receptor kinase inhibitor to the failing heart reverses cardiac dysfunction. Circulation 2001; 103(9): 1311-6.
[http://dx.doi.org/10.1161/01.CIR.103.9.1311] [PMID: 11238278]

[47] Schumacher SM, Gao E, Zhu W, *et al.* Paroxetine-mediated GRK2 inhibition reverses cardiac dysfunction and remodeling after myocardial infarction. Sci Transl Med 2015; 7(277): 277ra31.
[http://dx.doi.org/10.1126/scitranslmed.aaa0154] [PMID: 25739765]

[48] Gao MH, Lai NC, Roth DM, *et al.* Adenylylcyclase increases responsiveness to catecholamine stimulation in transgenic mice. Circulation 1999; 99(12): 1618-22.
[http://dx.doi.org/10.1161/01.CIR.99.12.1618] [PMID: 10096940]

[49] Lai NC, Roth DM, Gao MH, *et al.* Intracoronary adenovirus encoding adenylyl cyclase VI increases left ventricular function in heart failure. Circulation 2004; 110(3): 330-6.
[http://dx.doi.org/10.1161/01.CIR.0000136033.21777.4D] [PMID: 15249510]

[50] Gwathmey JK, Copelas L, MacKinnon R, *et al.* Abnormal intracellular calcium handling in myocardium from patients with end-stage heart failure. Circ Res 1987; 61(1): 70-6.
[http://dx.doi.org/10.1161/01.RES.61.1.70] [PMID: 3608112]

[51] Miyamoto MI, del Monte F, Schmidt U, *et al.* Adenoviral gene transfer of SERCA2a improves left-ventricular function in aortic-banded rats in transition to heart failure. Proc Natl Acad Sci USA 2000; 97(2): 793-8.
[http://dx.doi.org/10.1073/pnas.97.2.793] [PMID: 10639159]

[52] del MonteF , Harding SE, Schmidt U, *et al.* Restoration of contractile function in isolated cardiomyocytes from failing human hearts by gene transfer of SERCA2a. Circulation 1999; 100(23):

2308-11.
[http://dx.doi.org/10.1161/01.CIR.100.23.2308] [PMID: 10587333]

[53] Sakata S, Lebeche D, Sakata N, *et al.* Restoration of mechanical and energetic function in failing aortic-banded rat hearts by gene transfer of calcium cycling proteins. J Mol Cell Cardiol 2007; 42(4): 852-61.
[http://dx.doi.org/10.1016/j.yjmcc.2007.01.003] [PMID: 17300800]

[54] Lyon AR, Bannister ML, Collins T, *et al.* SERCA2a gene transfer decreases sarcoplasmic reticulum calcium leak and reduces ventricular arrhythmias in a model of chronic heart failure. Circ Arrhythm Electrophysiol 2011; 4(3): 362-72.
[http://dx.doi.org/10.1161/CIRCEP.110.961615] [PMID: 21406682]

[55] Hadri L, Bobe R, Kawase Y, *et al.* SERCA2a gene transfer enhances eNOS expression and activity in endothelial cells. Mol Ther 2010; 18(7): 1284-92.
[http://dx.doi.org/10.1038/mt.2010.77] [PMID: 20461063]

[56] Wahlquist C, Jeong D, Rojas-Muñoz A, *et al.* Inhibition of miR-25 improves cardiac contractility in the failing heart. Nature 2014; 508(7497): 531-5.
[http://dx.doi.org/10.1038/nature13073] [PMID: 24670661]

[57] Ghadge SK, Mühlstedt S, Ozcelik C, Bader M. SDF-1α as a therapeutic stem cell homing factor in myocardial infarction. Pharmacol Ther 2011; 129(1): 97-108.
[http://dx.doi.org/10.1016/j.pharmthera.2010.09.011] [PMID: 20965212]

[58] Suckau L, Fechner H, Chemaly E, *et al.* Long-term cardiac-targeted RNA interference for the treatment of heart failure restores cardiac function and reduces pathological hypertrophy. Circulation 2009; 119(9): 1241-52.
[http://dx.doi.org/10.1161/CIRCULATIONAHA.108.783852] [PMID: 19237664]

[59] Nicolaou P, Rodriguez P, Ren X, *et al.* Inducible expression of active protein phosphatase-1 inhibitor-1 enhances basal cardiac function and protects against ischemia/reperfusion injury. Circ Res 2009; 104(8): 1012-20.
[http://dx.doi.org/10.1161/CIRCRESAHA.108.189811] [PMID: 19299645]

[60] Ziaeian B, Fonarow GC. Epidemiology and aetiology of heart failure. Nat Rev Cardiol 2016; 13(6): 368-78.
[http://dx.doi.org/10.1038/nrcardio.2016.25] [PMID: 26935038]

[61] Hajjar RJ, Zsebo K, Deckelbaum L, *et al.* Design of a phase 1/2 trial of intracoronary administration of AAV1/SERCA2a in patients with heart failure. J Card Fail 2008; 14(5): 355-67.
[http://dx.doi.org/10.1016/j.cardfail.2008.02.005] [PMID: 18514926]

[62] Jessup M, Greenberg B, Mancini D, *et al.* Calcium upregulation by percutaneous administration of gene therapy in cardiac disease (CUPID): a phase 2 trial of intracoronary gene therapy of sarcoplasmic reticulum Ca2+-ATPase in patients with advanced heart failure. Circulation 2011; 124(3): 304-13.
[http://dx.doi.org/10.1161/CIRCULATIONAHA.111.022889] [PMID: 21709064]

[63] Greenberg B, Butler J, Felker GM, *et al.* Calcium upregulation by percutaneous administration of gene therapy in patients with cardiac disease (CUPID 2): a randomised, multinational, double-blind, placebo-controlled, phase 2b trial. Lancet 2016; 387(10024): 1178-86.
[http://dx.doi.org/10.1016/S0140-6736(16)00082-9] [PMID: 26803443]

[64] Penn MS, Mendelsohn FO, Schaer GL, *et al.* An open-label dose escalation study to evaluate the safety of administration of nonviral stromal cell-derived factor-1 plasmid to treat symptomatic ischemic heart failure. Circ Res 2013; 112(5): 816-25.
[http://dx.doi.org/10.1161/CIRCRESAHA.111.300440] [PMID: 23429605]

[65] Beltrami AP, Urbanek K, Kajstura J, *et al.* Evidence that human cardiac myocytes divide after myocardial infarction. N Engl J Med 2001; 344(23): 1750-7.
[http://dx.doi.org/10.1056/NEJM200106073442303] [PMID: 11396441]

[66] Aguirre A, Sancho-Martinez I, Izpisua Belmonte JC. Reprogramming toward heart regeneration: stem cells and beyond. Cell Stem Cell 2013; 12(3): 275-84.
[http://dx.doi.org/10.1016/j.stem.2013.02.008] [PMID: 23472869]

[67] Garbern JC, Lee RT. Cardiac stem cell therapy and the promise of heart regeneration. Cell Stem Cell 2013; 12(6): 689-98.
[http://dx.doi.org/10.1016/j.stem.2013.05.008] [PMID: 23746978]

[68] Website of the American Society of Gene and Cell Therapy. Available from: http://www.asgct.org/general-public/educational-resources/gene-therapy-and-cell-therapy-for-diseases/cardiovascular-diseases 2015.

[69] Alrefai MT, Murali D, Paul A, Ridwan KM, Connell JM, Shum-Tim D. Cardiac tissue engineering and regeneration using cell-based therapy. Stem Cells Cloning 2015; 8: 81-101.
[PMID: 25999743]

[70] Fuentes T, Kearns-Jonker M. Endogenous cardiac stem cells for the treatment of heart failure. Stem Cells Cloning 2013; 6: 1-12.
[PMID: 24426784]

[71] Martinez-Fernandez A, Nelson TJ, Yamada S, *et al.* iPS programmed without c-MYC yield proficient cardiogenesis for functional heart chimerism. Circ Res 2009; 105(7): 648-56.
[http://dx.doi.org/10.1161/CIRCRESAHA.109.203109] [PMID: 19696409]

[72] Houtgraaf JH, den Dekker WK, van Dalen BM, *et al.* First experience in humans using adipose tissue-derived regenerative cells in the treatment of patients with ST-segment elevation myocardial infarction. J Am Coll Cardiol 2012; 59(5): 539-40.
[http://dx.doi.org/10.1016/j.jacc.2011.09.065] [PMID: 22281257]

[73] Barile L, Gherghiceanu M, Popescu LM, *et al.* Human cardiospheres as a source of multipotent stem and progenitor cells Stem Cells Intl 2013.
[http://dx.doi.org/10.1155/2013/916837]

[74] Hare JM, Fishman JE, Gerstenblith G, *et al.* Comparison of allogeneic *vs* autologous bone marrow–derived mesenchymal stem cells delivered by transendocardial injection in patients with ischemic cardiomyopathy: the POSEIDON randomized trial. JAMA 2012; 308(22): 2369-79.
[http://dx.doi.org/10.1001/jama.2012.25321] [PMID: 23117550]

[75] Fish KM, Hajjar RJ. Mesenchymal Stem Cells & Endothelial Function. EBioMedicine 2015; 2(5): 376-7.
[http://dx.doi.org/10.1016/j.ebiom.2015.04.015] [PMID: 26137582]

[76] Thomas CE, Ehrhardt A, Kay MA. Progress and problems with the use of viral vectors for gene

therapy. Nat Rev Genet 2003; 4(5): 346-58.
[http://dx.doi.org/10.1038/nrg1066] [PMID: 12728277]

[77] Chen IY, Matsa E, Wu JC. Induced pluripotent stem cells: at the heart of cardiovascular precision medicine. Nat Rev Cardiol 2016; 13(6): 333-49.
[http://dx.doi.org/10.1038/nrcardio.2016.36] [PMID: 27009425]

SUBJECT INDEX

A

B

Panagiotis Georgoulias (Ed.)

D

E

F

G

H

I

Q

R

Made in United States
North Haven, CT
04 November 2026

21730356R00210